Authoritative Guide
to Self-Help Resources
in Mental Health

REVISED EDITION

D1441662

Authoritative Guide to Self-Help Resources in Mental Health

REVISED EDITION

John C. Norcross, PhD

John W. Santrock, PhD

Linda F. Campbell, PhD

Thomas P. Smith, PsyD

Robert Sommer, PhD

Edward L. Zuckerman, PhD

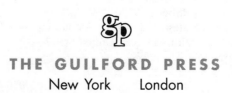

THE GUILFORD PRESS

New York   London

© 2003 The Guilford Press
A Division of Guilford Publications, Inc.
72 Spring Street, New York, NY 10012
www.guilford.com

The information in this volume is not intended as a substitute for
consultation with healthcare professionals. Each individual's health
concerns should be evaluated by a qualified professional.

Printed in the United States of America

This book is printed on acid-free paper.

Last digit is print number: 9 8 7 6 5 4 3 2 1

Library of Congress Cataloging-in-Publication Data

Authoritative guide to self-help resources in mental health /
    John C. Norcross . . . [et al.]. — Rev. ed.
        p. cm.
    Includes bibliographical references and index.
    ISBN 1-57230-896-6 (cloth) — ISBN 1-57230-839-7 (pbk.)
        1. Mental health—United States—Indexes. 2. Mental illness—United
    States—Indexes. 3. Mental health services—United States—
    Directories.   I. Norcross, John C., 1957–
    RA790.6.A94 2003
    362.2'0973—dc21   2003002772

John C. Norcross, PhD, is a professor and former chair of psychology at the University of Scranton, editor of *In Session: Journal of Clinical Psychology,* and a clinical psychologist in part-time practice. Author of more than 150 scholarly publications, he has cowritten or edited 12 books, including the *Insider's Guide to Graduate Programs in Clinical and Counseling Psychology, Psychotherapy Relationships That Work, Psychologists' Desk Reference,* and *Systems of Psychotherapy* (5th ed.). He has served as president of the American Psychological Association's Division of Psychotherapy and the International Society of Clinical Psychology, and on the editorial boards of a dozen journals. Dr. Norcross's many professional awards include being named the Pennsylvania Professor of the Year by the Carnegie Foundation and being elected a Distinguished Practitioner in the National Academies of Practice.

John W. Santrock, PhD, taught at the University of Charleston and the University of Georgia before joining the psychology department at the University of Texas at Dallas, where he is a professor and former department chair. He was recently a member of the editorial board of *Developmental Psychology.* Dr. Santrock has authored multiple textbooks, including *Psychology* (7th ed.), *Life-Span Development* (9th ed.), *Child Development* (10th ed.), *Children* (7th ed.), *Adolescence* (9th ed.), and *Human Adjustment* (2nd ed.), and is the coauthor of *Your Guide to College Success* (3rd ed.).

Linda F. Campbell, PhD, is an associate professor and director of the training clinic in the Department of Counseling and Human Development at the University of Georgia. She is coauthor of several books and scholarly publications, editor of *The Psychotherapy Bulletin* (a publication of the American Psychological Association's Division of Psychotherapy), and a member of several editorial boards. A member of the American Psychological Association's Ethics Committee and Council of Representatives, and president-elect of the Division of Psychotherapy, she has received several awards for service to her state association and for excellence in teaching from the University of Georgia.

Thomas P. Smith, PsyD, is a clinical psychologist in the Counseling Center at the University of Scranton and in independent part-time practice. He has worked in the fields of mental health and substance abuse for 25 years in both outpatient and inpatient settings. An adjunct faculty member for 12 years at Marywood University, he is currently an adjunct faculty member in the Counseling and Human Services Department at the University of Scranton. He has presented at conferences on such topics as cognitive therapy and self-help resources in psychotherapy. He is coauthor of several chapters and articles.

Robert Sommer, PhD, is a professor and former chair of psychology at the University of California, Davis. Author of 11 books and numerous articles, he has done research on autobiographies of mental health clients for over four decades. He is a past president of the American Psychological Association's Division of Population and Environmental Psychology. Dr. Sommer received a Fulbright Fellowship to Estonia, a Career Research Award from the Environmental Design Research Association, a Research Award from the California Alliance for the Mentally Ill, the Kurt Lewin Award, and an honorary doctorate from Tallinn Pedagogical University.

Edward L. Zuckerman, PhD, was in full-time independent practice of clinical psychology for almost 20 years and taught psychology courses at the University of Pittsburgh and Carnegie Mellon University for a total of 25 years. Dr. Zuckerman is currently a consultant to the Social Security Disability Determination Division and editor of The Clinician's Toolbox series for The Guilford Press. He is the author of the *Clinician's Thesaurus* (5th ed.), a guidebook for writing reports, and *The Paper Office* (3rd ed.), a manual for improving ethical and legal practices.

ACKNOWLEDGMENTS

This massive project required the generous contributions of a number of people over the years. First, we acknowledge the 3,000-plus clinical and counseling psychologists who took the time from their busy schedules to complete the lengthy questionnaires associated with our eight national studies. Second, we genuinely appreciate the diligent assistance of our research assistants at the University of Scranton who shepherded the three latest national studies through their entire development—from gathering prodigious lists of books and films, through creating the questionnaires, to stuffing and mailing 5,000 envelopes, inputting all the returns, and conducting the data analyses. Jessica Angela, Dennis Reidy, and Jennifer Simansky survived and thrived throughout the nine-month ordeal.

We each would also like to acknowledge the individuals and organizations who assisted us personally. John Norcross appreciates the continuing financial support of the University of Scranton, specifically, the Department of Psychology and the Student Summer Research Program. John Santrock is grateful to the many students who tracked down books, references, and reviews. Linda Campbell expresses her appreciation to her husband and her mother for their continued support, and to her departmental colleagues who pursue and value scholarship. She is also grateful to Betty Tanner for her assistance in accessing materials for this book. Tom Smith appreciates the expert library guidance of Joseph Fennewald and the word processing marvels of Sandy Toy. Bob Sommer credits Sheila Layton for helping him collect information on many autobiographies.

Last, but not least, a rousing thanks to the good folks at The Guilford Press. Seymour Weingarten, Editor-in-Chief, and Kitty Moore, Executive Editor, continually expressed confidence in the project and translated their enthusiasm into concrete suggestions that improved the final product.

CONTENTS

CHAPTER 1

Introduction to Self-Help in Mental Health

You have probably heard about or read several of the following self-help books:

Feeling Good by David Burns
Self Matters by Philip McGraw
What Color Is Your Parachute? by Robert Bolles
Who Moved My Cheese? by Spencer Johnson
Dianetics by L. Ron Hubbard
Infants and Mothers by T. Berry Brazelton
The Courage to Heal by Ellen Bass and Laura Davis
Ageless Body, Timeless Mind by Deepak Chopra
The Dance of Connection by Harriet Lerner
When Bad Things Happen to Good People by Harold Kushner
Your Perfect Right by Robert Alberti and Michael Emmons
The Silent Passage by Gail Sheehy
How to Win Friends and Influence People by Dale Carnegie
Men Are from Mars, Women Are from Venus by John Gray
What to Expect When You're Expecting by Arlene Eisenberg and others
Winning through Intimidation by Robert Ringer
You Just Don't Understand by Deborah Tannen
10 Stupid Things Couples Do to Mess Up Their Relationship by Laura Schlessinger
Don't Sweat the Small Stuff . . . and It's All Small Stuff by Richard Carlson
The Power of Positive Thinking by Norman Vincent Peale
Emotional Intelligence by Daniel Goleman
Dr. Atkins' New Diet Revolution by Robert C. Atkins
The 7 Habits of Highly Effective People by Steven Covey

You have probably also seen several of the following films on family relationships and mental health topics:

Traffic	*Grumpy Old Men*
In the Bedroom	*Eyes Wide Shut*
The Color Purple	*The Prince of Tides*
Cat on a Hot Tin Roof	*Days of Wine and Roses*
The War of the Roses	*As Good As It Gets*
9½ Weeks	*Good Will Hunting*
Ordinary People	*Baby Boom*
Rain Man	*When Harry Met Sally*
Field of Dreams	*A Beautiful Mind*
Dead Poets Society	*The Piano*

Each of these books has been at or near the top of national best-seller lists, and each of the films has been seen by millions of people. Are they good self-help books and films? That is, do they provide accurate information? Do they help individuals cope effectively with problems? The consensus of mental health experts in the United States is that one-third of these self-help books and films are *not* effective self-help resources; even though they were best sellers and top-grossing films, most mental health experts view them negatively. The other two-thirds of the books and movies on this list are excellent self-help materials. In this book, we tell which are the good ones and which are the bad ones.

SELF-HELP RESOURCES

Self-help materials have become an indispensable source of psychological advice for millions of Americans. Whether we want to improve our relationships, control our anger, gain self-fulfillment, overcome depression, become better parents, lose weight, solve sexual problems, cope with stress, recover from addictions, or tackle another problem, there is a self-help book.

Our preoccupation with self-improvement is nothing new; it's been around since the Bible. Although not exactly known as a self-help author, Benjamin Franklin dispensed self-improvement advice in *Poor Richard's Almanac*: "Early to bed, early to rise, makes a man healthy, wealthy, and wise." In the 19th century, homemakers read *Married Lady's Companion* for help in managing their houses and families. In the 1930s, Dale Carnegie's *How to Win Friends and Influence People* made him the aspiring businessman's guru. And the 1950s brought us Maxwell Maltz's *Psychocybernetics* and dozens of marriage manuals.

Interest in understanding the human psyche and how to improve it heated up in the 1960s and 1970s, and was accompanied by a glut of self-help books. *I'm OK, You're OK* and *Your Erroneous Zones* were read by millions of Americans and made fortunes for their authors. They turned out to be only the tip of the iceberg.

The advent of popular films, the information revolution, and the ascendancy of the Internet have given rise to a dizzying diversity of self-help resources. Millions routinely go to the movies, surf the net, and attend self-help groups for edification and assistance. This book is designed to guide you through this morass of self-help information—and misinformation—by providing quality ratings and brief descriptions of five types of self-help materials: self-help books, autobiographies, films, Internet sites, and self-help/support groups.

1. Self-Help Books

The self-help book market has yielded an overwhelming, bewildering array of choices. Self-help books appear at the rate of about 2,000 a year (Rosen, 1993), and they routinely occupy prominent places on best-seller lists. Books are written on every conceivable topic, as the following list of titles vividly demonstrates:

> *Dance Naked in Your Living Room*
> *How to Juggle Women Without Getting Killed or Going Broke*
> *I Lost 600 Pounds: I Can Sure Help You Lose 30*
> *Change Your Underwear, Change Your Life*
> *Dated Jekyll, Married Hyde*
> *Boldly Live as You Have Never Lived Before: Life Lessons from Star Trek*
> *The Fairy Godmother's Guide to Dating and Mating*
> *Celestial 911—Call with Your Right Brain for Answers*
> *Don't Bite the Apple 'til You Check for Worms*

The soaring volume of self-help books makes the question of quality—which one will work?—increasingly urgent. More than 95% of self-help books are published without any research documenting their effectiveness (Rosen, 1987, 1993). Buyers hope that they will work, but we do not have any systematic evidence to indicate that they do.

So how do people select self-help books? Until this book—the *Authoritative Guide to Self-Help Resources in Mental Health*—people have largely relied on the opinions of friends, ministers, doctors, therapists, talk shows, or the promotional information on the book's cover. But even personal contact with professionals, such as physicians and psychologists, provides limited information about which book to purchase. Self-help books have been published at such an astonishing pace that even the well-intentioned professional has difficulty keeping up with them. The professional may be well informed about books in one or two areas, such as depression or anxiety, but may know little about books in other areas, such as eating disorders, women's issues, relaxation, and parenting.

Some self-help books have been written by professionals who have masterful insights about who we are and how we can improve our lives. Others, to put it mildly, leave a lot to be desired. As a concerned psychologist lamented, "Many self-help books are not worth the paper they are printed on." With literally thousands of titles on the market, we wanted to know what the leading psychologists in the United States think are the best and the worst self-help books.

After all, restaurant critics inform us which restaurants are superb and which ones to avoid; automobile guides educate us about the gems and the lemons; and consumer magazines dispense advice on which refrigerators, computers, and VCRs to buy. A guide to self-help resources based on professional judgments by mental health experts is sorely needed. This book is that guide.

The good news from research is that self-help programs can be quite effective. Several reviews of the literature have determined that the effectiveness of a self-help program substantially exceeds that of no treatment (Kurtzweil, Scogin, & Rosen, 1996; Scogin, Bynum, & Calhoun, 1990). For example, in one analysis of the effectiveness of 40 self-help studies, effect sizes for self-help were nearly as large as those for therapist-assisted treatments (Gould & Clum, 1993). Fears, depression, headaches, and sleep disturbances were especially amenable to self-help.

Similarly, *bibliotherapy*—a fancy term for using self-help books—has been shown to be valuable for many, but not all, adults. In one thorough review (Marrs, 1995), bibliotherapy was as effective as therapist-administered treatments. Comparable findings have been reported for the effectiveness of self-help books for specific disorders, such as sexual dysfunctions (van Lankveld, 1998), depression (Cuijpers, 1997), anxiety (Weekes, 1996), alcohol problems (Walters, 2000; Watson & Sher, 1998), panic (Carlbring, Westling, & Andersson, 2000), and geriatric depression (Scogin, 1998; Scogin, Hamblin, & Beutler, 1987).

Self-help books come in many guises. In this book, we do not evaluate books that are primarily religious in nature or medical in content. Books that focus on physical health and disease, be it AIDS, cancer, or heart disease, were not included. Our target is self-help books on mental health topics.

Others have compiled personal recommendations of self-help books (e.g., Fried & Schultis, 1995; Joshua & DiMenna, 2000; Zaccaria & Moses, 1968); however, our compilation is unique and, we believe, superior, because our ratings are based on the collective wisdom of thousands of mental health experts. In our national studies, we asked mental health professionals to rate more than 700 self-help books. We chose these books by examining the shelves of major national bookstore chains, by perusing the wares of large Internet book dealers (Amazon.com, bn.com), by discussing self-help books with fellow psychologists, by consulting the best-seller lists, and by reading numerous articles.

2. Autobiographies

People love personal, compelling stories of self-transformation. Autobiographies provide an inside view of life's problems, drawing on the human capacity for self-description and self-analysis. Memoirs complement research and case studies performed from the outside looking in. Written in the person's own words, an autobiography emphasizes issues that the writer, as distinct from a therapist or researcher, considers important. Autobiographies describe disorders in family and environmental context, provide interesting narratives with strong story lines, and, in the end, typically reveal a successful outcome.

Autobiographical authors and their credentials vary tremendously. Some authors are celebrities, already the subject of public interest; others are writers, poets, and artists capable of portraying their inner worlds in words, songs, and drawings. Many accounts are written by ordinary people whose first contact with publishing is writing about their disorder. Some earlier accounts have become classics in mental health education; other books by Kay Jamison (*An Unquiet Mind*), William Styron (*Darkness Visible*), and Mark Vonnegut (*The Eden Express*) are likely to become future classics. Several autobiographies have been made into major films, bringing them to a wide public audience.

The books have been used in training mental health professionals and as part of therapy for mental health consumers.

Autobiographies cover virtually all diagnostic categories. There have been at least 100 published bibliographies and book-length anthologies of first-person accounts of mental disorder (Sommer, Clifford, & Norcross, 1998).

The autobiographies listed and evaluated in this book were selected specifically for their availability. Our earlier research articles on autobiographies contained many historical accounts, often very difficult to obtain. For this book, we focused on first-person accounts still in print that covered mental health problems and life challenges. We visited bookstores and checked electronic booksellers to make sure that the book was still available. The date listed is that of the most recent edition, often in paperback. Even so, it is likely that some books will no longer be available by the time this book is published. However, it is likely that an out-of-print title can be obtained on the used book market.

An autobiographical account presents a personal view of the disorder and its treatment. When an author says that a mood disorder was relieved by Prozac or blames a family member for some transgression, this represents the person's view of the situation. Most of the autobiographies were written by the person with the disorder, but occasionally there is a book by a family member, which provides another perspective on the disorder and the treatment.

The self-help industry is virtually unregulated. The people with the most influence on which autobiographies are published and marketed are the publishers, the owners of large bookstore chains, and a hodgepodge of authors with a vast range of credentials, knowledge, and competencies. We hope our studies and this book help exert a corrective influence. Systematic research and informed mental health professionals are superior to the merchandisers.

3. Films

Films are a powerful and pervasive part of our culture. The widespread availability of movie theaters, VCRs, videotapes, and DVDs allows most Americans ready access to movies. Gallup polls indicate that watching movies at home and in theaters are among adults' favorite pastimes (along with reading, watching television, and participating in family activities). Domestic box office revenues top, according to *Variety*, a staggering $14 billion for the 100 top-performing films. And movies frequently touch us emotionally more than books. Psychologist Ken Gergen (1991) opines that the movies have become one of the most influential rhetorical devices in the world: "Films can catapult us rapidly and effectively into states of fear, anger, sadness, romance, lust, and aesthetic ecstasy—often within the same two-hour period. It is undoubtedly true that for many people film relationships provide the most emotionally wrenching experiences of the average week" (pp. 56–57).

Films possess a number of advantages over books and computers. Films are fun to watch, require only a small investment of time, appeal to more people than reading, and are already part of many clients' usual routines. Instead of spending days or weeks reading a book, people get the thrust in a few hours. As a result, people may be more open to recommendations for movies, which are more accessible, fun, and familiar.

Movies are a hot new prescription in mental health these days. The use of films for treatment purposes can be traced back to the 1930s, but more and more professionals are recommending or prescribing specific films to enhance the effects of psychotherapy. Whether its called cinematherapy, movie treatment, or reel therapy, the objective is to improve health and happiness.

We are not the first to recommend specific films to enhance self-help, but we may well be the most systematic. Several mental health professionals have penned fine compilations of popular movies to use in understanding psychopathology (Wedding & Boyd, 1999), to use in psychotherapy (Hesley & Hesley, 2001), to help with life's problems (Solomon, G., 1995), and to illustrate how psychiatry is depicted in the American cinema (Gabbard & Gabbard, 1999). But all of their books essentially present the opinions of one or two individuals. By contrast, in this book, we present the consensus of thousands of mental health experts.

In preparation for our national studies, we compiled a large list of healing films by reviewing movie books (including those listed above), tracking the top-grossing films from the past decade, and throwing in some of our personal favorites. We also used the excellent Internet Movie Database (http://www.imdb.com) and Amazon.com to search for reviews. We conducted small pilot studies of colleagues to identify films that a sizable proportion had actually seen. The result was a list of popular, commercially available films that have played in theaters or, in a few cases, only on television. These were then evaluated by thousands of psychologists.

The movies portray healing stories. The best of them typically increase awareness about a disorder or treatment; *As Good As It Gets* comes immediately to mind for its accurate and humorous depiction of obsessive–compulsive disorder (OCD). The best films also show flawed, yet effective role models struggling realistically with problems and ultimately resolving them; two cases in point are *The Color Purple*, about overcoming childhood abuse, and *On Golden Pond*, about accepting the ravages of aging and healing family rifts. The favorably rated films typically generate hope and inspiration, and perhaps give us a new perspective on ourselves and our relationships.

As with all of the self-help resources in this book, using films requires certain warnings and preparation. Viewers are asked to enter a fantasy world, but not to overidentify or overgeneralize from a single cinematic episode. The young and the squeamish should be directed away from stark, frightening portrayals. People suffering from debilitating psychiatric disorders should be forewarned of possible negative consequences of dramatic films, and those who recently suffered from trauma depicted in films should be careful not to be retraumatized.

4. Internet Resources

The Internet has opened a whole new world for people seeking information and advice. Recent estimates put the number of web pages at 2.4 billion (and growing), and there are online sites for every aspect of human life and type of psychological suffering. Researchers estimate that 70% of all Internet users have already sought health care information there. And mental health topics are the most frequently searched topics on the Internet (Davis & Miller, 1999).

But which sites and which information should be trusted? Internet sites are unregulated, and their quality varies enormously. Research studies suggest that the quality of mental health sites is not impressive; almost half are judged to be inadequate in terms of accuracy and practicality (DiBlassio et al., 1999), and information is typically slanted to favor the site's sponsor or owner (Lissman & Boehnlein, 2001). Gleaning trustworthy information on the Internet is like taking a two-year-old on a walk: The toddler picks up a few pretty pebbles but also lots of garbage and dirt (Skow, 1999) Professionals may know when a beguiling irrelevancy can be dismissed with a click of the mouse, but the average person rarely does. And any single search engine indexes no more than 16% of the public web (Lawrence & Giles, 1999).

Dr. Edward Zuckerman, in July and August 2002, visited approximately 3,500 Internet sites that seemed related to the chapters in this book and that might provide assistance to people struggling with mental health problems and life challenges. He chose the 600 or so listed sites on the belief that they would assist people—with or without psychotherapy—by fulfilling two major functions. First, these Internet sites would support persons or clients with evidence that they are not alone, that others have overcome similar difficulties, and that much is known about their conditions. Second, the online resources would provide education for patients or families concerning symptoms and diagnoses, the logic and methods of treatment, and other aspects of treatment.

Subsequently, two psychologists—Drs. Linda Campbell and Thomas Smith—independently reviewed and evaluated the 600 or so sites listed in this book. They provided their own ratings on the websites and then conferred with Ed Zuckerman on the final rating. In this manner, each website was independently evaluated and rated by at least two psychologists/book coauthors.

These Internet resources can be used in different ways and toward different ends. Some resources can be used as homework to save time, increase accuracy and completeness of education, enhance adherence and motivation, and provide instruction in the self-administration of some techniques. Online materials can also empower people and raise their self-confidence, encourage socializing, enhance lifestyle changes, maintain changes after treatment, reduce the number of sessions, reinforce points or strategies of a session, and the like.

A mental health professional should *always* read the online materials, because their contents may frighten rather than educate some clients, may conflict with a particular treatment plan, or may have changed since the evaluations described in this book. In the seven months between preparing this book and its publication, fully 18% of the URLs changed.

You should assume that all materials on the net are copyrighted. If you find them of value, someone worked hard to make them valuable, and that person deserves credit. Generally, for multiple copies, educational uses, or commercial distribution, you must get permission from the copyright holder. Therefore, obtain permission to use any of these materials unless they specifically indicate that they are available for reprinting. You must include the copyright holder's information if you reproduce materials.

In selecting Internet sites, we included those that provide information, explanations, and introductions to treatments beyond what the clinician could easily supply. The material had to be current; we estimate that more than 90% of the sites listed here were written in the last three years. All sites were visited as the book was being published and were working at that time.

We excluded sites from this book for a number of reasons. About 2,500 sites were excluded because they

- Are purely commercial, pushing a book, seminar, drug, treatment center, or private practice.
- Are not concerned with the psychology or treatment of a disorder.
- Are essentially popular magazines of loosely related but superficial contents presented for their entertainment value.
- Possess strong religious tones or messages (that may not fit many clients).
- Represent only a nonprofessional author's opinions or experiences.
- Consist of listserves, mailing lists, and bulletin boards on which anyone can post anything—recommendations, gossip, rumors, diatribes, and suggestions, as well as accurate information.
- Are a chat, or real-time equivalent of the mailing lists, chat rooms, and discussion groups. Chat is live, simultaneous typed statements by all those who signed in. They appear in sequential order on the viewer's screen. Anyone can join in, and the statements are off-the-cuff, usually unmonitored, and contain irrelevant messages from people without providing real names or identities. Professionals are usually not present and often are not welcome.

In each chapter, Internet sites are listed under the following headings:

Metasites. These are rich collections of links (underlined and/or in blue print on the computer screen) to materials or collections at other sites on the Internet. Generally, nonprofessionals would be overwhelmed by being referred to metasites because they offer hundreds of links. However, for those needing specifics not available through a search engine (because a good question cannot be generated), metasites are a boon. Also, because metasites were created by someone viewing, evaluating, and creating links to multiple sites, there has been some thoughtful selection, so that the materials are all of relevance to the topic.

Psychoeducational Materials for Clients and Families. This is where most of the sites appear. When there are large numbers of good sites, subheadings have been added to simplify searching. Where an author's name does *not* appear, we could find no author. This does not mean that the material is not copyrighted; it is.

Online Support Groups. Only when these are particularly applicable have they been offered. For those seeking local or real-world meetings of support groups, see the American Self-Help Clearinghouse Sourcebook, which is online at http://www.mentalhelp.net/selfhelp (and is also available in print).

Our compilation of online listings is not exhaustive. If you desire additional or different sites, we heartily recommend that you refer to other practical sources. An excellent printed resource is John Grohol's latest *Insider's Guide to Mental Health Resources Online.* Another source would be *The Therapist's Internet Handbook* (Stamps & Barach, 2001). The CMHC corporation (http://www.cmhc.com) supports two immense and wonderfully rich sites: Mental Health Net's Disorders and Treatments at http://mentalhelp.net/poc/view_index.php?idx=centers is the most comprehensive metasite for the problems and disorders addressed in this book. Dr. Ladd's book, *Psychological Self-Help,* at http://www.mentalhelp.net/psyhelp explains most problems in ordinary language, gives practical directions for about 100 self-change methods, and cites 2,000 references. In 15 chapters, Clayton E. Tucker-Ladd, PhD, offers information on all kinds of psychological problems and their treatments. The book can be downloaded or sections can be read online.

Two sites, in addition, provide many patient handouts. Internet Mental Health's site at http://www.mentalhealth.com/book/p40.html lists hundreds of booklets. Manisses Communications at http://www.psychlink.com/resource/Hand.html has posted about 40 brief handouts.

If we have missed an Internet site that you have found useful for yourself or patients, please send an e-mail to edzuckerma@aol.com, so that we can share it with others in the next edition of this book.

5. Self-Help/Support Groups

A self-help group is a supportive, educational, mutual-aid group that addresses a single life problem or condition shared by its members (Kurtz, 1997). Participation is voluntary, members serve as leaders, and professionals rarely play an active role in the group's activities. All forms of self-help groups have one thing in common: promotion of the member's inner strengths. The groups do so by imparting information, emphasizing self-determination, providing mutual support, and by mobilizing the resources of the person, the group, and the community (Reissman & Caroll, 1995).

Millions of Americans have come to rely on self-help or support groups for assistance with virtually every human challenge. The most recognizable of these are the 12-step groups patterned after Alcoholics Anonymous (AA) that address a wide spectrum of addictive disorders, such as those to drugs, food, and sex. But self-help groups encompass much more than addictions. There are groups for dealing with death, Alzheimer's, attention deficit disorder, difficult children, and abusive partners, as even a casual glance of the blue pages of a telephone directory will confirm. In fact, 5% of American adults attended a self-help group in the past year (Eisenberg et al., 1998).

The popularity of self-help groups is easy to understand: They are typically free, widely available, and surprisingly effective. Although research studies on these groups are infrequent and plagued with methodological problems, they do generally show positive results. Sophisticated analyses (Kownacki & Shadish, 1999; Tonigan, Toscoova, & Miller, 1995) have found that participation in AA and reduction in drinking are positively related, especially in outpatient populations. Several large and well-controlled evaluations of 12-step programs for addictive disorders have shown that they generally perform as effectively as professional treatment, including at follow-up (Morgenstern, Labouvie, McCrady, Kahler, & Frey, 1997; Ouimette, Finney, & Moos, 1997; Project MATCH Research Group, 1997).

Research on other self-help mutual aid groups generally concludes that participation is beneficial. Attending self-help groups produces higher rates of patient improvement (Barlow, Burlingame, Nebeker, & Anderson, 1999). And participants frequently evaluate self-help groups to be as helpful as psychotherapy (Seligman, 1995).

At the end of most chapters of this book, we alphabetically list prominent self-help/support groups for that particular challenge or disorder. These are listed without ratings—and for good reason. The effectiveness of self-help groups largely depends on the local members and leaders, so it is impossible to make general claims about the quality of any particular group. We provide contact numbers for the national office and online sites, so that you can identify the mission of the organization and determine whether there is a group in your locale.

The American Self-Help ClearinghouseAmerican Self-Help Clearinghouse's *Self-Help Sourcebook* at http://mentalhelp. net/selfhelp/ serves "as your starting point for exploring real-life support groups and networks that are available throughout the world and in your community." The similar National Mental Health Consumers' Self-Help Clearinghouse at http://www. mhselfhelp.org/ is a consumer-run association to connect mental health consumers with peer-run groups and to offer technical assistance with self-help groups. We strongly recommend that you visit these sites, particularly if you are searching for a support group on a topic or disorder not covered in this guide.

EIGHT NATIONAL STUDIES

We have conducted a series of national studies over the past 10 years to determine the most useful self-help resources. In each study, the methodology and the samples were very similar: a lengthy survey mailed to clinical and counseling psychologists residing throughout the United States. Across the eight studies, nearly 3,500 psychologists contributed their expertise and judgment to evaluate self-help books, autobiographies, and movies. Appendix A presents the methodological details of these studies.

These mental health professionals are all members of the clinical or counseling divisions of the American Psychological Association. To be a member of these divisions, mental health professionals are required to have obtained a doctorate from an accredited university and have been recommended for membership by their colleagues. Their ratings on the books, autobiographies, and films are based on many years of experience in helping people with particular problems and are an invaluable resource for sorting through the bewildering maze of self-help materials.

Our studies are probably the earliest and the most thorough to be conducted on a large-scale, national basis. A number of the mental health professionals who participated in the studies spontaneously commented about the virtual absence of information available to the public about how to select good self-help materials. Their positive comments about the need for our studies and the extensiveness of the materials rated bolstered our motivation for writing this book.

The psychologists rated self-help resources with which they were sufficiently familiar on the same five-point scale:

+2	Extremely good	Outstanding; highly recommended book, best or among best in category
+1	Moderately good	Provides good advice, can be helpful; worth purchasing
0	Average	An average self-help book
−1	Moderately bad	Not a good self-help book; may provide misleading or inaccurate information
−2	Extremely bad	This book exemplifies the worst of the self-help books; worst, or among worst in its category

The wording was slightly modified for rating autobiographies and films—for example, "an average autobiographical account" and "outstanding; highly recommended film." Mental health professionals rated self-help materials in the following 36 categories:

Abuse
Addictive Disorders
Adult Development
Aging
Anger
Anxiety Disorders
Assertiveness
Attention-Deficit/Hyperactivity Disorder
Bipolar Disorder (Manic–Depression)
Borderline and Narcissistic Personality Disorders
Career Development
Child Development and Parenting
Communication and People Skills
Death and Grieving
Dementia/Alzheimer's
Depression
Divorce
Eating Disorders
Families and Stepfamilies
Infant Development and Parenting
Love and Intimacy
Marriage
Men's Issues
Obsessive–Compulsive Disorder
Posttraumatic Stress Disorder
Pregnancy
Schizophrenia
Self-Management and Self-Enhancement
Sexuality
Spiritual and Existential Concerns
Stress Management and Relaxation
Suicide
Teenagers and Parenting
Weight Management
Women's Issues
Violent Youth

ONE TO FIVE STARS AND A DAGGER

We analyzed the responses to our national studies by computing how often the self-help resources were rated and how high or low the ratings were. All resources not listed at least 10 times were eliminated from the final ratings. Then, based on how often and how high they were rated, books and films with positive ratings were given one to five stars. The rare self-help books and films receiving a negative rating were given a dagger. Specifically:

★★★★★ Average rating of 1.25 or higher and rated by 30 or more mental health professionals

★★★★ Average rating of 1.00 or higher and rated by 20 or more mental health professionals

★★★ Average rating of .50 through .99 and rated 10 or more times

★★ Average rating of .25 through .49 and rated 10 or more times

★ Average rating of .00 through .24 and rated 10 or more times

† Average negative rating and rated by 10 or more mental health professionals

The sole exception to this rating system was the autobiographies. There, we used a cutoff of 8 or more ratings, as opposed to 10, simply because fewer psychologists were sufficiently familiar with autobiographies than with self-help books or films, and because we had previously used 8 as the minimum number of raters. Thus, the rating system for autobiographies was:

★★★★★ Average rating of 1.25 or higher and rated by 24 or more mental health professionals

★★★★ Average rating of 1.00 or higher and rated by 16 or more mental health professionals

★★★ Average rating of .50 through .99 and rated 8 or more times

★★ Average rating of .25 through .49 and rated 8 or more times

★ Average rating .00 through .24 and rated 8 or more times

† Average negative rating and rated by 8 or more mental health professionals

Internet resources, as previously noted, were individually evaluated and independently rated by at least two psychologists. The Internet sites were not part of the national studies. But we use a similar system to rate their quality and utility:

★★★★★ Quality interactive materials and/or lots of readings with value for patient education; accessible, accurate, current, clearly presented, and pitched at a common reading level

★★★★ Some readings or other material of high quality

★★★ A limited number of readings that can help extend a client's understanding

★★ One small reading that was, however, all that was available on the Internet on that topic

★ Of limited value for self-help or patient education; sites with this rating have been excluded from the book

In this book, the four-star and five-star self-help resources are Strongly Recommended; the three-star resources are Recommended; the one-star and two-star books are Not Recommended; and the daggered books are Strongly Not Recommended. In addition to these ratings, some self-help books, autobiographies, and films received high ratings but were rated infrequently. These resources were assigned to the Diamonds in the Rough category (♦). They have the potential to become four-star or five-star books if they become more widely known.

HOW THIS BOOK IS ORGANIZED

The following chapters present the self-help categories alphabetically, beginning with "Abuse" and ending with "Violent Youth." Each chapter opens with a brief description of the life challenge or disorder and of the audiences to which the self-help resources are addressed. We then provide our Recommendation Highlights for that chapter, which includes all five-star resources, most four-star resources, and many Diamonds in the Rough. Next, we present the expert ratings and our profiles of, in order, self-help books, autobiographies, films, and Internet sites. Descriptions and contact information are provided for self-help/support groups; however, we do not offer evaluative information or expert ratings on these groups. Not every chapter provides listings of all resources, either because there were too many resources available for that disorder or, conversely, there were too few. Our profile of each resource entails a terse review of its contents, objectives, and organization. In the final chapter, we feature 11 strategies for selecting a self-help resource.

The four appendixes contain statistical and methodological data. Appendix A details the methodology of our eight national studies. Appendix B presents the experts' average ratings for all the self-help books evaluated by five or more psychologists. Appendix C presents the average ratings for all the autobiographies evaluated by five or more respondents, and in turn, Appendix D does likewise for all the films.

USING THIS BOOK EFFECTIVELY

The *Authoritative Guide to Self-Help Resources in Mental Health* is intended for both mental health professionals and the general public.

Psychotherapists increasingly recommend self-help resources to their clients. In one of our studies involving 1,229 psychologists, 82% were recommending self-help groups to their psychotherapy patients, and 85% were recommending self-help books. Almost one-half were prescribing particular films to patients, and about one-fourth recommended autobiographies.

Moreover, psychotherapists are increasingly convinced of the effectiveness of self-help resources in conjunction with psychotherapy. Table 1.1 summarizes the results of one of our studies; it clearly demonstrates that psychologists find self-help materials to be somewhat helpful or very helpful in 70–90% of psychotherapy cases. Psychologists report that these self-help resources exerted a harmful effect on only 2–3% of their patients, a deterioration rate lower than professional treatment. Indeed, careful review of

TABLE 1.1. Psychologists' Estimated Effects of Self-Help Resources on Patients as Part of Psychotherapy

Effect	Self-help books (N = 571)	Autobiographies (N = 192)	Movies (N = 295)
Very harmful	1%	0%	1%
Somewhat harmful	2%	2%	1%
No effect	4%	29%	30%
Somewhat helpful	74%	60%	61%
Very helpful	19%	9%	7%

the evidence on self-administered treatments shows that negative outcomes are rare (Scogin et al., 1996).

Mental health professionals can use the *Authoritative Guide to Self-Help Resources in Mental Health* for information about the quality of self-help resources on a wide-ranging set of behavioral disorders and life transitions. The evaluative ratings and concise reviews will increase therapists' knowledge of more than 1,000 resources that can be used with or without professional treatment. Because all this information is packed into a single volume, books, autobiographies, films, and Internet resources can be quickly compared to determine their appropriateness.

Laypersons can also use the *Authoritative Guide* to become knowledgeable about a large number of self-help resources and to learn which ones are helpful and which are not. This is a self-help book on self-help resources. Chapter 38, Strategies for Selecting Self-Help Resources, can help you evaluate self-help more effectively.

Now that we have introduced self-help materials, our national studies, and the organization of this book, let's turn to the ratings in specific areas of mental health, beginning with Abuse.

CHAPTER 2

Abuse

Experiencing abuse can transform a person's life forever. Once victimized, many individuals never again feel quite as strong or trusting. Determining the scope of abuse is difficult because many abused individuals never reveal their experiences. Especially disturbing in the available figures are the abuses perpetuated by close friends and family members. Acquaintances of the victim are implicated in almost 50% of child sexual assaults, romantic partners in 50–75% of sexual assaults reported by college-age and adult women. The burden of abuse falls on women unequally: More than 75% of the reported cases of child sexual abuse involve girls, and more than 90% of adult rape victims are women.

Over the past decade, a professional and legal controversy has erupted over the reality of childhood abuse uncovered during psychotherapy. On the one side are those mental health professionals who regularly encounter clients who report being physically or sexually abused as children but who have repressed these traumatic memories because they were too painful. On the other side are some mental health professionals, memory researchers, and accused parents who contend that the "recovered" memories of abuse are frequently fictitious accounts subtly prompted by suggestive and hypnotic therapy techniques and by social hysteria. The storm has spilled over into the professional literature and into the nation's courtrooms. But all sides of the debate agree on two fundamental propositions: First, abuse of children is all too common and devastating; and second, the matter of recovered or false memories deserves serious scientific attention.

The following is a capsule summary of the self-help books, autobiographies, films, and Internet sites that our experts recommend on the national epidemic of abuse. But first, our Recommendation Highlights.

RECOMMENDATION HIGHLIGHTS

Self-Help Books

- On adult women's recovery from child sexual abuse:

  ★★★★★ *The Courage to Heal* by Ellen Bass and Laura Davis

  ★★★★★ *Healing the Incest Wound* by Christine A. Courtois

  ★★★ *Healing the Trauma of Abuse*
  by Mary Ellen Copeland and Maxine Harris

- On adult men's recovery from child sexual abuse:

  ★★★★ *Victims No Longer* by Michael Lew

- For the partners of adult survivors of child sexual abuse:

  ★★★★ *Allies in Healing* by Laura Davis

- On battered women who have been abused by their partners:

  ★★★★ *The Battered Woman* by Lenore Walker

  ★★★★ *Getting Free* by Ginny NiCarthy

- On date or acquaintance rape:

  ★★★ *I Never Called It Rape* by Robin Warshaw

- For women who have endured verbal abuse:

  ★★★ *The Verbally Abusive Relationship* by Patricia Evans

  ★★★ *The Secret of Overcoming Verbal Abuse*
  by Albert Ellis and Marcia Grad-Powers

- On the effect of sexual abuse on sexuality:

  ★★★ *The Sexual Healing Journey* by Wendy Maltz

- For parents of a child who has been molested:

  ★★★ *When Your Child Has Been Molested*
  by Kathryn B. Hagans and Joyce Case

Autobiographies

- On sexual abuse and incest:

  ★★★ *Daddy's Girl* by Charlotte Vale Allen

- On physical and sexual abuse:

  ★★★★ *The Lost Boy* by Dave Pelzer

  ★★★★ *A Man Named Dave* by Dave Pelzer

  ★★★ *A Child Called "It"* by Dave Pelzer

- On sexual obsessions following sexual molestation:

  ★★★ *Secret Life* by Michael Ryan

Films

- On domestic abuse and triumphant survival:
    - ★★★★ *The Color Purple*
    - ★★★★ *This Boy's Life*
    - ★★★★ *Radio Flyer*
- On sexual abuse of children:
    - ★★★★ *A Thousand Acres*
    - ★★★ *Dolores Claiborne*
- On spousal abuse:
    - ★★★ *What's Love Got to Do with It?*

Internet Resources

- On sexual assault:
    - ★★★★★ *Sexual Assault Issues* http://danenet.wicip.org/dcccrsa/saissues.html
    - ★★★★★ *Violence Against Women Office* http://www.ojp.usdoj.gov/vawo
- On domestic violence:
    - ★★★★★ *Domestic Violence* http://www.katesfeminist.info/dv
    - ★★★★★ *Domestic Abuse* http://www.police.nashville.org/bureaus/investigative/domestic/default.htm
    - ★★★★★ *Shattered Love, Broken Lives* http://www.s-t.com/projects/DomVio
    - ★★★★★ *Trust Betrayed* http://meb.marshall.edu/trust/trust-toc.htm
    - ★★★★★ *When Love Hurts: A Guide for Girls on Love, Respect and Abuse in Relationships* http://www.dvirc.org.au/whenlove
    - ★★★★★ *Domestic Violence Resources* http://www.daniel-sonkin.com/
    - ★★★★ *Why Women Stay* http://www.prevent-abuse-now.com/domviol.htm
- On date rape:
    - ★★★★ *"Friends" Raping Friends—Could It Happen to You?* http://www.eon.anglia.ac.uk/DOVI/articles/article13.htm
- On those who batter and abuse others:
    - ★★★★ *Blain Nelson's Abuse Pages* http://www.blainn.cc/abuse
- On child abuse:
    - ★★★★ *Child Abuse FAQs* http://www.law-faqs.org/nat/v-chi-en.htm
- On preventing self-abuse and self-injury:
    - ★★★★★ *Self-Injury: You Are NOT the Only One* http://www.palace.net/~llama/psych/injury.html
- On elder abuse:
    - ★★★★ *National Center on Elder Abuse* http://www.elderabusecenter.org
    - ★★★★ *NY Elder Abuse Coalition* http://www.ianet.org/nyeac/

SELF-HELP BOOKS

Strongly Recommended

★★★★★ *The Courage to Heal* (third ed., 1994) by Ellen Bass and Laura Davis. New York: Harper Perennial.

This outstanding self-help book has become a bible for many women who were sexually abused as children. Originally published in 1988, a third edition appeared in 1994. Ellen Bass realized how little help was available to adult survivors of child sexual abuse when she was teaching creative writing workshops in the 1970s. Although not trained as a psychologist, she decided to offer groups for survivors and developed the I Never Told Anyone workshops, creating a safe context where women could face their own pain and anger and begin to heal. Laura Davis was sexually abused as a child and turned to Ellen Bass for help. *The Courage to Heal* begins with a brief introduction about how healing is possible. Readers answer a series of 14 questions that help them determine if they were victims of child sexual abuse. The bulk of the book is divided into five parts: Taking Stock, The Healing Process, Changing Patterns, For Supporters of Survivors, and Courageous Women. Two sections toward the end of the book focus on counseling and healing resources. Any woman who knows she was sexually abused as a child will probably benefit from this book. The writing is clear, the survivors' stories are artfully woven through the book, the writing exercises are valuable tools, and the authors' compassion and insight are apparent. Unlike some recovery books that dwell too extensively on the past, this resource moves on in positive ways to help women heal and recover.

As a visible and best-selling book on sexual abuse of children, *The Courage to Heal* has been drawn into the repressed versus false memory storm. The authors contend that women who strongly sense that they were sexually abused but do not have specific memories of it were probably abused. Although this position fosters an acceptance and trust toward women whose abuse may have been denied by others, it simultaneously may generate or perpetuate false "memories" of abuse that never occurred. Critics contend that specific memories of early childhood abuse are notoriously unreliable and that encouraging rhetoric might create false memories and thus false accusations against innocent family members. In this specific respect, some psychologists are unhappy that this self-help resource was the top-rated book on abuse in our national studies.

The Courage to Heal Workbook (1990) was authored by Laura Davis to provide in-depth exercises for both women and men who were sexually abused as children. The workbook includes a combination of checklists, open-ended questions, writing exercises, art projects, and activities that take the adult survivor through the healing process. This book is a helpful companion to *The Courage to Heal* and is organized into four main sections: Survival Skills, Taking Stock, Aspects of Healing, and Guidelines for Healing Sexually.

★★★★★ *Healing the Incest Wound: Adult Survivors in Therapy* (1996) by Christine A. Courtois. New York: Norton.

This sensitive guide to understanding and treating incest gives the reader a poignant view of the suffering of survivors and a hopeful view of recovery. The text is comprehensive in range of information and could be used as a textbook, a practitioner's guide, a self-discovery book, or a training guide. The topics focus first on understanding incest by citation of demographics and characteristics (e.g., types of behavior, age and sex of victims and perpetrators, family structure), dynamics of incestuous family, and parent–child patterns. Then, symptoms and secondary elaborations are differentiated among young children, adolescents, and adults. Various theories of incest are reviewed, and an important chapter details how these individuals present in therapy and how assessment and diagnostic patterns often manifest. The third section attends to treatment goals, strategies, and techniques. Attention is given to group screening, ground rules, and process issues in group therapy. This is a highly rated self-help resource on a controversial topic but a book that might be too academic for some patients.

★★★★ *The Battered Woman* (1979) by Lenore Walker. New York: Harper & Row.

This excellent self-help book is written for women who have been or continue to be abused by their husbands or romantic partners. Lenore Walker is widely recognized as a leading therapist who studies and counsels battered women. The book is divided into three main parts: Psychology of the Battered Woman includes valuable information about the myths and realities of abuse, as well as psychological theories that help explain the victimization of the battered woman; Coercive Techniques in Battering Relationships provides vivid, heart-wrenching stories told by battered women themselves; and The Way Out examines not only the dark side of legal, medical, and psychological systems that tend to keep battered women as victims, but also the services battered women themselves say would be more helpful. Walker asserts that battered women undergo a process of victimization, acquiring a sense of learned helplessness that leaves them prey to abuse, unable to fault their abusers, and unwilling to leave them. The case studies unabashedly present battering from a woman's perspective; indeed, Walker acknowledges that the book is written from a woman's point of view. *The Battered Woman* was written in 1979 and has not been revised. One of its few shortcomings is its age, but a woman in an abusive relationship with a man will likely benefit from this excellent self-help book.

★★★★ *Allies in Healing* (1991) by Laura Davis. New York: Harper Perennial.

The partners of survivors are an overlooked group. This book by one of the coauthors of *The Courage to Heal* is written for partners who may not have been abused themselves, but who are living with the effects of abuse. The question and answer format makes the book highly readable, with each question at the top of a page. Questions are organized under basic topics, including My Needs and Feelings, Dealing with Crisis, Intimacy, Family Issues, and Realistic Expectations. Sensitive and difficult questions are asked, and the answers are candid and informative. A significant part of the book describes the stories of eight partners and their struggles and triumphs.

★★★★ *Getting Free: You Can End Abuse and Take Back Your Life* (3rd ed., 1997) by Ginny NiCarthy. Seattle, WA: Seal.

This book is intended for women and is about battering. It is divided into six sections: Making the Decision to Leave or Stay, Getting Professional Help, Helping Yourself to Survival, After You Leave, The Ones Who Got Away, and New Directions. The final section examines topics that do not appear in the other books on battered women listed here and provides valuable analysis and recovery advice for abused teens and abused lesbians. *Getting Free* has an extensive number of exercises for readers and is thus virtually a combination of narrative and workbook.

★★★★   *Victims No Longer: Men Recovering from Incest and Other Sexual Child Abuse* (1990) by Michael Lew. New York: Harper & Row.

Whereas the previous books in this category were designed for women, this splendid self-help book was written for men who experienced childhood incest and other sexual abuse. The focus section lends special emphasis or specific experience to the chapter subject (e.g., defining victim and survivor, debt to the women's movement, myths that interfere with recovery). Personal accounts from survivors are sprinkled between chapters. Topics are clustered into myths and realities of abuse, messages about masculinity, surviving abuse, and recovery. This book provides an emotional journey for the reader and tells the story of courageous recoveries.

Recommended

★★★   *The Sexual Healing Journey* (2001) by Wendy Maltz. New York: Harper Perennial.

The healing journey is intended to augment psychotherapy or to prepare for change at the reader's own pace. The reader is helped to understand how sexuality has been affected by sexual abuse, a realization that most survivors don't make on their own and that is often at the root of sexual difficulties. Types of sexual abuse, fears of acknowledgment, and the impact of abuse on sexuality are informatively described. Healing steps to take with one's partner are suggested, and techniques for relearning touch and solving specific sexual problems are explained. The text effectively includes exercises and exploratory questions. The interactive format in each chapter allows the reader to participate. A highly valued but infrequently rated book in our studies, thus designated as a three-star resource.

★★★   *I Never Called It Rape* (1994) by Robin Warshaw. New York: Harper Perennial.

A major study conducted by *Ms.* magazine and the National Institute of Mental Health, as well as interviews of 150 women conducted by the author are cited throughout this book in describing acquaintance rape. Author Warshaw presents a road to recovery for those sexually assaulted by an acquaintance. The denial of acquaintance rape in our culture and the uphill battle of survivors are thoughtfully chronicled. The book focuses on acquaintance rape on the college campus, in the workplace, and in other settings. The intended audience is not only the survivors of acquaintance rape but also family, parents, educators, counselors, and those in the legal system. The book is not widely known among experts in our studies, but those who do know it accord it high ratings. It is probably the best self-help book available on date rape. Any female who has experienced date rape can benefit from Warshaw's portrayal of the healing process; any dating female can benefit from the book's detailed observations about how and why date rape happens; and males can benefit from the book's description of the devastating aftereffects of date rape.

★★★   *Healing the Trauma of Abuse: A Women's Workbook* (2000) by Mary Ellen Copeland and Maxine Harris. Oakland, CA: New Harbinger.

This book is a step-by-step guide for women who have been abused sexually, emotionally, or physically. The material is designed as a self-help book to be read sequentially: The format of each chapter entails a beginning and an ending ritual of identifying positive experiences in the person's current life, reading about and understanding the problem in question (e.g., emotional abuse, physical abuse), recommendations for coping, optional activities to be practiced, and things to remember about oneself (e.g., positive affirmations). Chapter subjects lend themselves to self-exploration and prepare the reader to conduct change activities. The latter chapters identify ways of making life changes through understanding family myths, making better decisions, and understanding blame and acceptance. The book closes with a self-inventory that was also done at the beginning of the book, with the goal of contrasting the perceptual changes the reader has made through these exercises. A highly valued book in our national studies, had it been more frequently rated, it would have probably reached four- or five-star status.

★★★   *The Secret Trauma* (1999) by Diana E. H. Russell. New York: Basic Books.

This book is based on an extensive study conducted by the author to investigate incestuous abuse, extrafamilial child sexual abuse, rape, and other types of sexual assault perpetrated against females. Personal interviews were conducted with 930 randomly chosen women. The methodology of the study and the extensive results are reported. The findings are clustered into initial descriptions of the problem of incest, including reporting trends, characteristics of incest abuse, and social factors. A major part of the book is devoted to understanding victims: who they are and how they cope, revictimization, long-term effects, and several case studies. Also, different than other books on abuse, this book presents information on the perpetrators: who they are, father–daughter incest, biological versus stepfather incest, and other familial incidences of incest. Myths versus realities of the findings are outlined in an attempt to portray more accurately incestuous abuse. This book was highly but infrequently rated, perhaps due to its more scholarly orientation.

★★★   *When Your Child Has Been Molested* (1998) by Kathryn B. Hagans and Joyce Case. San Francisco: Jossey-Bass.

This informative guide on child molestation provides a series of observations and recommendations called "reality checks" that will assist parents in making decisions and in attending to the needs of their child. Topics include Believing your child's reality, understanding the child's continued fears, the grief process, dealing with guilt, healing the communication process in the family, the child's appearance in court, and what to say to others. The reality checks are helpful questions to ask or observations to make: ways to talk with your child, signs of possible molestation, how shock and denial are expressed in the grief process, questions to ask a potential therapist, preparing your child for court. This book is unique in providing information about the court process and what to expect. A glossary of terms is helpful and covers legal and psychological expressions. A final checklist can determine whether the family is getting better and what to do about it. This is another book that would have merited more stars had it been more widely known and thus more frequently rated in our studies.

★★★   *Battered Wives* (revised ed., 1989) by Del Martin. Volcano, CA: Volcano.

This book is intended for women who have been in an abusive relationship with a man or who continue to be abused in the relationship. Although the book is titled *Battered Wives*, Martin says that her book applies equally to unmarried women who live with violent men; many of the examples she uses involve unmarried cohabitants. In Martin's view, the underlying problem that has led to the battering of so many women is found

not in the husband–wife interaction or immediate triggering events but rather in the institution of marriage itself, historically negative attitudes toward women in society, the
economy, and inadequacies in legal and social services. The book is at its best in its
scathing feminist critiques of a society that discriminates against women and, in this respect, is more a sociological analysis of battered women than an in-depth psychological
analysis. The textbook style of writing makes for difficult reading in many places. The
riveting case studies and more personal tone in Walker's book will be more attractive to
most readers, and even the 1989 revision of *Battered Wives* is dated.

★★★ *The Secret of Overcoming Verbal Abuse* (2000) by Albert Ellis and Marcia Grad-
        Powers. Hollywood, CA: Wilshire.

The story of verbal abuse is told from a woman's perspective—of sadness, of disrespect,
of the personality change of Prince Charming, and of the loss of a relationship that was
not to be. The abuse syndrome and accompanying dynamics are richly described for
the reader who may feel unique and alone. The authors effectively present the typical
feelings and thoughts of the abuse victim and signs that one is in an abusive relationship. Rational–Emotive Behavioral Therapy (REBT) is explained and applied to the verbal abuse syndrome, with attention to the role of cognitive distortions and the importance of moving toward unconditional self-acceptance. The fears of aloneness, change,
and the unknown are discussed as obstacles to change. Skill development, relaxation,
and other techniques are presented as additional therapeutic interventions. Resolving
the fears that keep individuals stuck is a focus of the therapeutic intervention.

★★★ *Healing the Shame That Binds You* (1988) by John Bradshaw. Deerfield Beach, FL:
        Health Communications.

This book appeared on the *New York Times* best-seller list and sold more than half a million copies. Bradshaw believes that people with a wide array of problems, including addictions, compulsions, and codependencies, developed their problems because of toxic
shame. What is toxic shame? Bradshaw never gives a clear definition, but he does provide some hints about its nature. He says that toxic shame is present when people believe that things are hopeless and feel that they themselves are worthless. They feel de-
fective, flawed, and inadequate as people. Individuals with toxic shame perceive that
they lack power. How can people get rid of shame-based feelings? Bradshaw believes
that the healing process involves getting the shame out of hiding and externalizing it.
This involves liberating the lost inner child, integrating disowned parts, loving the self,
healing memories, improving self-image, confronting and changing inner voices, coping with toxic shame relationships, and awakening spiritually. Bradshaw describes a
number of therapy strategies that can be used to help individuals externalize their toxic
shame. Although popular with the public, this book received tepid and mixed evaluations by the mental health experts in our national studies.

★★★ *Wounded Boys, Heroic Men: A Man's Guide to Recovering from Child Abuse* (1992) by
        Daniel Jay Sonkin. Stamford, CT: Longmeadow.

The step-by-step material in this book is designed for men who were abused physically,
sexually, or psychologically when they were boys, as well as for their partners, friends,

and family members. Special focus is given to the gender-based roadblocks that men face, including not seeking help, being expected to pull themselves up by their bootstraps, thinking and not feeling, and taking punishment like a real man. Topics are how to begin the journey, types of abuse, breaking the pattern of denial, and healing through attitude and behavior change. Bullet points highlight the message of each chapter (e.g., knowing you're on the right track, how abuse affects you today). This book provides a hopeful and demythologizing message about recovery.

★★★　*Beginning to Heal: A First Book for Survivors of Child Sexual Abuse* (1993) by Ellen Bass and Laura Davis. New York: Harper Perennial.

Beginning to Heal, a condensed version of *The Courage to Heal*, reviewed above, is designed for those who are just starting to face the abuse they experienced earlier in life. The approach offers an empathic and validating perspective that involves healing, believing it happened, grieving, anger, change, and moving on. Inserts, including quotes and observations in boxed form, contribute to clarity on subjects such as surviving the panic stage, how most people begin to remember, breaking the silence, and how to change. A significant section of the book recalls the stories of five women who were abused as children and how they moved through the healing process. This book serves as an invitation and introduction to recovery from child sexual abuse.

★★★　*The Verbally Abusive Relationship* (1996) by Patricia Evans. Holbrook, MA: Adams Media.

The stories in this book were told to the author by women who were verbally abused. Their experiences serve as validation for abused women who have questioned the legitimacy and reality of their experiences. Forty verbally abused women between the ages of 21 and 66 were interviewed. Verbal abuse is discussed from the perspective of power and dominance. The first part of the book presents a self-evaluation questionnaire, and the second part characterizes categories of verbal abuse (e.g., withholding, discounting, accusing, trivializing, denial), using illustrations of typical scenarios. A valuable aspect of the book is that it addresses how to respond effectively to verbal abuse. Examples provide clear ways to interpret and deal with abusive communication. This edition includes a chapter for therapists that considers verbal abuse from the therapeutic standpoint, and chapters on children in abusive environments. The book received a stellar rating of 1.61 in one of our national studies but was rated by only 13 experts, thus leading to its three-star rating and to an underestimation of its probable usefulness.

Diamond in the Rough

◆　*You Are Not Alone: A Guide for Battered Women* (2000) by Linda P. Rouse. Holmes Beach, FL: Learning Publications.

This book is written for women who have experienced battering at the hands of a man who is not a stranger to them. The book provides a straightforward self-evaluation to help women determine where their relationships are. The profile of battering men is described, and the societal and familial roots of battering men are explored, including low self-esteem, traditional sex-role expectations, jealousy and control focus, abusive family background, and failure to acknowledge the need for change. The authors provide valuable information regarding contacting a shelter, the importance of medical care, the centrality of psychological services, and a flowchart on navigating the legal system. Factors in deciding to stay or not to stay are concluding topics. Helpful resources in the appendices include worksheets on fears in leaving, secondary gains, and strength resilience. This book, infrequently rated in our national studies, was rated very highly by those who did read it.

Not Recommended

★★ *Toxic Parents: Overcoming Their Hurtful Legacy and Reclaiming Your Life* (1989) by Susan Forward. New York: Bantam.

★★ *Abused No More: Recovery for Women from Abusive or Co-Dependent Relationships* (1989) by Robert Ackerman and Susan E. Pickering. Blue Ridge Summit, PA: TAB Books.

★ *Reclaiming the Inner Child* (1990) edited by Jeremiah Abrams. Los Angeles: Jeremy P. Tarcher.

AUTOBIOGRAPHIES

Recommended

★★★★ *The Lost Boy: A Foster Child's Search for the Love of a Family* (1997) by Dave Pelzer. Deerfield Beach, FL: Heath Communications.

This is the second book of a trilogy, whose first volume, *A Child Called "It,"* describes the author's harrowing early life with an extremely abusive mother. This book covers the author's subsequent nine years in the foster care system, moving from one home to another, until the he finally lands in a home that can give him the love he so desperately craves. It is emotionally wrenching to read, not only because of the past abuse but also because of the shame, insecurity, and loneliness of kids moved from one household to another. On the positive side, the book underscores the fact that resilient kids can come through. An excellent book for foster parents interested in the inner worlds of their children, and for foster children who want to know how others have survived the combination of abuse and foster care.

★★★★ *A Man Named Dave: A Story of Triumph and Forgiveness* (2000) by Dave Pelzer. New York: Plume.

Pelzer's trilogy begins with his life in an abusive household, his nine years in various foster homes, and now his life as an adult. This is a story of survival, resilience, willpower, coming to terms with a horrific past, incorporating that information in one's life, and moving on. Pelzer enlisted in the Air Force at age 18 and served in Operations Desert Shield and Desert Storm. While in the Air Force, he worked with at-risk youth and since retiring has become a child advocate whose work received national and international recognition. Some readers may be put off by the graphic descriptions of abuse, but if they have gotten through the two earlier books, this one will provide a degree of closure, especially when the author describes his positive relationship with his young son and his reconciliation with his father. The lessons are clear— abuse can be survived and surmounted, and even gruesome experiences can form the basis for a productive career and a satisfying life.

★★★ *A Child Called "It": One Child's Courage to Survive* (1995) by Dave Pelzer. Deerfield Beach, FL: Health Communications.

This is the first book of a trilogy describing different periods in the author's life. It is a horrifying account of his abuse as a child by a sadistic and alcoholic mother who nearly killed him. She referred to him as "it" and starved and burned him. Eventually, Dave was rescued by an alert schoolteacher. This best-selling book demonstrates how hope and love can overcome extreme adversity in childhood. The account of abuse is so horrifying as to shock sensitive readers, but the books contains underlying themes of hope and recovery.

★★★ *Daddy's Girl* (1995) by Charlotte Vale Allen. New York: Berkeley.

A professional writer struggles to free herself from memories of her father's incestuous demands, which began when she was seven years old and continued until she was 17, and from her image of herself as ugly and unlovable. The author is now active in behalf of victims of child abuse and domestic violence. A compelling autobiography, it is a good discussion of the connection between childhood abuse and adult relationships.

★★★ *Sleepers* (1996) by Lorenzo Carcaterra. New York: Ballantine.

As a young man growing up in a poor neighborhood, the author and his friends engaged in petty crimes. When they were caught, the young men were sent to a juvenile home, where they were assaulted and raped by brutal guards. Years later, the men took revenge against their tormenters. The book was made into a popular movie of the same name. (Also reviewed in Chapter 37 on Violent Youth.)

★★★ *Secret Life* (1996) by Michael Ryan. New York: Vintage.

Poet Michael Ryan attributes the sexual obsessions of his adult years to having been molested at age five by a neighbor and being physically abused by an alcoholic father. He bares his soul to the reader in this searing autobiography. It is an excellent and disturbing portrait of sex addiction, the compulsive drive for sex regardless of the consequences for self and others.

FILMS

Strongly Recommended

★★★★ *The Color Purple* (1986) directed by Steven Spielberg. PG-13 rating. 152 minutes.

This unforgettable movie depicts a magnificent triumph of the human spirit over endless and vile cruelties—physical and sexual—brought about by family separation, abuse, and ignorance. Despite her sufferings, Celie, a poor, unloved, unlovely, African American woman in the turn-of-the-century South, discovers her beauty, courage, and potential. If she can do it, we all can. The movie is notable for its superb performances and the Oscars it won.

★★★★ *This Boy's Life* (1994) directed by Michael Caton-Jones. R rating. 115 minutes.

A mother takes her son and heads west after divorce to the little town of Concrete. Desperate for marriage, she weds a pathetic bully. The heart of the story is the war between a nice kid and his sadistic, lying, con-artist stepfather, who is perfectly portrayed as a sick adult child, always feeling cheated and misunderstood, and blaming the boy. The film illustrates the boy's growth in confidence and hope to escape, the mother's passivity, and the loathsome man's character weaknesses. As such, it demonstrates hope and growth despite a terrible childhood.

★★★★ *Radio Flyer* (1992) directed by Richard Donner. PG-13 rating. 120 minutes.

This beautiful but painful film illustrates the denial patterns of a codependent wife and her physically and verbally abusive alcoholic husband. The two boys, who are the focus of the story, try to protect her and each other from his beatings. Although the movie offers no usable guidance for coping with or overcoming the abuse or its denial, the nature of the pathology is clearly displayed.

★★★★ *A Thousand Acres* (1997) directed by Jocelyn Moorhouse. R rating. 105 minutes.

An aging farmer transfers ownership to the family farm to his grown daughters and their husbands. The film sensitively traces the generational struggle for control and power—*King Lear* set on an Iowa farm—but is riveting in gradually revealing the secrets of the father's physical and sexual abuse years earlier. He beat the children and forced himself sexually on two daughters, who together protected their younger sibling from him. The discovery and confrontation of incest in a family of origin are frighteningly realistic and, in the end, only partially effective as minimization prevails. The father never expresses remorse or achieves understanding. An effective (and potentially painful) film for those who have been physically or sexually abused.

Recommended

★★★ *Dolores Claiborne* (1995) directed by Taylor Hackford. R rating. 132 minutes.

Dolores, a maid working in remote Maine, is accused of murdering her wealthy employer. Dolores's daughter, Selena, returns to her mother's side after 15 years of estrangement and anger. We discover that Dolores's alcoholic husband beat her and sexually molested Selena. Although initially idealizing her father and resenting her mother, Selena eventually realizes that her father molested her and that her mother protected her the best she could. It is a poignant and realistic film for women who were abused by spouses, for adults who were sexually abused as children, and for those wanting to understand the complicated dynamics of abusive relationships.

★★★ *What's Love Got to Do with It?* (1994) directed by Brian Gibson. R rating. 119 minutes.

A true and completely believable story of a seductive, charming, abusive husband and his talented wife, who stays with him long beyond what reason or love would require. He beats her, flaunts his girlfriends, and abuses cocaine. She excuses him, believes his apologies, and gives him many more chances. The movie is an unflinching and honest look at how such patterns can exist in any family.

★★★ *The Apostle* (1997) directed by Robert Duvall. PG-13 rating. 134 minutes.

A fundamentalist preacher in the South showers love and concern on his congregation but violence and infidelity on his marriage. Sonny (Robert Duvall) is a complex man— good and bad, loving and abusing, saintly and devilish—and an ambiguous apostle. Viewers with no experience in the southern Pentecostal culture might find the film confusing, but it is a strong story of a fatally flawed, religiously militant man who abuses his spouse.

★★★ *Sleeping with the Enemy* (1991) directed by Joseph Ruben. R rating. 98 minutes.

A battered trophy wife fakes her own death in order to break away from the total dominance and control of her husband. She runs away to restart her life; he finds her and threatens her again. That is all the film has to offer. It is best used to illustrate the characters and dynamics of the couple.

Not Recommended

★★ *Thelma and Louise* (1992) directed by Ridley Scott. R rating. 129 minutes.

★★ *Mommie Dearest* (1981) directed by Frank Perry. PG rating. 129 minutes.

★★ *Matilda* (1996) directed by Danny DeVito. PG rating. 98 minutes.

Strongly Not Recommended

† *The Prince of Tides* (1992) directed by Barbra Streisand. R rating. 132 minutes.

INTERNET RESOURCES

There are an enormous number of resources available online about all kinds of abuse. The sites described here focus on sexual assault and abuse, domestic violence, child abuse, abused males, and abuse by professionals. Excluded are materials primarily about workplace violence; the legal side (prosecution, suits, advocacy); sexual harassment; sex offenders; ritual abuse and torture; and sites that combine abuse with materials on dissociation. Reading some of these sites may trigger memories in those who have experienced abuse. Please exercise caution.

Metasites

★★★★★ *Sexual Assault Issues* http://danenet.wicip.org/dcccrsa/saissues.html

This website contains many fact sheets, articles, and a good booklet. Well written and displayed, they cover all aspects, such as male victims, medical and legal issues, offenders, child victims, safety, and information about therapy.

★★★★★ *Domestic Violence* http://www.katesfeminist.info/dv

An excellent general site with lists of Internet sites with help for victims, fact sheets, what you can do, and so on.

★★★★★ *Office of Violence Against Women* http://www.ojp.usdoj.gov/vawo/

This federal government site offers links, hotlines, laws, toolkits, grants, and much more on all aspects of abuse, violence, stalking, and battering.

Psychoeducational Materials for Clients and Families

Sexual Assault and Abuse

★★★★ *Coercion, Rape, and Surviving*
    http://ub-counseling.buffalo.edu/violence.shtml

The site offers about 10 pages of solid information including a sexual rights questionnaire and what men can do. It is excellent for raising consciousness.

★★★★ *Sexual Abuse* http://soulselfhelp.on.ca/

There are about 10 pages on definitions, effects, memory recovery, anger, obesity, and getting support. The section on Tools in Recovery is a good set of tips and advice on relapse prevention, helpful slogans, definitions, and so forth.

★★★★ *Becoming Whole Again: Healing from Sexual Assault*
    http://www.utexas.edu/student/cmhc/booklets/rape/rape.html

The site provides definitions and information on immediate responses, coping, recovering, and self-care, plus suggestions for family—all in five pages. Designed for a college audience, it is an excellent starting point.

★★★★ *Rape Victim Advocacy Program* http://www.uiowa.edu/~rvap/contents.html

This is a counseling center in Iowa, but its online readings for victims include Facts about Sexual Assault, If You Have Been Assaulted, What To Do If My Child Has Been Assaulted, and What to Say to a Rape Survivor.

★★★★ *Information for Victims of Sexual Assault and Their Families*
    http://www.connsacs.org/library/infocsa.htm

A comprehensive and informative 10-page brochure that addresses both legal and medical concerns.

★★★★ *"Friends" Raping Friends—Could It Happen to You?* by Jean O'Gorman Hughes
       and Bernice R. Sandler
       http://www.eon.anglia.ac.uk/DOVI/articles/article13.htm

Although from 1987, this is a superb overview in 16 packed pages.

★★★★ *STDs and Sexual Assault: Information on HIV/AIDS, Hepatitis B, and Other Sex-
       ually Transmitted Diseases*   http://www.connsacs.org/library/hivbook.html

Seven pages of facts.

★★★ *Frequently Asked Questions* http://www.mincava.umn.edu/faqs.asp

This set of questions and answers is useful as a beginning point, primarily because of its
links to data sources.

Domestic Violence

★★★★★ *Domestic Abuse*   http://www.police.nashville.org/bureaus/investigative/do-
         mestic/default.htm

This remarkable series of brief but realistic checklists (from the Nashville Police De-
partment) should make the reader much less vulnerable. They are headed Potential
Indicators of Domestic Abuse, Stress Related Problems in Children of Abuse, Pro-
gression of Violence, How Abusers Stage a Return, Signs of Rehabilitation, Common
Characteristics of the Battered and the Batterer, Similar Stories of Battered Spouses,
Dangers after Separation, Long-Term Effects of Abuse, and Make a Separation Safety
Plan.

★★★★★ *Shattered Love, Broken Lives* http://www.s-t.com/projects/DomVio

Here are 60 integrated newspaper articles examining all aspects of domestic violence.
They could provide both specific and background information for all readers.

★★★★★ *Trust Betrayed* http://meb.marshall.edu/trust/trust-toc.htm

A superb booklet of about 20 pages teaches what are healthy and controlling relationships and ways of dealing with abusive relationships.

★★★★★ *When Love Hurts: A Guide for Girls on Love, Respect and Abuse in Relation-
         ships* http://www.dvirc.org.au/whenlove

A superb and stylish booklet of about 20 pages that provides information on abusive relationships, help in thinking about respect, and ideas about changing.

★★★★★ *Domestic Violence Resources* by Daniel Jay Sonkin, PhD
         http://www.daniel-sonkin.com/

Under Online Articles and then General Public Information are five sections totaling
about 15 pages with solid information, techniques, and advice for abusers.

★★★★★　*AWARE: Arming Women Against Rape and Endangerment*
　　　　http://www.aware.org

A fine introduction to "effective self-protection for intelligent women who want help, not hype."

★★★★★　*Domestic Violence Information Manual*
　　　　http://www.uwm.edu/~edari/resdocs/DVIM1.doc

This Internet book from Australia covers myths blaming the victim, theories, programs, and links.

★★★★　*Why Women Stay* by Nancy Faulkner, PhD
　　　　http://www.prevent-abuse-now.com/domviol.htm

In 13 pages, the author describes the 13 types of persons who stay and their reasons for staying. Well done and clear, the site could help clarify the issues for a victim.

★★★★　*Family Life Library*
　　　　http://www.oznet.ksu.edu/library/famlf2/#family%20living

Page down to Violence Hits Home for six articles suitable as handouts and brochures from a Kansas State University program. The articles have to be downloaded and opened using Adobe Acrobat.

★★★★　*Domestic Violence Brochure*
　　　　http://www.noda.new-orleans.la.us/source/dv_bro1.html

From the District Attorney of New Orleans, this site offers definitions, myths, information on the legal processes, a checklist of what to take when leaving, and victim's rights, all in about eight pages. A good starting place for advice.

★★★★　*Blain Nelson's Abuse Pages*　http://www.blainn.cc/abuse

Nelson offers two long questionnaires, which are consciousness raising. Not all abuse is simple or physical.

★★★★　*Is Your Relationship Heading into Dangerous Territory?*
　　　　http://www.utexas.edu/student/cmhc/booklets/relatvio/relaviol.html

Six pages of checklists raise awareness, comparing violent and nonviolent relationships, the cycle of domestic violence, and what to do.

Child Abuse

★★★★　*Child Abuse FAQs*
　　　　http://www.law-faqs.org/nat/v-chi-en.htm

About 25 brief, well-written, and clear answers to questions.

Abused Males

★★★★ *The National Organization on Male Sexual Victimization*
      http://www.nomsv.org

The 7 Myths about Male Sexual Abuse is valuable, and the links on that page offer many very relevant articles about all aspects of male victims, a bibliography, poetry, names of therapists, and so on.

Self-Injury

★★★★★ *Self-Injury: You Are NOT the Only One*
      http://www.palace.net/~llama/psych/injury.html

This is a high-quality, rich site. The Quick Primer is very educational, as is Self-Help. There are a questionnaire, quotes, references, chat, and more. Much of it can be used with Linehan's Dialectical Behavior Therapy.

Abuse by Professionals

★★★★★ *H.O.P.E. (Help Overcoming Professional Exploitation)*
      http://www.advocateweb.org/hope/default.asp

This excellent resource contains links to all the major groups and resources. It includes dozens of informative readings under Articles, on the left.

★★★★ *SNAP (Survivors Network of those Abused by Priests)*
      http://www.survivorsnetwork.org

This is a self-help, online support group with many resources listed. See also the support group SOSA: Survivors of Spiritual Abuse at http://www.sosa.org.

Other Aspects of Abuse

★★★★★ *WHOA (Women Halting Online Abuse)* http://www.haltabuse.org

This site provides readings, technical suggestions, and support for those harassed or stalked in the online world.

★★★★ *Information for Mothers and Other People Concerned about Children Who Witness Domestic Violence* http://www.dvirc.org.au/publications/childrendv.htm

A brief, factual overview and many good articles and links.

★★★★ *National Center on Elder Abuse* http://www.elderabusecenter.org

The best site for FAQs, definitions, and readings.

NATIONAL SUPPORT GROUPS

Batterers Anonymous
1041 South Mt. Vernon Avenue
Suite G-306
Colton, CA 92324
Phone: 909-355-1100

For men who wish to control their anger and eliminate their abusive behavior.

Child Help USA Hotline
15757 North 78th Street
Scottsdale, AZ 85260
http://www.childhelpusa.org
Phone: 480-922-8212

General information on child abuse and related issues, and some crisis counseling. Referrals to local agencies for child abuse reporting.

Domestic Violence Anonymous
DVA, c/o BayLaw
PO Box 29011
San Francisco, CA 94129
Phone: 415-681-4850
E-mail: Baylaw1@ix.netcom.com
http://www.baylaw.com

Twelve-step spiritual support for men and women who are recovering from domestic violence.

False Memory Syndrome Foundation
1955 Locust Street
Philadelphia, PA 19146
Phone: 215-940-1040
E-mail: mail@fmsfonline.org
http://www.fmsfonline.org

Research-oriented organization for persons falsely accused of childhood sex abuse based on recovered or repressed memories.

National Child Abuse Hotline
Phone: 800-422-4453;
    800-222-4453 (TDD)

National Domestic Violence Hotline
http://www.ndvh.org
Phone: 800-799-SAFE (7233);
    800-787-3224 (TDD)

Information and referrals for victims of domestic violence.

Network for Battered Lesbians and Bisexual Women
E-mail: advocate@thenetwork.lared.org
http://www.thenetwork.lared.org
Phone: 617-423-7233

Parents Anonymous
675 West Foothill Boulevard, Suite 220
Claremont, CA 91711-3416
Phone: 909-621-6184
E-mail: parentsanonymous@
    parentsanonymous.org
http://www.parentsanonymous.org

Professionally facilitated, peer-led group for parents who are having difficulty and would like to learn more effective ways of raising their children.

Parents United International
615 15th Street
Modesto, CA 95354-2510
Phone: 209-572-3446
E-mail: parents.united@usa.net

Provides treatment for child sexual abuse.

RAINN (Rape Abuse and Incest National Network)
Phone: 800-656-4673
http://www.rainn.org

Offers a national hotline network for victims and survivors of sexual abuse who cannot get to a local rape crisis center.

SAFE (Self-Abuse Finally Ends) Alternative Information Line
Phone: 800-DONT-CUT

Provides information on dealing with self-abuse and self-mutilation, and the treatment options.

SESAME (Survivors of Educator Sexual Abuse and Misconduct Emerge)
PO Box 905
Pahrump, NV 89041
E-mail: babe4justice@aol.com
http://www.sesamenet.org

Support and information network for families of children (K–12) who have been sexually abused by a school staff member.

S.I.A. (Survivors of Incest Anonymous) World Service Office
PO Box 190
Benson, MD 21018-9998
Phone: 410-282-3400 or 410-893-3322
http://www.siawso.org

Self-help, 12-step program for men and women who have been victims of child sexual abuse and want to be survivors.

SNAP (Survivors Network of Those Abused by Priests)
PO Box 6416
Chicago, IL 60680
Phone: 312-409-2720

http://www.survivorsnetwork.org

Support for men and women who were sexually abused by any clergy person.

Violence Against Women Office
Phone: 800-799-7233 or 800-787-3244 (TDD)
http://www.ojp.usdoj.gov/vawo

From the U.S. Department of Justice, this site offers, under "VAW Online Resources," lots of information on interventions, advocates, and resources concerning domestic violence, from rape to stalking to child abuse and custody. There is also an up-to-date list of hotlines and local groups.

VOCAL (Victims Of Child Abuse Laws)
Phone: 513-777-8940
http://www.nasvo/nashville.org
E-mail: marygoff@juno.com

To protect the rights of persons falsely and wrongly accused of child abuse. Referrals to psychologists.

See also Posttraumatic Stress Disorder (Chapter 26) and Violent Children (Chapter 37).

CHAPTER 3

Addictive Disorders

Most self-help authorities, as well as psychotherapists, realize the immense difficulty of recovering from an addiction. Virtually all authors of self-help books, autobiographies, and Internet sites on addiction recognize that some form of treatment or ongoing self-help group is needed for recovery. Therefore, reading a self-help book or watching a film on addictions is unlikely, by itself, to conquer or control an addiction. However, good self-help materials can assist in the identification of an addictive disorder, can direct a person to the optimal form of self-help group or therapy, can serve as an effective adjunct to treatment, and can support family and friends of a person with an addictive disorder.

In defining the range of addictive disorders for this chapter, we choose to focus on substance abuse (alcohol and drugs). Some mental health professionals would also consider sex or eating disorders as addictions, but these are located in the chapters on Sexuality (Chapter 30) and Eating Disorders (Chapter 19).

In addition to materials on alcohol and drugs, we consider a handful of self-help books devoted to the controversial concept of codependency. Although codependency originally referred to the problems of people married to alcoholics, it spread rapidly, perhaps indiscriminately, to include a host of other circumstances. Agreement on a precise definition of codependency has not been forthcoming, but those who write about the topic agree that the number of women who are codependent is staggering. And they agree that women who are codependent have low self-esteem, grew up in a dysfunctional family, and should focus more on their own inner feelings instead of catering to someone else's needs. In the language of codependency, many women stay with an unreliable partner, usually a male, because they are addicted to the relationship dynamics of being subservient to a male.

In this chapter, we present the experts' consensual ratings on self-help books, autobiographies, films, and Internet resources on addictive disorders and codependency. The titles and contact information for prominent self-help organizations are included as well.

RECOMMENDATION HIGHLIGHTS

Self-Help Books

- On Alcoholics Anonymous and related strategies of recovery:
    - ★★★★ *Alcoholics Anonymous* by Alcoholics Anonymous
    - ★★★★ *Twelve Steps and Twelve Traditions* by Alcoholics Anonymous

- On maintaining sobriety with or without AA:
    - ★★★ *The Addiction Workbook* by Patrick Fanning and John O'Neill
    - ★★★ *Sober and Free* by Guy Kettelhack
    - ★★★ *When AA Doesn't Work for You* by Albert Ellis and Emmett Velton

- On adult children of alcoholics:
    - ★★★★ *A Time to Heal* by Timmen Cermak
    - ★★★ *It Will Never Happen to Me* by Claudia Black

Autobiographies

- On the descent into alcohol abuse and recovery:
    - ★★★★ *A Drinking Life* by Pete Hamill
    - ★★★★ *Getting Better* by Nan Robertson

- On struggling with codependency and substance abuse:
    - ★★★★ *Codependent No More* by Melodie Beattie

- On a teenager's polydrug abuse:
    - ★★★★ *Go Ask Alice* by Anonymous

- On the challenges of fetal alcohol syndrome:
    - ★★★★ *The Broken Cord* by Michael Dorris

Films

- On the depressing descent into alcoholism:
    - ★★★★★ *The Lost Weekend*
    - ★★★★★ *Days of Wine and Roses*
    - ★★★★ *Ironweed*

- On inspiring recovery and the founding of AA:
    - ★★★★ *My Name Is Bill W.*

- On surrendering and recovering from cocaine addiction:
    - ★★★★ *Clean and Sober*

- On substance abuse in families:
    - ★★★★ *Traffic*
    - ★★★★ *When a Man Loves a Woman*
    - ★★★ *Cat on a Hot Tin Roof*

Internet Resources

- On all addictions:

  ★★★★★ *Web of Addictions* http://www.well.com/user/woa

- On alcohol:

  ★★★★★ *HabitSmart* http://www.cts.com/crash/habtsmrt

- On other drugs:

  ★★★★ *National Institute on Drug Abuse* http://www.nida.nih.gov

  ★★★★ *National Inhalant Prevention Coalition* http://www.inhalants.org

- On codependency:

  ★★★★ *The Issues of Codependency*
  http://www.soulselfhelp.on.ca/coda.html

SELF-HELP BOOKS

Strongly Recommended

★★★★ *Alcoholics Anonymous* (4th ed., 2001). New York: Alcoholics Anonymous World
Services.

In our national studies, this and the Cermak book (listed below) emerged as the highest
rated self-help books for alcoholism. Revised three times since the first edition was published in 1939, the book is the basic text for Alcoholics Anonymous (AA) self-help
groups. The principles of AA have been revised and adapted by a number of self-help
groups, such as Narcotics Anonymous, Gamblers Anonymous, and Al-Anon (for people
with a variety of addictions and their families). Called the Big Book by AA, *Alcoholics
Anonymous* is divided into two parts. The first part describes the AA recovery program,
which relies heavily on confession, group support, and spiritual commitment to help individuals cope with alcoholism. Extensive personal testimonies by AA members from
different walks of life make up the latter two-thirds of the book. Successive editions of
the book have expanded the case histories to include examples of alcoholics from a variety of backgrounds in the hope that alcoholics who read the book can identify with at
least one of them. Brief appendixes include AA's Twelve Steps and Twelve Traditions,
and several testimonials to AA by ministers and physicians. The book also explains how
to join AA and attend meetings.

★★★★ *Twelve Steps and Twelve Traditions* (pocket ed., 1995). New York: Alcoholics
Anonymous World Services.

This book is devoted to detailed discussions of the Twelve Steps and Twelve Traditions
used in AA. The Steps and Traditions represent the heart of AA's principles, providing
a guide for members to use in recovery. The strong religious nature of the Twelve Steps
and Traditions is apparent in the first five steps:

1. We admitted we were powerless over alcohol . . . that our lives had become unmanageable.
2. We came to believe that a Power greater than ourselves could restore us to sanity.
3. We made a decision to turn our will and our lives over to the care of God as we understood Him.
4. We made a searching and fearless moral inventory of ourselves.
5. We admitted to God, to ourselves, and to another human being the exact nature of our wrongs.

Almost 200 pages are devoted to elaborating the basic principles of the Twelve Steps. Like its sister book, *Alcoholics Anonymous*, *Twelve Steps and Twelve Traditions* earned a four-star Recommended rating in the national studies.

Because the Twelve Steps have become so widely used, mental health experts have carefully analyzed them. Criticisms focus mainly on their spiritual basis. Unhappy with the strong religious flavor, some mental health experts have recast the steps in nonreligious terms to appeal to a wider range of people. Before his death, the famous behaviorist B. F. Skinner put together a psychological alternative to AA's Twelve Steps. Here are the first five steps:

1. We accept the fact that all our efforts to stop drinking have failed.
2. We believe that we must turn elsewhere for help.
3. We turn to our fellow men and women, particularly those who have struggled with the same problem.
4. We have made a list of the situations in which we are most likely to drink.
5. We ask our friends to help us avoid those situations.

★★★★   *A Time to Heal: The Road to Recovery for Adult Children of Alcoholics* (1988) by Timmen L. Cermak. Los Angeles: Jeremy P. Tarcher.

This book attempts to carry the promise of hope. Along with a time to heal will come a time to belong. Each chapter addresses a specific time along the path of healing, which includes a time to heal, to see, to remember, to feel, to separate, to be honest, to trust, to belong, and a time for courage. Included are case histories of the trauma and emotional pain adult children of alcoholics (ACOAs) lived with as kids and currently as adults. Two important points made are that healing begins with honesty and that the flaws of an ACOA's lifestyle can only be dissolved by making the discipline of recovery a part of daily life. This is a helpful book for ACOAs, especially with their current relationships, and for the professionals who work with them.

Recommended

★★★   *It Will Never Happen to Me* (reissued 1991) by Claudia Black. New York: Ballantine.

Unlike the AA books that are directed at alcoholics themselves, Black's book was written to help children—as youngsters, adolescents, and adults—cope with the problem of having an alcoholic parent. Black has counseled many alcoholic clients who were raised in alcoholic families, as well as wives of alcoholics. She comments that virtually every one of them said, "It will never happen to me"; hence, the title of her book. Black believes that when people grow up in alcoholic homes, they learn to not talk, not trust, and not feel, whether they drink or not. This book received an impressive rating, but by only a small number of people who were familiar with it, which is why it has a three-star rating. Black's book is a superb self-help book for children and spouses of alcoholics. She does a good job of describing the alcoholic cycle, paints a vivid picture of the pitfalls faced by those related to alcoholics, and is upbeat in giving them hope for recovery and positive living. In the final chapter, Black tells readers about a number of resources for relatives of alcoholics.

★★★ *The Addiction Workbook: A Step-By-Step Guide to Quitting Alcohol and Drugs* (1997) by Patrick Fanning and John O'Neill. New York: Fine.

Prolific self-change author Fanning and drug counselor O'Neill collaborate on this comprehensive workbook for quitting alcohol and drugs. It is, as the subtitle declares, a step-by-step self-change manual, starting with "Do You Have a Problem?" in Chapter 2 and ending with "Relapse Prevention" in Chapter 12. In between is an assortment of awareness and action methods that include finding help, nutrition, relaxation, spirituality, emotional expression, communication, and making amends. *The Addiction Workbook* is ecumenical and compatible with Twelve Step programs, medications, cognitive-behavioral treatments, and the evolving sciences of addictions. Several experts in our national studies praised it for its balanced and integrative approach; in fact, had it been known and rated by more professionals, it would have achieved a four-star designation.

★★★ *One Day at a Time in Al-Anon* (1988). New York: Al-Anon Family Group Headquarters.

Originated by a group of women with alcoholic husbands, Al-Anon is a support group for relatives and friends of alcoholics. Like a number of self-help support groups for alcoholics and their relatives, Al-Anon members follow AA's Twelve Steps of recovery. This book reflects an important principle of Al-Anon: Focus on one day at a time when living with an alcoholic. Each day is viewed as a fresh opportunity for self-realization and growth rather than for dwelling on past problems and disappointments. Like the other AA books, *One Day at a Time in Al-Anon* has a strong spiritual emphasis. Each page is devoted to one day—from January 1 to December 31—and consists of two parts: a message and a daily reminder. Religious quotations are used frequently throughout the book.

★★★ *Sober and Free: Making Your Recovery Work for You* (1996) by Guy Kettelhack. New York: Simon & Schuster.

This book primarily focuses on maintaining sobriety, with tips on managing slips and on relearning to create significant relationships. The author stresses the importance of finding one's own way of maintaining sobriety, with help from support groups, psychotherapy, medication, family, and friends. For those in conventional programs who are looking for more, or for people who do not feel that conventional programs will work for their recovery, this book could be a helpful resource.

★★★ *The Recovery Book* (1992) by Al J. Mooney, Arlene Eisenberg, and Howard Eisenberg. New York: Workman.

This book is designed like a road map from active addiction to recovery and then to relapse prevention. Topics covered are understanding recovery, deciding to quit, picking the right treatment and support group, knowing the facts and feelings about treatment and support groups, maintaining sobriety and dealing with temptations, relationships (families and social life), dentistry, physical fitness, financial and medical concerns, mind, emotions and spiritual issues, and relapse prevention. A section is devoted to dependency as a family disease. This book is a blend of medical knowledge and practical wisdom. It is also a comprehensive source for patients, families, and professionals dealing with the recovery process.

★★★ *A Day at a Time* (1976). Minneapolis: CompCare.

This book of daily reflections, prayers, and catchy phrases is intended to offer inspiration and hope to recovering alcoholics. The book is based on the spiritual aspects of AA, especially the Twelve Steps and Twelve Traditions. Like Al-Anon's *One Day at a Time in Al-Anon*, each page is devoted to a day—from January 1 through December 31. Each page is divided into three parts: Reflection for the Day, Today I Pray, and Today I Will Remember. The brief daily messages come from poets, philosophers, scholars, psychologists, and AA members.

★★★ *When AA Doesn't Work for You: Rational Steps to Quitting Alcohol* (1992) by Albert Ellis and Emmett Velton. Fort Lee, NJ: Barricade.

The authors acknowledge that AA works for many people, but not for everyone. The beginning chapters help readers determine whether they have a drinking problem and introduces Rational–Emotive Therapy as the best strategy for recovery. A number of helpful step-by-step methods, including the use of a daily journal and homework assignments, are provided in later chapters. The authors focus on maladaptive thought patterns and specific ways to replace them with more adaptive ones. Unlike many of the books in the addiction category, Ellis and Velton's book does not include spiritual commitment in the recovery process. In fact, Ellis and Velton believe that AA's notion of the alcoholic's powerlessness is an irrational idea. Rational Recovery (RR), one of an increasing number of nonreligious self-help groups formed in recent years for recovering alcoholics, traces its roots directly to the ideas of Albert Ellis and his Rational–Emotive Therapy. RR teaches that what leads to persistent drinking is a person's belief that he or she is powerless and incompetent. Using Ellis's approach, a moderator (usually a recovered RR member) helps guide group discussion and gets members to think more rationally and act more responsibly. Whereas AA stresses that alcoholics can never fully recover, RR tells members that recovery is not only possible but that it can also happen in a year or so.

★★★ *Codependent No More: How to Stop Controlling Others and Start Caring for Yourself* (2nd ed., 1996) by Melodie Beattie. Center City, MN: Hazelden.

This is Melodie Beattie's personal narrative about being addicted to a codependent relationship and how she recovered from it. In addition to describing her own personal struggles, she discusses the nature of codependency and how to recover from it. Beattie estimates that upwards of 80 million Americans are emotionally involved with an addict or are addicted themselves, not necessarily to alcohol or drugs but also to sex, work, food, or shopping. What kind of characteristics do codependents have? Beattie says that they are sufferers who feel anxiety, pity, and guilt when other people have a problem and that they overcommit themselves. How do codependents get out of this mess? Beattie endorses insight about the nature of codependent relationships and a version of the Twelve Step recovery popularized by AA. Another theme of Beattie's recovery strategy is to begin having a love affair with yourself instead of with someone else to whom you have given too much.

This volume received a three-star rating and a very mixed reception in our national studies. Some respondents called it a great book; others an awful book. Although *Codependent No More* was on the *New York Times* best-seller list for 115 weeks and has sold upwards of 4 million copies, mental health professionals are not uniformly enthusiastic about it—thus, the rather tepid three-star rating.

★★★ *Beyond Codependency* (1989) by Melodie Beattie. New York: Harper & Row.

This sequel to Beattie's *Codependent No More* elaborates the self-sabotaging behavior patterns of codependency in which a codependent person overcares for an unreliable, addictive person. Beattie addresses healthy recovery, the role of recycling (falling into old bad habits) in recovery, and how positive affirmations can counter negative messages. Testimonials from people who have used this method to break away from addictive relationships are liberally interspersed throughout the book. This book, too, received a three-star rating in the national studies, and virtually the same plaudits and criticisms that characterize reviews of Beattie's earlier work apply to *Beyond Codependency* as well.

★★★ *The Truth about Addiction and Recovery* (1992) by Stanton Peele, Archie Brodsky, and Mary Arnold. New York: Fireside.

Drawing on recent research and case studies, the authors conclude that addictions are not diseases, and they are not necessarily lifelong problems. Instead of medical treatment or a Twelve Step program, Peele, Brodsky, and Arnold recommend a life process program that emphasizes coping with stress and achieving one's goals. The book is a calm and reasoned alternative to the disease model of addiction that can prove very helpful. Although it does include a number of case studies, it is more like a textbook than the other books in this category. A number of research studies and academic sources are cited to support the authors' interpretations and recommendations. The book is well-documented but somewhat difficult to digest. It is particularly applicable to people seeking or valuing an alternative to the Twelve Step approach.

★★★ *Out of the Shadows: Understanding Sexual Addiction* (3rd ed., 2001) by Patrick Carnes. Minneapolis: Hazelden Foundation.

This book is a guide to understanding sexual addictions using a Twelve Step program as a means to recovery. Important milestones are discovered, for example, the moment that comes for every addict, the cycle and levels of the addictive process, and the family's relationship to the world of a person and his or her addiction. Charts and diagrams are used to elucidate the system's levels, beliefs, and the Twelve Steps of AA and their adaptation to sexual addiction. The author states that, like other addictions, sexual addiction is also rooted in a complex web of family and marital relationships, and that part of therapy is to discover the role of the previous generation in the addiction. The author examines the tangled web of love, addictive sex, hate, fear, and relationships. Ultimately, this book is about hope. If you are a sex addict or suspect you are, and have the courage to face yourself, this book is intended for you.

★★★ *Addiction and Grace* (1988) by Gerald C. May. New York: HarperCollins.

This volume combines spiritual and psychological principles to help combat any type of addiction, whether to alcohol, drugs, sex, food, work, or gambling. Reflecting his belief in the roles that relationships with others and spirituality play in addiction, May has subtitled his book *Love and Spirituality in the Healing of Addictions.* He states that the deepest human need is to be in a loving relationship with God and others. However, says May, our freedom to satisfy this need is restricted by many different addictions (including fame as well as drugs) that use up our desire. This book may particularly appeal to individuals with a strong spiritual orientation, but many people will find its writing style too abstract and technical to benefit them.

★★★ *Adult Children of Alcoholics* (expanded ed., 1990) by Janet Woititz. Deerfield Beach, FL: Health Communications.

Janet Woititz, the "mother" of the ACOA (adult children of alcoholics) movement, describes basic problems and vulnerabilities of ACOAs. Woititz says that reading her book can be the first step to recovery, along with Al-Anon and its Twelve Step program. The key to recovery is learning the principle of detachment. In her view, because ACOAs received inconsistent nurturing as children, as adults they hunger for nurture and are too emotionally dependent on their parents. They have to separate themselves from their parents in the least stressful way possible. Although this book was on the *New York Times* best-seller list for more than 45 weeks and has sold more than 2 million copies, the ratings by the mental health experts in our studies were mixed.

Diamond in the Rough

♦ *Sex, Drugs, Gambling, and Chocolate: A Workbook for Overcoming Addictions* (1998) by A. Thomas Horvath. San Luis Obispo, CA: Impact.

This notable workbook on addictions is distinguished by three features: It covers multiple addictions as a whole instead of a single one; it advances a cognitive-behavioral model instead of a medical or Twelve Step model; and it is based on scientifically supported methods of change. The book is replete with specific exercises and self-study questions, and covers many topics ignored by competing self-help resources, such as the research on cue reactivity, natural recovery, relapse prevention, and harm reduction. The workbook format and easy reading make it attractive to consumers, although many adherents of Twelve Step models will find the book contrary to their established beliefs. We missed listing this book in our latest national study but add it here.

Not Recommended

★★ *The Alcoholic Man* (1990) by Sylvia Carey. Los Angeles: Lowell House.

★★ *How to Break Your Addiction to a Person* (1982) by Howard Halpern. New York: McGraw-Hill.

★ *Love Is a Choice* (1989) by Robert Helmfelt, Frank Minirth, and Paul Meier. Nashville, TN: Thomas Nelson.

★ *Co-Dependence: Healing the Human Condition* (1991) by Charles Whitfield. Deerfield Beach, FL: Health Communications.

Strongly Not Recommended

† *Healing the Addictive Mind* (1991) by Lee Jampolsky. Berkeley, CA: Celestial Arts

† *The Miracle Method: A Radically New Approach to Problem Drinking* (1995) by Scott D. Miller and Insoo Kim Berg. New York: Norton.

AUTOBIOGRAPHIES

Strongly Recommended

★★★★ *The Broken Cord: A Family's Ongoing Struggle with Fetal Alcohol Syndrome* (1990) by Michael Dorris. New York: HarperCollins.

This book first brought fetal alcohol syndrome (FAS) to public attention. The author, a member of the Modoc tribe, was in graduate school working on his dissertation when he decided to adopt Adam, a three-year-old Native American child. He was aware that Adam was developmentally disabled but did not know why. After the child showed a succession of serious health, behavioral, and learning problems, Adam was diagnosed with FAS. Dorris, by this time a successful author and professor, made FAS into a research project. He traveled across the nation collecting stories of native children with FAS (Adam's natural mother had died from drinking antifreeze) and interviewing FAS experts. The tone of the book varies among love, compassion, and rage directed at women who drink during pregnancy. There are sections by Dorris's wife, writer Louise Erdrich, and by Adam, then 20 years old. The ending is tragic, with Dorris committing suicide. It is a very good book about FAS, the risks of adoption, and the urgent need for substance abuse education in native communities.

★★★★ *Go Ask Alice* (1995) by Anonymous, edited by Beatrice M. Sparks. New York: Aladdin.

This best-selling reprinted edition of a yearlong diary in the life of a 15-year-old girl starts from her first introduction to LSD at a party, the following week's experimentation with marijuana and methamphetamine, and subsequent struggles to bring her drug use and life under control. Stark realism strips the glamour and romance from drugs as the author becomes a liar, thief, runaway, dealer, rape victim, and street person. This is a great book for teens wondering about the effects of drugs, not simply on tonight's mood, but on their lives. Good book for parents, too.

★★★★ *A Drinking Life: A Memoir* (1995) by Pete Hamill. Boston: Little, Brown.

A gritty description of growing up in a tough New York neighborhood and becoming a tough guy, brawler, drunk, rebel, and finally a writer. Noted journalist and novelist Hamill, now sober for two decades, discusses without sentimentality the critical role alcohol played in his life. Drinking was a crucial part of his early life and wrecked his first marriage. He argues that alcohol is not necessary to stimulate literary creativity. This is the book that inspired Caroline Knapp, author of *Drinking: A Love Story* (listed below), to sober up. It is an excellent resource for showing the effects of a person's family and neighborhood on his/her alcohol use and how a determined person can stop drinking on his/her own.

★★★★ *Codependent No More: How to Stop Controlling Others and Start Caring for Yourself* (2nd ed., 1996) by Melodie Beattie. Center City, MN: Hazelden.

The second edition of the author's best-selling *Codependent No More*, this edition updates Beattie's views on how to break away from destructive codependent relationships. She tried various self-help groups, including AA, Al-Anon, and Sex Addicts Anonymous, and she advocates their use for those in codependent relationships. Beattie describes her previous drinking problem, recovery, and work as an alcohol counselor. In an engaging writing style, she emphasizes the effects of addiction on family and friends. Also reviewed in this chapter as a self-help book.

★★★★ *Getting Better: Inside Alcoholics Anonymous* (1988) by Nan Robertson. New York: William Morrow.

The author chronicles the growth of AA, provides descriptions of meetings, and recounts her own struggle with alcoholism. This is one of the best accounts of the founding and evolution of AA, still one of the most successful and probably one of the most spiritual self-help programs. It is a movement history, as well as a compelling autobiography.

Recommended

★★★ *Note Found in a Bottle: My Life as a Drinker* (1998) by Susan Cheever. New York: Simon & Schuster.

The daughter of a famous writer with serious drinking problems, Susan Cheever discusses the role that alcohol played in her own life and in her three failed marriages. She started early in life identifying cocktails with sophistication and sociability, but soon alcohol controlled her life. Now in recovery, Cheever reflects on social aspects of alcohol use in our society. A particularly good book for a person crossing the line from social drinking to addiction. Highly rated by our mental health professionals but not widely known, thus accounting for its three stars.

★★★ *Terry: My Daughter's Life-and-Death Struggle with Alcoholism* (1997) by George S. McGovern. New York: Dutton.

In the winter of 1994, police found the body of Teresa McGovern, daughter of presidential candidate and Senator George McGovern, frozen in a snowbank after an evening of drinking. This is the heartbreaking account of Terry's descent into oblivion. The book draws heavily from her diary and from personal recollections of family members. Terry was genetically vulnerable, with alcoholism on her father's side and depression on her mother's. She started on alcohol at age 13, took marijuana and LSD in high school, spent time on the locked ward of a psychiatric hospital, almost went to jail, and attempted suicide. There was a brief respite of sobriety in her 30s, with marriage and two daughters, but the marriage ended and the daughters went to live with their father. After this, she was in and out of detox and treatment programs. The diary makes it clear she knew what was happening to her but was unable to prevent it. The family blames itself for not doing more, yet the reader can see from the journals that little could be done when Terry blew off all attempts at treatment. This is not a hopeful book, because the tragic ending is known at the beginning, but it is a gripping account of a family's continued efforts to battle a daughter's addiction that all could see but no one save Terry could stop. Especially recommended for parents of young alcoholics and for teens who deny the ravages of alcohol addiction. The mental health professionals in our studies highly but infrequently rated this book, accounting for its three-star rating.

★★★ *Drinking: A Love Story* (1997) by Carolyn Knapp. New York: Delta.

Daughter of a psychoanalyst, the author grew up in a well-to-do family. She graduated *magna cum laude* from Brown University before becoming a reporter and later an editor. She was an anorexic and a high-functioning alcoholic who kept her addiction hidden from her associates. She bottomed out, checked into a rehab center, joined AA, and started on the slow path to recovery. Knapp had been inspired to quit drinking by Pete Hamill's book (see above). She describes in stylish prose her complex relationship to alcohol, her self-destructive behaviors, and early powerlessness. A book especially suitable for female alcohol abusers.

★★★ *Now You Know* (1990) by Kitty Dukakis with J. Scovell. New York: Simon & Schuster.

The wife of a former governor of Massachusetts and presidential candidate discusses her bouts with bipolar disorder and her addiction to alcohol and pills. Although out of print and difficult to obtain, the book is a good account of the author's two-decade battle with substance abuse and bipolar disorder.

FILMS

Strongly Recommended

★★★★★ *The Lost Weekend* (1945) directed by Billy Wilder. Not rated. 101 minutes.

This classic film stars Ray Milland as a writer and chronic alcoholic struggling to overcome his addiction. He goes on multiday benders and literally loses a weekend. In a classic line, the bartender chides Milland: "One's too many and a hundred's not enough." He engages in typical addictive behaviors, including hiding his stash, according alcohol first priority, and rationalizing his slips. He refuses help from significant others and draws his girlfriend into his massive denial. Eventually, he accepts responsibility and treatment for his drinking. Several scenes were filmed at Bellevue Hospital in New York City, and the withdrawal symptoms are convincing indeed. The treatment methods are dated—and clients should be reassured that they will not suffer the severe delirium tremens pictured in the movie—but the addictive process and consequences are timeless. Widely considered one of the best films ever made about alcoholism.

★★★★★ *Days of Wine and Roses* (1962) directed by Blake Edwards. Not rated. 108 minutes.

This film is a portrait of a successful, middle-class couple's agonizing struggles with progressive alcoholism in the 1950s. The husband recovers with AA, but the wife cannot, and he must leave her. The movie is depressing, with its depiction of job loss, repeated lapses, descent into ugliness, and the eventual dissolution of the marriage. It is particularly useful as a warning and illustration of the patterns of alcoholic couples.

★★★★ *My Name Is Bill W.* (1989) directed by Daniel Petrie. Not rated. 100 minutes.

This superbly acted television movie is the true story of the founder of AA, Bill W, a successful financial manager who gradually lost his job, friends, self-respect, and all he valued to alcoholism. Finally, he met Dr. Bob, and they kept each other sober and invented AA. Nothing is held back, and their success is highly inspirational.

★★★★ *Clean and Sober* (1988) directed by Glenn Gordon Caron. R rating. 124 minutes.

To escape the police for a murder he did not commit and a large theft from his employer, a young cocaine-addicted real estate salesman enters a drug rehabilitation program. He is in massive denial, but despite valiant attempts, he cannot escape the insights, confrontations, and caring of the counselors. The process of surrender and recovery by an ordinary and less-than-perfect client is well illustrated and believable.

★★★★ *When a Man Loves a Woman* (1994) directed by Luis Mandoki. R rating. 124 minutes.

This film about alcoholism and families is not overly simple, stereotyped, or designed with a happy ending. After extensive drinking and denial, the wife enters treatment and recovery, and that is when her loving and accepting husband, a born enabler, must also change. He must give up handling all the responsibilities and making the decisions. His world is thus shaken up, too. No quick or final fixes are offered, but the movie portrays treatment adequately and recovery from denial with rare realism.

★★★★ *Traffic* (2000) directed by Steven Soderbergh. R rating. 140 minutes.

Three riveting, intertwined stories about drug abuse: two DEA agents in pursuit of drug kingpins; a crooked constable south of the border in pursuit of his integrity; and a U.S. drug czar in pursuit of his heroin-addicted daughter. The film accurately shows the complexity of the drug trafficking—from its origins in foreign countries to its terminals in city streets—and the victimization of the young and weak. *Traffic* delves into the dark and personal corners of drug abuse, particularly the privileged daughter's descent into hopeless addiction. One of the most realistic portrayals of drugs' collective ravages on American families.

★★★★ *Ironweed* (1987) directed by Hector Babenco. R rating. 143 minutes.

Meryl Streep and Jack Nicholson are compelling as homeless alcoholics during the depression. It is difficult film to watch: The two have hit rock bottom, struggle daily to survive on the streets, and trade their self-esteem and bodies for food and alcohol. The film's cold and depressing photography add to the ambience. Although a lengthy and brutal film, it unforgettably presents the harsh realities of alcohol-consumed, homeless existence.

Recommended

★★★ *Cat on a Hot Tin Roof* (1958) directed by Richard Brooks. 108 minutes.

A superb writer's portrayal of the greedy family of a dying Southern patriarch. The family members all try to please him for their selfish benefits, except for the guilt-ridden ex-jock son and his sexually frustrated wife. The film is the classic story of family conflict and confrontation.

★★★ *Bright Lights, Big City* (1988) directed by James Bridges. R rating. 110 minutes.

Michael Fox's character suffers the death of his mother and being dumped by his wife, and resorts to self-medicating with alcohol, cocaine, and promiscuous sex in the Big Apple. Based on Jay McInerney's acclaimed novel of New York's sex and drug scene, the film shows Fox hitting rock bottom and confronting his inner demons before they destroy him. An exceptional soundtrack and grainy photography add to the chilling effect, but many viewers will experience difficulty in accepting cuddly Fox as a desperate coke-snorter. Particularly applicable for younger clients into the party scene of urban life.

★★★ *Mask* (1986) directed by Peter Bogdanovich. PG-13 rating. 120 minutes.

A teenager, horribly disfigured by a rare disease, remains unbowed in the face of cruelties with the love and help of his gutsy, albeit addicted mother. He succeeds at school, begins a relationship with a blind girl, relates normally to his mother's boyfriend, and lectures his mother on drug abuse. She protects and loves him so intensely that you believe he will somehow survive his fatal condition. The film makes the love between a mother and son palpable and inspirational.

★★★ *Leaving Las Vegas* (1995) directed by Mike Figgis. R rating. 112 minutes.

In a poignant film about doomed losers, he is irretrievably dedicated to drinking himself to death, and she is a prostitute, abused and misused daily. He has no choices left, but she chooses to stay with him and care for him because he is her redemption. The film illustrates her unselfish love, charity, and gentleness despite the hardness of their lives and the weaknesses of their characters.

★★★ *Blow* (2001) directed by Ted Demme. R rating. 124 minutes.

Johnny Depp stars in the true story of George Jung, an insider in the Colombian cocaine cartel and one of the largest cocaine traffickers in the early 1970s. He makes bush-
els of money and becomes the target of a federal investigation. For all of his fabulous
wealth, the true costs of his own addiction and treacherous occupation are visited on
himself and his family. This is more of a cautionary historical tale than a self-help film
per se.

★★★ *Drugstore Cowboy* (1989) directed by Gus Van Sant, Jr. R rating. 100 minutes.

A junkie and his four-person "family" rob drugstores to support their habits, which
consume their empty lives. The excitement of drugs and the staged robberies alter-
nate with the ennui of their highs and the routines of moving around the country.
They are all sick and try ineffectively to help each other. After the death of a member of the group and a meeting with a haunted and haunting old addict, the junkie
plans to get into treatment. His wife cannot understand a world without drugs and
tries to pull him back. Utterly realistic, even to its junkie logic, and wonderfully
acted, this movie might help clients see what the road ahead looks like and the possibility of difficult change.

★★★ *28 Days* (2000) directed by Betty Thomas. PG-13 rating. 103 minutes.

A single woman in her late 20s, played by Sandra Bullock, involuntarily enters a 28-day,
inpatient rehabilitation program for her alcohol and pain-killer addictions. She passes
through classic denial, withdrawal symptoms, and into recovery. The movie realistically
illustrates the disease concept and Twelve Step treatment, including group therapy,
family confrontation, and eventual reevaluation of her relationships. An entertaining
and moving film.

★★★ *Postcards from the Edge* (1991) directed by Mike Nichols. R rating. 101 minutes.

A drug-addicted young actress is falling apart, barely surviving at work, sleeping around
with strangers, misplacing her days, and awaiting her next fix. Her mother, a famous actress, is addicted more acceptably to alcohol. The daughter enters rehab. Her mother
visits her but responds only to the attentions of her fans. Mother–daughter rivalry is
dramatized, and the ladies have many parallels. Well written and acted, the film drifts
and does not reveal much about recovery. It might illustrate a not uncommon mother–
daughter relationship for some clients.

★★★ *Jungle Fever* (1991) directed by Spike Lee. R rating. 132 minutes.

On its surface, this is a film about an interracial romance between a successful, middle-
class, married African American architect and a white, working-class temp in his office.
Lee, the director, calls this interracial attraction Jungle Fever and portrays it as based
on media-enhanced stereotypes and America's focus on skin color. However, the film is
much more. It portrays many of the effects of this relationship on the members of the
families and communities from which the lovers come. It might be a suitable film for exploring interracial relationships and their contexts.

★★★ *Gia* (1998) directed by Michael Cristofer. R rating. 120 minutes.

Angelina Jolie stars in this movie based on the life of supermodel Gia Marie Carangi. Originally shown on HBO television, the film follows her life, from a rebel working in her father's diner at the age of 17 to her death from AIDS at the age of 26. In between, Gia's life was a downward spiral of drug abuse and failed relationships. For the purposes of self-help, the film spends excessive time on Gia's modeling and bisexuality, but if viewers can focus on her problems with drugs and commitment, it has several important lessons about the short, drug-infested lives of the young and famous.

★★★ *The Gambler* (1974) directed by Karel Reisz. R rating. 111 minutes.

Despite his education and position as a college professor, the central character is a compulsive gambler sacrificing all to his addiction. He is pursued by the mob. Desperate, he gets money from his mother, which he then gambles away. He tries to end it all in one last attempt. This film might be useful to show gamblers or their families how compulsive and destructive this addiction is.

INTERNET RESOURCES

There are literally thousands of sites on these topics. Many are devoted to prevention; they are not cited here because only those about treatment are relevant to self-help.

Metasites

★★★★★ *Web of Addictions* http://www.well.com/user/woa

In this superb source of accurate information, The Facts offers links to hundreds of fact sheets from many trustworthy sources.

★★★★ *Hazelden* http://www.hazelden.org/resource_center.dbm

Under General Resources (the Alive & Free link) are about 100 short newspaper columns. The Search function under Professional Resources searches the entire Hazelden site. The Links to Helpful Resources guide you to two dozen rich sites about addictions.

Psychoeducational Materials for Clients and Families

Alcohol

★★★★★ *HabitSmart* http://www.cts.com/crash/habtsmrt

Using the best cognitive-behavioral therapy and harm reduction models, this site offers a dozen long essays and several interactive exercises for overcoming ambivalence, introducing cognitive-behavioral therapy ideas, and other solid materials by Robert Westermeyer.

★★★★ *Secular Organization for Sobriety/Save Our Selves*
        http://www.unhooked.com/toolbox/index.html

If you desire a nonreligious approach to sobriety, this page offers several fine long pieces for patients using the SOS model, the empirical evidence, and links to groups.

★★★★ *Alcohol Dependence* http://www.mentalhealth.com/dx/fdx-sb01.html

Although designed for professionals, the two rating scales, several booklets from the World Health Organization, and information on alcohol abuse may be especially helpful in some situations. This material is unique to Dr. Long's site.

★★★★ *Concerned about Your Drinking?* http://www.carebetter.com

The most obvious feature of this site is an interactive, anonymous test of drinking and confidential feedback of results. Plus, the information under FAQs is good. Both the FAQs and the Related Sites encourage self-control treatment models.

★★★★ *JACS—Jewish Alcoholics, Chemically Dependent Persons and Significant Others*
       http://www.jacsweb.org

The Library contains 10 articles that can be of help in breaking down denial and ignorance.

★★★ *Common Sense* http://www.pta.org/commonsense

This section of the Parent Teachers Association site, with material aimed at parents, contains solid information, support, and good advice.

★★★ *Adult Children of Alcoholics* http://www.couns.uiuc.edu/brochures/adult.htm

A three-page handout on adult children for college students; see also *Children of Alcoholics* (http://www.aacap.org/publications/factsfam/alcoholc.htm)

★★★ *What Is Alcoholism?*   http://www.mayoclinic.com/findinformation/
       diseasesandconditions/invoke.cfm?id=ds00340

This very well-written and comprehensive overview in about 10 pages might be the basis for further exploration with clients.

★★★ *SMART: Self-Management And Recovery Training* http://www.smartrecovery.org

Based on Ellis's Rational–Emotive Behavior Therapy, this approach eschews war stories, sponsors, and meetings for life with structured meetings run by trained advisors. Their Four-Point Program is (1) building and maintaining motivation to abstain; (2) coping with urges; (3) managing thoughts, feelings, and behavior; and (4) balancing momentary and enduring satisfactions.

★★★ *Al-Anon and Alateen* http://www.Al-Anon-Alateen.org

The usual AA literature in a dozen languages may serve as a good introduction to the naive or to those in denial.

★★★ *Drug/Alcohol Brochures*   http://www.uiuc.edu/departments/mckinley/
       health-info/drug-alc/drug-alc.html

Seven single-page handouts from a university counseling center with guidelines and facts. Basic information.

Drug Abuse

★★★★ *National Institute on Drug Abuse* http://www.nida.nih.gov

This site contains many publications that can be useful for patients. The Research Reports are large and sophisticated, but for a thorough overview, they are of high quality. The NIDA Infofax—Science Based Facts on Drug Abuse and Addiction contains three- to five-page summaries available online and by fax. There are a dozen summaries about different chemicals and four on treatments. The site links to club drugs, steroids, and marijuana information.

★★★★ *Public and Research Views of Dual-Diagnosis Explored* by Leslie Knowlton
     http://www.mhsource.com/pt/p950536.html

A four-page introduction written for an educated public that explains some of the interactions of substance use and mental illness.

★★★★ *Cocaine Abuse and Addiction*
     http://www.nida.nih.gov/researchreports/cocaine/cocaine.html

A comprehensive, fairly recent (May 1999) document from the National Institute on Drug Abuse.

★★★ *The Do It Now Foundation* http://www.doitnow.org/pages/pubhub.html

Here you will find readable and printable copies of approximately a hundred brochures about smoking, drugs, alcohol, street drugs, and drugs and kids. The style is often hip and striking.

★★★ *Commonly Abused Drugs: Street Names for Drugs of Abuse*
     http://www.nida.nih.gov/DrugsofAbuse.html

A chart with current names, medical uses, periods of detection, and so forth.

Codependency

★★★★ *The Issues of Codependency* http://www.soulselfhelp.on.ca/coda.html

This site includes essays on boundaries, the codependent personality, and similar topics.

Compulsive Gambling

★★★ *National Council on Problem Gambling* http://www.ncpgambling.org/

Under Resources, their links and publications are quite comprehensive.

★★ *Pathological Gambling*
     http://www.dhh.state.la.us/oada/gambing-directory/path-gambling.htm

This site contains the entire section of the DSM-IV on all aspects of this disorder.

Other Resources

★★★★ *National Inhalant Prevention Coalition* http://www.inhalants.org

About a dozen brief informational resources, with well-done information about a growing area of abuse.

★★★ *Software for Recovering People* http://christians-in-recovery.org/software

Mainly Bible study and 12 steps, but also journaling, references, and goal setting.

★★★ *Addiction Resource Guide* http://www.addictionresourceguide.com

To assist with choosing a rehabilitation program, this guide has descriptions of about 100 inpatient programs, guidelines, and definitions.

NATIONAL SUPPORT GROUPS

Adult Children of Alcoholics World Services Organization
PO Box 3216
Torrance, CA 90510
Phone: 310-534-1815
http://www.adultchildren.org
E-mail: info@adultchildren.org

A Twelve Step and Twelve Tradition program of recovery for adults raised in a dysfunctional environment that included alcohol or other family dysfunctions.

Alateen and Al-Anon Family Groups
1600 Corporate Landing Parkway
Virginia Beach, VA 23454-56127
Phone: 757-563-1600 or 888-425-2666
E-mail: wso@al-anon.org
http://www.al-anon.org

A fellowship of young persons whose lives have been affected by someone else's drinking.

Alcoholics Anonymous
Box 459, Grand Central Station
New York, NY 10163
Phone: 212-870-3400
http://www.AA.org

American Council on Alcoholism
Hotline: 800-527-5344
Referrals to treatment centers and DWI classes.

Chemically Dependent Anonymous
PO Box 423
Severna Park, MD 21146-0423
Phone: 888-CDA-HOPE
http://www.cdaweb.org

Twelve Step program for friends and relatives of people who are chemically dependent.

Cocaine Anonymous
3740 Overland Avenue, Suite C
Los Angeles, CA 90034-6337
For local chapters, call 800-347-8998 or 310-559-5833
E-mail: cawso@ca.org
http://www.ca.org

Debtors Anonymous
PO Box 920888
Needham, MA 02492-0009
Phone: 781-453-2743
E-mail: new@debtorsanonymous.org or mem@debtorsanonymous.org
http://www.debtorsanonymous.org

Fellowship that follows the AA Twelve Step program for mutual help in recovering from compulsive indebtedness.

Gamblers Anonymous
PO Box 17173
Los Angeles, CA 90017
Phone: 213-386-8789
E-mail: isomain@gamblersanonymous.org
http://www.gamblersanonymous.org

Gam-Anon Family Groups
PO Box 157
Whitestone, NY 11357
Phone: 718-352-1671
http://www.gam-anon.org

Twelve Step program of recovery for relatives and friends of compulsive gamblers.

Marijuana Anonymous (MA)
PO Box 2912
Van Nuys, CA 91404
Phone: 800-766-6779
E-mail: office@marijuana-anonymous.org
http://www.marijuana-anonymous.org

Twelve Step program of recovery from marijuana addiction.

Mothers Against Drunk Driving
511 E. John Carpenter Freeway, Suite 700
Irving, TX 75062
Phone: 800-438-6233
http://www.madd.org

This large organization provides support though local chapters, education, political activism, and victim assistance.

Moderation Management (MM)
22 West 27th Street
New York, NY 10001
Phone: 212-871-0974
E-mail: mm@moderation.org
http://www.moderation.org

Emphasizes self-management and moderation of alcohol abuse. Intended for early-stage problem drinkers, not those severely dependent on alcohol.

Narcotics Anonymous
PO Box 9999
Van Nuys, CA 91409
Phone: 818-773-9999
E-mail: info@na.org
http://www.na.org

Nar-Anon World Wide Service
302 West 5th Street, Suite 301
San Pedro, CA 90731
Phone: 310-547-5800

Twelve Step program of recovery for families and friends of addicts.

National Clearinghouse for Alcohol and Drug Information
PO Box 2345
Rockville, MD 20847-2345
E-mail: info@health.org
Hotline: 800-788-2800 (Touch-Tone); 800-729-6686 (rotary)

Information on alcohol and drug abuse, prevention, and treatment centers.

National Institute on Alcohol Abuse and Alcoholism
6000 Executive Boulevard
Bethesda, MD 20892-7003
Phone: 301-443-3860
http://www.niaaa.nih.gov

Rational Recovery (RR)
PO Box 800
Lotus, CA 95651
http://www.rational.org
Phone: 530-621-2667 or 530-621-4374

Founded 1986. Abstinence-based.

Self Management and Recovery Training (SMART)
7537 Mentor Avenue, Suite 306
Mentor, OH 44060
E-mail: srmail1@aol.com
http://www.smartrecovery.org
Phone: 440-951-5357

An abstinence-based, cognitive-behavioral approach.

See also Eating Disorders (Chapter 19).

CHAPTER 4

Adult Development

For too long, psychologists believed that development was something that happens only to children. To be sure, growth and development are dramatic in the initial decades of life, but development goes on in the adult years, too. In this chapter, we consider self-help resources for people in the middle adult years.

Several topics tend to emerge repeatedly during the middle years in the self-help literature. Prominent among these are midlife crises, menopause, and retirement planning.

The adult years are important not only to the adults who are passing through them but also to their children, who often want to understand their parents better and improve their relationships with them. Changes in body, personality, and ability can be considerable during the adult years. Adults want to know how to adjust to these changes to make the transitions smoothly.

Here, then, are the evaluative ratings and reviews of self-help books, autobiographies, films, and Internet sites devoted to adult development. We begin with a snapshot of our primary recommendations.

SELF-HELP BOOKS

Strongly Recommended

★★★★ *Necessary Losses* (reprint ed., 1998) by Judith Viorst. New York: Fireside.

This book, on best-seller lists for more than a year, describes how we can grow and change through the losses that are an inevitable part of our lives. When we think of loss, we often think of the death of people we love. But Viorst talks about loss as a far more encompassing theme of life. She says we lose not only through death but also by leaving and being left, by changing and letting go and moving on. Viorst also describes the losses we experience as a result of impossible expectations, illusions of freedom and

RECOMMENDATION HIGHLIGHTS

Self-Help Books

- For adult daughters seeking to understand and improve relationship with their mothers:

    ★★★★ *Necessary Losses* by Judith Viorst

- For young adults looking to understand and improve relationships with their parents:

    ★★★ *How to Deal with Your Parents When They Still Treat You Like a Child* by Lynn Osterkamp

- For men wanting to learn about stages of adult development:

    ★★★★ *Seasons of a Man's Life* by Daniel J. Levinson

- For women wanting to learn about stages of adult development:

    ★★★ *Passages* by Gail Sheehy

- For those seeking to understand menopause:

    ★★★ *The Silent Passage* by Gail Sheehy

Autobiographies

- For a tutorial on life's (and death's) lessons:

    ★★★★★ *Tuesdays with Morrie* by Mitch Albom

- For dealing with a midlife crisis:

    ★★★ *Fly Fishing through the Midlife Crisis* by Howell Raines

Films

- For living with adult children while maintaining one's independence and goals:

    ★★★★★ *The Trip to Bountiful*

- For becoming a caring patient and partner:

    ★★★★★ *The Doctor*

- For inspiring fables on life paths and second chances:

    ★★★★ *It's a Wonderful Life*

    ★★★★ *Mr. Holland's Opus*

Internet Resources

- For a different perspective on a common problem:

    ★★★★ *The Mid-life Crisis: An Opportunity in Disguise*
    http://www.clarian.org/content/rodales/166.jhtml

- For probably the largest collection of information on aging on the net:
    ★★★★ *Friendly4Seniors* http://www.friendly4seniors.com/

- For awareness raising on a subtle prejudice:
    ★★★★★ *Ageism* http://garnet.berkeley.edu/%7Eaging/ModuleAgeism.html

- For understanding aging in a fuller context:
    ★★★★★ *Social Gerontology* http://www.trinity.edu/~mkearl/geron.html

---

power, illusions of safety, and the loss of our own younger self, the self we always thought would be unwrinkled, invulnerable, and immortal. Although most of us try to avoid loss, Viorst gives a positive tone to our emotional struggles. She believes that through the loss of our mother's protection, the loss of impossible expectations we bring to relationships, and the loss of loved ones through separation and death, we gain a deeper perspective, true maturity, and fuller wisdom about life. This fine self-help book was the highest rated book in the adult development category. Viorst writes extraordinarily well, and her sensitive voice comes through clearly. Most adults can benefit from reading *Necessary Losses* and will relate to its many examples.

★★★★ *Seasons of a Man's Life* (reissued ed., 1986) by Daniel J. Levinson. New York: Ballantine.

This national bestseller is an adult development book that outlines the stages adults pass through, with a special emphasis on the midlife crisis. The book's title accurately reveals that *Seasons of a Man's Life* is more appropriate for men than for women. In this book, Levinson and his colleagues summarize the results of their extensive interviews with 40 middle-aged men. Conclusions are bolstered with biographies of famous men and memorable characters from literature. Although Levinson's main interest is midlife change, he describes a number of stages and transitions in the life cycle between ages 17 and 65. Levinson believes that successful adjustment requires mastering developmental tasks at each stage. He sees the 20s as a novice phase of adult development. At the end of the teenage years, people need to make a transition from dependence to independence, a transition marked by the formation of a dream—an image of the desired life, especially in terms of career and marriage. From about 28 to 33, people go through a transition period in which they must face the more serious question of determining their development. In the 30s, individuals enter the phase of "becoming one's own man" (or BOOM). By age 40, they have reached a stable location in their careers and now must look forward to the kind of lives they will lead as middle-aged adults. Levinson reports that 70–80% of the men he interviewed found the midlife transition (ages 40 to 45) tumultuous and psychologically painful. This book is one of several that helped form the American public's image of a midlife crisis. The book is three decades old now and tends to overdramatize the midlife crisis. However, it remains a classic self-help resource.

Recommended

★★★   *Making Peace with Your Parents* (reissued 1996) by Harold Bloomfield. New York: Random House.

This book is about adults' relationships with their parents. According to Bloomfield, to become a fulfilled and competent person, you need to resolve the conflicts surrounding your relationship with your parents. Drawing on insights from his clinical practice, research in the area of adult children–parent relationships, and personal experiences in his own family, Bloomfield describes the problems many adults encounter in expressing love and anger toward their parents. *Making Peace with Your Parents* contains exercises and case studies that help adults improve their communication with their parents; cope effectively with difficult parents; unravel parental messages about love, sex, and marriage; and deal with parents' aging and death. The author especially believes that adults have to become their own best parent by nurturing themselves and engaging in self-responsibility instead of relying on their parents to satisfy important needs. This book just missed making the four-star category. It is an excellent book for adults who have a great deal of anger toward their parents. The message of self-responsibility and the clear examples can help individuals become aware of how their relationships with their parents have continued to shape their lives as adults.

★★★   *The Silent Passage* (revised ed., 1998) by Gail Sheehy. New York: Random House.

This bestseller concerns menopause, the time in middle age—usually in the late 40s or early 50s—when a woman's menstrual periods and childbearing capability cease and production of estrogen drops considerably. Journalist Gail Sheehy is also the author of the widely read adult development book, *Passages*, reviewed below. To better understand menopause, Sheehy interviewed many middle-aged women and talked with experts in a number of fields. Sheehy argues that the passage through menopause is seldom easy for women because of distracting symptoms, confusing medical advice, unsympathetic reactions from loved ones, and the scornful attitudes of society. For these reasons, menopause has been a lonely and emotionally draining experience for many women. Sheehy's goal is to erase the stigma of menopause and help women understand that it is a normal physical process. She describes her own difficult experiences and reports the frustrations of many women she interviewed. Sheehy's optimism comes through in her hope that menopause will come to be known as "the gateway to a second adulthood" for women. She is a masterful writer, and the book is quick and easy reading (it is a small-format book, only about 150 pages long). Few self-help writers' books ring with the clear-toned prose that Sheehy's do. At the same time, many medical and psychological experts simply don't believe that menopause is the widespread problem Sheehy thinks it is. Critics contend that just as Sheehy overdramatizes midlife as a crisis, she has done the same with menopause.

★★★   *Passages: Predictable Crises of Adult Life* (1976) by Gail Sheehy. New York: Dutton.

Like *Seasons of a Man's Life*, *Passages* is about the stages of adult development. In the mid-1970s, Sheehy's book was so popular that it topped the *New York Times* best-seller list for 27 weeks. Sheehy argues that we all go through developmental stages roughly bound by chronological age. Each stage brings problems people must solve before they can progress to the next stage. The periods between the stages are called passages. Sheehy uses catchy phrases to describe each stage: "the trying 20s," "catch 30," "the deadline decade" (35 to 45 years of age), and "the age 40 crucible." Sheehy's advice never waivers: Adults in transition may feel miserable, but those who face up to agonizing self-evaluation, who appraise their weaknesses as well as their strengths, who set goals for the future, and who try to be as independent as possible will find happiness more often than those who do not fully experience these trials. Sheehy believes that these passages earn people an authentic identity, one that is not based on the authority of one's parents or on cultural prescriptions. Not surprisingly, given its popularity with the public, this was one of the most frequently rated books in our national studies.

But the experts' evaluations, while largely positive, were mixed. On the positive side, some mental health experts believe the book has given people in their 30s, 40s, and 50s new insights about the transitions in adult development. On the negative side, some experts believe that Sheehy's book describes midlife as too much of a crisis and does not adequately consider the many individual ways people go through midlife. Dilemmas in adult development do not spring forth at 10-year intervals as Sheehy implies.

★★★ *When You and Your Mother Can't Be Friends* (1990) by Victoria Secunda. New York: Delacorte.

As the title of this book suggests, Secunda writes about the problems that can unfold in mother–daughter relationships when daughters become adults—daughters who have not resolved unhappy childhood attachments to their mothers and who continue to have unhappy relationships with them. Secunda believes that many adult women won't admit or explore their emotional confusion about their mothers. Yet honesty is exactly what is needed to go beyond mother–daughter bitterness, she says. One problem is that many adult daughters may not recognize how their relationships with their mothers have skewed their adulthood. Such women may play out their unresolved disaffection with husbands and lovers, coworkers and friends, and especially with their own children. Adult daughters can resolve unhappy relationships with their mothers and develop affectionate truces. Excerpts from 100 interviews with adult daughters are interspersed throughout the book to help adult daughters come to know, understand, and accept their mothers. This is an excellent book for adult daughters who have problematic relationships with their mothers. It is also easy to read, with an optimistic tone and many real-life examples. On the other hand, some mental health professionals marked down the book, citing it as stereotyping adult daughter–mother relationships and giving too little attention to individual variations.

★★★ *How to Deal with Your Parents When They Still Treat You Like a Child* (1992) by Lynn Osterkamp. New York: Berkley.

This book was written for adult children who want to understand and improve their relationships with their parents. Author Osterkamp helps the reader answer several important questions:

- Why are so many adults still worrying about what their parents think?
- Why can't I talk to my parents the way I talk to other people?
- Why do we keep having the same arguments?

- How can I stop feeling guilty?
- How can I change family gatherings and holidays?
- What role would I like for my parents to play in my life today?

Osterkamp's analysis of adult children–parent relationships can especially benefit adults in their 20s and 30s who want to get along better with their parents. Osterkamp suggests ways to communicate more effectively with parents. And she motivates the reader to develop a step-by-step action plan to accomplish relationship goals. Well written and well researched, this book is full of helpful examples and wise advice.

Diamond in the Rough

♦ *Your Renaissance Years* (1991) by Robert Veninga. Boston: Little, Brown.

This volume, subtitled *Making Retirement the Best Years of Your Life,* begins by describing the secrets of successful retirement and urging the reader to consider early retirement. Subsequent parts of the book focus on the following retirement concerns: money, housing, health, leisure, relationships, and spirituality. Case histories of 135 retirees are interspersed throughout. *Your Renaissance Years* was positively rated in our national studies, but by only five psychologists; few of the mental health professionals were familiar with it. Nonetheless, it is a valuable, well-written, in-depth resource for coping effectively with retirement (also reviewed in Chapter 5 on aging).

Not Recommended

★ *The 50+ Wellness Program* (1990) by Harris McIlwain, Debra Fulghum, Robert Fulghum, and Robert Bruce. New York: Wiley.

AUTOBIOGRAPHIES

Strongly Recommended

★★★★★ *Tuesdays with Morrie: An Old Man, a Young Man, and Life's Greatest Secrets* (1997) by Mitch Albom. New York: Doubleday.

Sportswriter Albom had been a student of sociology professor Morrie Schwartz 20 years earlier. Reunited after he saw Schwartz on *Nightline*, Albom finds that his former professor is dying from Lou Gehrig's disease. The book describes 14 Tuesday visits Albom made to his dying mentor and the content of their conversations. It is a moving best-seller.

Recommended

★★★ *Fly Fishing through the Midlife Crisis* (1994) by Howell Raines. New York: Doubleday.

Similar in approach to Robert Pirsig's *Zen and the Art of Motorcycle Maintenance*, Pulitzer Prize–winning journalist Raines uses fly fishing as a metaphor for midlife, reflecting on being a son, brother, and husband tutored by older men. He started as an acquisitive

"Redneck Fisher," determined to catch and keep it all. From his Uncle Erskine, he learned the higher order of fly fishing, which was more about attitude, contemplation, elegance, and friendship than catching fish. The book is about life, death, and what comes in between, at the borderline between sport and reflection. Fly fishing, more than a release or therapy for the author, has been a way of coping with family problems, divorce, and death, a metaphor for a reflective life. You don't have to be an angler to appreciate this book.

FILMS

Strongly Recommended

★★★★★   *The Trip to Bountiful* (1985) directed by Peter Masterson. PG rating. 106 minutes.

A country woman forced by circumstances to live with her son and daughter-in-law in a small city apartment is surprised to discover how old she has become and decides to revisit her girlhood home in Bountiful, Texas. She stubbornly persists, evading her family's fears about this trip, and makes the journey to reminisce and imagine her parents in the old house. In a subplot, she relates to a young girl during the brief bus trip to Bountiful, and we see her learn to accept her life and choose to make the best of it. This film illustrates (but does not resolve) conflicts between people of different generations and demonstrates what adult development is like.

★★★★★   *The Doctor* (1991) directed by Randa Haines. PG-13 rating. 125 minutes.

A pompous surgeon develops throat cancer and experiences what it is like to be a patient in an uncaring and mechanical system. He discovers his disconcerting mortality, and gets a reprieve to lead a life of caring and compassion. This may be useful for all those lacking empathy, struggling with what the health care system has become, or needing an example of how to communicate with a spouse made distant.

★★★★   *It's a Wonderful Life* (1946) directed by Frank Capra. 129 minutes.

A man who has done the right thing all his life, living by his values and those of his neighbors, is brought low by a relative's accidental misplacement of bank funds and contemplates suicide. An angel appears and shows him how badly his town, its families, and its ordinary citizens would have suffered had he not been there to lend them funds and give advice. The movie works as an inspiring fable, encouraging people to examine their lives, gain perspective, and take a second chance.

★★★★   *Mr. Holland's Opus* (1996) directed by Stephen Herek. PG rating. 142 minutes.

Mr. Glen Holland is a composer who accepts a temporary teaching position to pay the rent while he composes a memorable piece of music to leave his mark on the world. However, his temporary job turns into a lifetime commitment to his students and music education. His definition of success grows over the course of his career to encompass assisting his students and his family. It is a powerful film for addressing the meaning of success, the midlife reevaluation of career choices, and the personal sacrifices made for family gains.

Recommended

★★★   *Field of Dreams* (1989) directed by Phil Alden Robinson. PG rating. 106 minutes.

A couple choose a simple farming lifestyle instead of the hectic modern world. The husband then hears a voice telling him to "build it and he will come." Despite his doubts, the threat of foreclosure, and family opposition, with his wife's support he builds a baseball diamond in a cornfield, and the legends of a simpler time in professional baseball emerge and toss a few around. This movie may inspire self-doubters to cling to their dreams and others to take the risk of supporting their loved ones' dreams. At the same time, it is important to recognize the fantasy and insubstantiality of the plot.

★★★   *A Christmas Carol* (1938) directed by Edwin L. Marin. Not rated. 69 minutes.

The film is a ideal for reminding those too focused on making money that family can provide enormous satisfaction. But this theme can be expanded to include examining any of one's values: relationships, seeking fame, accepting invitations to become different, and generally looking at the future outcomes of current choices (the three ghosts' visits).

INTERNET RESOURCES

Although there are vast numbers of sites on aging, medical problems, and menopause, there is much less on self-help. These are the most clinically useful sites.

Metasites

★★★★   *Friendly4Seniors* http://www.friendly4seniors.com/

Very likely the largest site for finding information or resources on the net regarding aging. After the 10 major sections, the thousands of sites are listed alphabetically, so finding a particular resource may be difficult.

★★★★   *Geropsychology Central* http://www.premier.net/~gero/geropsyc.html

Slow loading because of graphics, the Senior's Corner offers the best short lists of links about health, retirement, news, and bulletin boards. The next section offers many valuable links to professional resources.

Psychoeducational Materials for Clients and Families

★★★★★   *Social Gerontology* http://www.trinity.edu/~mkearl/geron.html

Written for the college educated, this page offers an introductory context and connections for understanding aging from a social-psychological perspective. The sections and the links allow one to come to understand aging in a fuller context than is presented anywhere else.

★★★★★ *Ageism* by Barrie Robinson
http://garnet.berkeley.edu/%7Eaging/ModuleAgeism.html

Prepared as resources for college courses, the exercises in the Appendices and the other contents can help anyone become more aware of this subtle prejudice, its crippling myths, and the liberating truths.

★★★★★ *Attitudes: Key to Health, Happiness and Longevity*
http://www.attitudefactor.com/

The 20-item questionnaire asks about feelings of well-being, happiness, and hopefulness. The site then scores and returns information on the longevity consequences of your answers. This could be useful feedback for unhappy persons who cannot commit to therapy or change. The site offers the empirical support citations for this relationship and many readings on this issue.

★★★★ *Seniors-Site* http://seniors-site.com

About 30 message boards on all topics of relevance to seniors, their children, and caregivers.

★★★ *The Mid-life Crisis: An Opportunity in Disguise*
http://www.clarian.org/content/rodales/166.jhtml

A good brief overview to raise awareness and offer some direction.

★★ *Educational Resources Information Center/Clearinghouse on Adult, Career, and Vocational Education* http://ericacve.org/pubs.asp

Although designed for educators, the materials under Myths & Realities and Practice Application Briefs are valuable for solid information on training, work, and career paths.

See also Aging (Chapter 5), Death and Grieving (Chapter 15), Men's Issues (Chapter 24), and Women's Issues (Chapter 36).

CHAPTER 5

Aging

More than a century ago, Oliver Wendell Holmes said, "To be seventy years young is sometimes far more cheerful and hopeful than to be forty years old." In Holmes's day, being 70 years young was unusual, as the average life expectancy was less than 45 years. In the ensuing century, we have gained an average of more than 30 years of life, mainly because of improvements in sanitation, nutrition, and medical knowledge.

For too long, the aging process was thought of as an inevitable, irreversible decline. Aging involves both decline and growth, loss and gain. The previous view of aging was that we should passively live out our final years. The new view stresses that, although we are in the evening of our lives, we are not meant to live out our remaining years passively. Everything we know about older adults suggests that the more active they are, the happier and healthier they are.

In this chapter, we present self-help books, autobiographies, films, Internet resources, and national support groups for people who are in their older years and, in some cases, for their children and caregivers.

SELF-HELP BOOKS

Recommended

★★★ *Aging Well (2002)* by George Vaillant. Boston: Little, Brown.

This book describes the most recent results from longitudinal studies of aging conducted by psychiatrist George Vaillant. Inspirational messages reveal how men and women can lead happier, more fulfilling, healthier lives as they grow older. Vaillant does a wonderful job of interspersing case studies and research results to provide an in-depth look at the mechanisms of aging well. He concludes that individual lifestyles play a greater role than genetics, wealth, or ethnicity in determining how happy people are as older adults. He describes in step-by-step fashion how people can change their life-

RECOMMENDATION HIGHLIGHTS

Self-Help Books

- On aging in general, with emphasis on the medical and physical dimensions:
    - ★★★ *Complete Guide to Health and Well-Being after 50* by Robert Weiss and Genell Subak-Sharpe
    - ★★★ *Aging Well* by James Fries

- On aging successfully, with emphasis on lifestyle dimensions:
    - ★★★ *Aging Well* by George Vaillant
    - ★★★ *It's Better to Be over the Hill Than under It* by Eda LeShan

- On making environmental changes to improve life quality:
    - ★★★ *Enjoy Old Age* by B. F. Skinner and M. E. Vaughan

Autobiographies

- On conversations about life and death:
    - ★★★★ *Tuesdays with Morrie* by Mitch Albom

- On remaining active and contributing to society:
    - ★★★★ *The Virtues of Aging* by Jimmy Carter
    - ★★★ *The Last Gift of Life* by Carolyn G. Heilbrun

- On turning 50 and passing through menopause:
    - ◆ *Getting Over Getting Older* by Letty Cottin Pogrebin

- On taking care of aging parents along with one's own family:
    - ★★★ *Changing Places* by Judy Kramer

Films

- On accepting the limitations of age and repairing relationships:
    - ★★★★★ *On Golden Pond*
    - ★★★ *Wrestling Ernest Hemingway*

Internet Resources

- On aging and geropsychology:
    - ★★★★ *National Institute on Aging*
      http://www.nia.nih.gov/data/publist.asp
    - ★★★★ *Geropsychology Central*
      http://www.premier.net/~gero/geropsyc.html
    - ★★★★ *Administration on Aging* http://www.aoa.dhhs.gov

- On the basics of geriatric care:
  - ★★★★★ *Multidisciplinary Education in Geriatrics and Aging*
    http://cpmcnet.columbia.edu/dept/dental/
    Dental_Educational_Software/
    Gerontology_and_Geriatric_Dentistry/introduction.html

- On publications for health concerns:
  - ★★★★ *Health Information Publications List*
    http://www.nia.nih.gov/data/publist.asp

- On resources for those 55 and older:
  - ★★★★★ *The American Association of Retired Persons (AARP)*
    http://www.aarp.org

---

style to lead a more fulfilling life as they age. This is an outstanding book, one that undoubtedly would have been given five stars had it been rated by enough psychologists in our national studies.

★★★ *Another Country: Navigating the Emotional Terrain of Our Elders* (2000) by Mary Pipher. New York: Riverhead.

Psychologist Pipher describes the transition into old age, which is what she means by "another country." She believes that the greatest shame of older adults is that they are not self-sufficient, and that they keep their feelings to themselves. The old must be valued and involved, must give back and be engaged in life. The book includes excerpts of sessions with Pipher's clients, interspersed with advice for sensitively communicating with the elderly. Pipher says that there is a huge cultural gap between baby boomers, who express their emotions openly, and their emotionally restrictive, aging parents. This is a curious argument, because, recently, researchers such as Laura Carstensen of Stanford University and others have found that older adults place a higher value on emotional satisfaction than do younger adults. Nonetheless, psychologists in our studies rate the book quite favorably but infrequently.

★★★ *It's Better to Be over the Hill Than under It: Thoughts on Life over Sixty* (1990) by Eda LeShan. New York: Newmarket.

This book consists of what LeShan believes are her best columns from *Newsday* on a wide range of aging topics related mainly to the social, psychological, and lifestyle aspects of aging. The articles are divided into three sections: Loving and Living, Memories, and Growing and Changing. The 75 essays range from "An Open Letter to the Tooth Fairy" to "Nothing Is Simple Anymore" and "Divorce after Sixty." Many life issues that have to be dealt with in old age are covered: money, love, sex, anger, facing mortality, work, marriage, friendship, retirement, holidays, grandparenting, children, and so on. Woven through the essays is hope for older adults, hope that will allow them to love and grow, and to keep their minds and bodies active and alive. The real test for older adults, LeShan says, is not looking back but rather dealing with the present, regardless of the inevitable aspects of aging, and anticipating each coming day. This three-star book was favorably reviewed, deserving of four stars were it not for the small number of experts evaluating it. LeShan is a masterful writer who mixes wit with sage advice. The book is especially good for older adults who feel caught in a rut and need their spirits lifted.

★★★ *Enjoy Old Age: A Program of Self-Management* (1983) by B. F. Skinner and M. E. Vaughan. New York: Norton.

Vaughan, a former Harvard research associate and well-known expert on aging, and Skinner, a pioneer in behaviorism, combine their talents to assist older adults in making environmental changes to improve the quality of their lives. Specific areas covered include forgetfulness, thinking clearly and creatively, doing something about old age, getting along better with people, and dealing with the new emotions of aging. Advanced planning and a positive approach can provide solutions to the problem of age. Skinner describes his own solutions, and Vaughan contributes selections from the literature on aging. The book is written in a nonscientific way, using everyday English. It is useful for people approaching or already in their 60s or 70s, or for those living or working with older people.

★★★ *The Fountain of Age* (1993) by Betty Friedan. New York: Simon & Schuster.

The book looks at new possibilities and new directions for aging of both men and women. Topics covered include women living longer than men; physical, emotional, and environmental changes; and age as adventure. The author encourages older people not to buy into the myth that aging is a problem, a plight, a time of rapidly declining faculties. Friedan provides research and anecdotal evidence that the older adult years may be a period of true creativity. She discusses the tragic practice of early retirement, myths about menopause, early preparation for death, and overprotectiveness of family, friends, professionals, and the government. Creative ideas about health care, housing, work, and relationships are discussed. A book for all adults but especially a critique of our society and aging that will definitely move the over-60 crowd.

★★★ *Ageless Body, Timeless Mind: The Quantum Alternative to Growing Old* (1993) by Deepak Chopra. New York: Harmony.

Chopra, a best-selling author, offers an Eastern philosophical approach to the problems of aging. He combines mind–body medicine with current antiaging research. He states that a prolonged fruitful life is not a question of mind over matter, but rather of mind and matter, mind and body, together as one with the universe. By intervening at the level where belief becomes biology, we can achieve our potential: Mental, social, and intellectual activity can keep people vital and alert as they age. Chopra offers step-by-step exercises to help create a healthy life. A separate chapter examines India's traditional medical system of Arurveda. The book reveals how we can learn to direct the way our bodies metabolize time and reverse the aging process. This volume is for the layperson and professional interested in a blend of Eastern philosophy and Western scientific research.

★★★   *Complete Guide to Health and Well-Being after 50* (1988) by Robert Weiss and Genell Subak-Sharpe. New York: Times Books.

The full title of this book is actually *The Columbia University School of Public Health Complete Guide to Health and Well-Being after 50*. The book was produced under the auspices of the Columbia University School of Public Health. The word *Complete* in the title is appropriate: The book provides information about an encyclopedic number of physical and mental health issues that older adults face. Topics range from medical and physical concerns, such as heart disease, arthritis, and cosmetic surgery, to psychological and lifestyle concerns, such as coping with stress and retirement. Most self-help books don't have elaborate charts and tables, but this one is filled with them, along with many illustrations, exercises, diets, and self-tests. This excellent guide provides solid descriptions of the health problems of the elderly and the best ways to deal with them. As would be expected in a book written by public health experts, *Complete Guide to Health and Well-Being after 50* is strongly tilted toward a presentation and exploration of physical health issues. Coverage of the psychological and social dimensions of aging is not as thorough and not as insightful.

★★★   *Aging Well* (1989) by James Fries. Reading, MA: Addison-Wesley.

Fries believes that we have the capability to age well, with grace, wisdom, energy, and vitality. Aging well is not an easy task, he says. It requires a basic understanding of the aging process, a good plan, work, and persistence. Part I, Vitality and Aging, communicates the value of pride and enthusiasm in preventing disease and provides a wealth of understanding about specific diseases such as arthritis and osteoporosis. Part II, General Concerns, describes five keys to a healthy senior lifestyle: selecting and dealing with doctors, sexual issues, retirement, chronic illness, and completing a plan that will ensure that your wishes are carried out after you die. Part III, Solutions, is a step-by-step guide to managing a full range of medical problems, including pain, urinary tract problems, and heart ailments. The book is optimistic, well-written, and thorough. Fries's expertise on aging clearly comes through. The book is especially helpful as a guide to consult when physical and medical problems arise.

★★★   *How to Live Longer and Feel Better* (1986) by Linus Pauling. New York: Freeman.

This book provides a regimen that the author believes will add years to your life and make you feel better. Linus Pauling, a two-time Nobel Prize winner, shows how vitamins work and how to make them work for you. Pauling especially believes that vitamin C is responsible for producing and maintaining the body's supply of collagen, which he calls the glue that holds the body together. He argues that megadoses of vitamin C and other critical vitamins can slow down the aging process, make us look younger, and help us feel better. This book received three stars in the national studies, barely making it into the Recommended category. In the past, Pauling's ideas clashed with those of the medical establishment, but, recently, researchers are finding that the antioxidant vitamins may help to slow the aging process and improve the health of older adults. Pauling portrays himself as a misunderstood, maligned maverick whose ideas will eventually be accepted by the medical community.

Diamond in the Rough

◆ *Your Renaissance Years* (1991) by Robert Veninga. Boston: Little, Brown.

This volume, subtitled *Making Retirement the Best Years of Your Life,* begins by describing the secrets of successful retirement and urging the reader to consider early retirement. Subsequent parts of the book focus on the following retirement concerns: money, housing, health, leisure, relationships, and spirituality. Case histories of 135 retirees are interspersed throughout. *Your Renaissance Years* was positively rated in the national study, but by only five psychologists; few of the mental health professionals were familiar with it. Nonetheless, it is a valuable, well-written, in-depth resource for coping effectively with retirement (also presented in Chapter 4 on adult development).

AUTOBIOGRAPHIES

Strongly Recommended

★★★★★ *Tuesdays with Morrie: An Old Man, a Young Man, and Life's Greatest Secrets* (1997) by Mitch Albom. New York: Doubleday.

Sportswriter Albom had been a student of sociology professor Morrie Schwartz 20 years earlier. Reunited after he saw Schwartz on *Nightline,* Albom finds that his former professor is dying from Lou Gehrig's disease. The book describes 14 Tuesday visits Albom made to his dying mentor and the content of their conversations. This moving best-seller deepens understanding of life and death, is both funny and sad, and is as much about Albom's life as about his subject, who speaks for himself in *Morrie: In His Own Words.*

★★★★ *The Virtues of Aging* (1998) by Jimmy Carter. New York: Ballantine.

The former President discusses aging in America, with special attention to the state of the Social Security system, health, exercise, and financial planning. Carter discusses the importance of family ties and describes ways in which older people can remain active and contribute to social betterment. Down to earth and easy to read, this book focuses on the wisdom that people accumulate over a lifetime and how it can be applied. President Carter personifies those whose reputation and good works increased following "retirement."

Recommended

★★★ *Changing Places: A Journey with my Parents into their Old Age* (2001) by Judy Kramer. New York: Berkley.

Originally written as a series of newspaper columns, the book describes the aging of journalist Cramer's parents, their move into a nursing home, and their deaths. While holding a full-time job and caring for her own family, Kramer becomes her parents' caregiver, grappling on a daily basis with their medical appointments, Medicare paperwork, and bills. The book portrays with realism and tenderness the transition from being one's parents' child to becoming their caregiver, and the sandwiched feeling of meeting demands of two families.

★★★   *The Last Gift of Life: Life beyond Sixty* (1998) by Carolyn G. Heilbrun. New York: Ballantine.

The author had it all—a fine education, career, family, and great recognition. She was an English professor at Columbia, a noted feminist critic, and author of a well-known mystery series under the pseudonym Amanda Cross. However, when she was young, Heilbrun had vowed to take her life at age 70, in the belief that life after that was not worth living. The realization of how enjoyable and productive life had been in her 50s and 60s changed her mind. Now safely past 70, she had not lost her spirit; describing herself as "still dancing for joy" and free from earlier constraints and the pushes and pulls of family and career. Now, she can fully be herself in a family context, as wife, mother, and grandmother. She is a great fan of e-mail and the Internet, describing how they expanded her universe. Heilbrun is a role model for younger women and an inspiration for older women.

★★★   *The Fountain of Age* (1994) by Betty Friedan. New York: Touchstone.

One of the major figures in the modern feminist movement and author of *The Feminine Mystique,* Friedan deconstructs current beliefs about aging while maintaining that it can be a time of adventure, exploration, fulfillment, and creativeness. Combining the personal and the political with research findings, this book is a trenchant critique of the decline model of aging. A good book for a socially conscious reader, it was also rated earlier in this chapter as a self-help book.

Diamonds in the Rough

♦   *I'm Not as Old as I Used to Be* (1998) by Frances Weaver. New York: Hyperion.

In a sprightly account of life after 70, NPR commentator and senior editor of the *Today Show* Frances Weaver describes her battle with alcoholism after her husband's death. She went to a detox center and eventually achieved sobriety. Weaver returned to school, traveled, and began writing. She employs her keen wit to demonstrate how to be active and productive during life's later years. A relatively recent book, probably not widely known by mental health experts—and thus classified as a Diamond in the Rough—this is a good account of developing new interests after the age of 70.

♦   *Getting Over Getting Older* (1997) by Letty Cottin Pogrebin. New York: Berkley.

Well-known feminist writer Pogrebin describes her reactions to turning 50 and her concerns about her appearance, health, relationships, sex, and going through menopause. The book conveys a sense of sisterhood and community among older women. Her playful tone and some very funny sections occasionally reduce the seriousness of some important points, but the book is a good and illuminating read.

FILMS

Strongly Recommended

★★★★★   *On Golden Pond* (1981) directed by Mark Rydell. PG rating. 109 minutes.

An 80-year-old retired teacher becomes preoccupied with death and losing his faculties as his birthday is celebrated. He becomes anxious, irritable, and difficult to live with, but his wife knows how to handle him and helps his alienated daughter make the connections needed by both for resolution before his death. All three principal actors received Oscars. This film might be most useful to those alienated from parents and trying to communicate with those parents. It might reinforce the fact that there may not be time for healing unless one acts now.

Recommended

★★★ *Wrestling Ernest Hemingway* (1993) directed by Randa Haines. PG-13 rating. 122 minutes.

In this character study of two lonely old men trapped in the emptiness of their own lives, Frank and Walter meet in a park and gradually become friends, but eventually separate after quarrels and misbehavior. In words and deeds, the two men discuss and accept the imminence of death. A sensitive film on a sensitive topic: aging and death.

★★★ *Cocoon* (1986) directed by Ron Howard. PG-13 rating. 117 minutes.

Disregard the subplot of visiting intergalactic aliens and focus on how the senior citizens of a Florida retirement community find an actual fountain of youth. They experience new vigor and possibilities. The movie is, of course, a fantasy and a denial of the negatives and losses of aging; nonetheless, it is an inspiring and perhaps helpful film about what may still be felt and lived.

Not Recommended

★★ *Space Cowboys* (2000) directed by Clint Eastwood. PG-13 rating. 130 minutes.

★★ *Grumpy Old Men* (1993) directed by Donald Petrie. PG-13 rating. 103 minutes.

INTERNET RESOURCES

Although there are vast numbers of sites on aging, medical problems, and geriatric information, there is much less self-help on the Internet. These are the most clinically useful sites.

Metasites

★★★★ *Friendly4Seniors* http://www.friendly4seniors.com

This is very likely the largest site for finding any information or resources on the Internet on the issues of aging. After the 10 major sections, thousands of sites are listed alphabetically, so finding a particular resource may be difficult.

★★★★ *Health Information Publications List*
http://www.nia.nih.gov/data/publist.asp

The National Institute on Aging has many useful publications, described in this catalog, and all are available by download. Take a look at the dozens of Age Page fact sheets, especially Talking with Your Doctor and The Resource Directory for Older People.

★★★★   *Geropsychology Central*   http://www.premier.net/~gero/geropsyc.html

Slow loading because of graphics, the Senior's Corner offers the best short lists of links on health, retirement, news, and bulletin boards. The next section offers many valuable links to professional resources.

★★★★   *National Institute on Aging*   http://www.nia.nih.gov/data/publist.asp

This list of about 100 publications includes the Age Page fact sheets, Connections newsletter, exercise videos, and materials on Alzheimers. For all needs and audiences.

★★★★   *Administration on Aging*   http://www.aoa.dhhs.gov

This is a federal site with lots of information. National Institute on Aging Age Pages offer many brochures with accurate information about health, alcohol, exercise, sexuality, and so on. Some 20 Fact Sheets provide facts and references designed for the educated reader.

★★★★   *Aging Internet Information Notes: Cultural and Racial Diversity and Aging*
     http://www.aoa.gov/NAIC/Notes/diversityaging.html

A magnificent collection of papers, programs, and training materials on the overlap between diversity and aging.

★★★   *ElderWeb*   http://www.elderweb.com

This research site for professionals and family members contains more than 4,500 links to eldercare and long-term care information, including legal, financial, medical, and housing issues, and policy, research, and statistics.

Psychoeducational Materials for Clients and Families

★★★★★   *Multidisciplinary Education in Geriatrics and Aging*
     http://cpmcnet.columbia.edu/dept/dental/Dental_Educational_Software/
     Gerontology_and_Geriatric_Dentistry/introduction.html

Although intended for professionals, this 12-module training program is an online textbook with wider uses. The modules on Normal Aging and Mental Health (mainly assessment) are perhaps the most relevant, but the others may be right for some caregivers and clients. "The purpose of this series of learning modules is to teach graduate and undergraduate students in the health sciences the basic concepts in geriatric care."

★★★★★   *Social Gerontology*   http://www.trinity.edu/~mkearl/geron.html

Written for the college-educated, this page offers an introductory context and links for understanding aging from a social-psychological perspective. The sections and the links allow one to come to understand aging in a fuller context than is presented elsewhere.

★★★★   *American Association of Retired Persons*
     http://www.aarp.org/indexes/health.html#stress

Over 100 very informative yet simply written articles are available here under headings of Staying Fit, Eating Well, Managing Stress, Preventing Disease, Aging Well, Caregiving, and End of Life.

★★★★ *Alcohol and the Elderly* http://alcoholism.about.com/library/weekly/
aa981118.htm?pid=2750&cob=home

This page has links to many others of relevance to alcohol and drug overuse in the elderly population. They may help overcome denial in clients or families. Similarly, the upstream site, http://alcoholism.about.com/cs/elder/, offers 10 links on different aspects of this issue.

★★★★ *Attitudes: Key to Health, Happiness and Longevity*
http://www.attitudefactor.com

The 20-item, 5-minute questionnaire asks about feelings of well-being, happiness, and hopefulness, and then provides information on the longevity consequences of your answers. This could be useful feedback for unhappy persons who cannot commit to change. The site offers empirical support citations for this relationship and many readings.

★★★ *Spirituality and Aging—Bibliography* http://www.usc.edu/isd/locations/
science/gerontology/MLA/mlabib_god.html

Lists about 40 books, without annotations.

★★★ *Alcohol, Medications and Aging: Use, Misuse and Abuse*
http://www.asaging.org/alcohol-shocked/adframe.html

A web-based training program designed for professionals but usable by anyone. It could be useful for those in denial or for the ninformed.

★★★ *If You're over 65 and Feeling Depressed . . . Treatment Brings New Hope*
http://www.nimh.nih.gov/publist/964033.htm

"Many older people believe that their age alone is responsible for feelings of exhaustion, helplessness, and worthlessness. This brochure discusses the causes of depression in the older years, symptoms, type of treatment, and where to go for help." About six pages of general information on depression.

★★★ *Curriculum Module on Aging and Ethnicity* by Andrew E. Scharlach, PhD, Esme
Fuller-Thomson, PhD, and B. Josea Kramer, PhD
http://garnet.berkeley.edu/~aging/ModuleMinority1.html

Each section of the module provides an overview, references, and an interview with an expert. Designed to flesh out college courses, contents specific and relevant to Native Americans, Africans, Asians, and Hispanics will help anyone understand minority issues in aging.

★★★ *Caregiving—Special Topics* http://www.usc.edu/isd/locations/science/gerontology/MLA/mlabib_care.html

An unannotated list of about 40 books.

NATIONAL SUPPORT GROUPS

American Association of Retired Persons (AARP)
601 East Street NW
Washington, DC 20049
Phone: 800-424-3410
E-mail: member@aarp.org
http://www.aarp.org

American Parkinson's Disease Association
1250 Hylan Boulevard, Suite 4B
Staten Island, NY 10305-1946
Phone: 800-223-APDA or 718-981-8001
E-mail: Apda@apdaparkinson.org
http://www.apdaparkinson.com

American Society on Aging
833 Market Street, Suite 511
San Francisco, CA 94103-1824
Phone: 415-974-9600
E-mail: info@asaging.org
http://www.asaging.org

Arthritis Foundation
PO Box 7669
Atlanta, GA 30357-0669
Phone: 800-283-7800
http://www.arthritis.org

Department of Veterans Affairs
http://www.va.gov
   Publishes a resource guide for working with older adults.

Gray Panthers
733 15th Street NW, Suite 437
Washington, DC 20005
Phone: 202-737-6637 or 800-280-5362
E-mail: info@graypanthers.org
http://www.graypanthers.org
   For young and old adults working together.

National Council on Aging
409 3rd Street SW, Suite 200
Washington, DC 20024
Phone: 202-479-1200 or 800-424-9046
http://www.ncoa.org

National Family Caregivers Association
10400 Connecticut Avenue, Suite 500
Kensington, MD 20895-3944
Phone: 800-896-3650
E-mail: info@nfcacares.org
http://www.nfcacares.org

National Hispanic Council on Aging
2713 Ontario Road NW
Washington, DC 20009
Phone: 202-265-1288
E-mail: nhcoa@worldnet.att.net
http://www.nhcoa.org

National Parkinson Foundation
1501 NW 9th Avenue
Bob Hope Road
Miami, FL 33136-1494
Phone: 305-547-6666 or 800-327-4545
E-mail: mailbox@parkinson.org
http://www.parkinson.org

National Stroke Association
9707 E. Easter Lane
Englewood, CO 80112
Phone: 303-649-9299 or 800-STROKES
http://www.stroke.org

Older Women's League
666 11th Street NW, Suite 700
Washington, DC 20001
Phone: 202-783-6686 or 800-825-3695
E-mail: owlinfo@owl-national.org
http://www.owl-national.org
   Membership organization that advocates on behalf of various economic and social issues for midlife and older women.

See also Adult Development (Chapter 4), Death and Grieving (Chapter 15), and Dementia/Alzheimer's (Chapter 16).

CHAPTER 6

Anger

Anger is a powerful emotion. People who have fiery tempers—who become furious when they are criticized, get angry when they are slowed down, say nasty things when they get mad, and feel like hitting someone when they are frustrated—hurt not only others but themselves as well. Everybody gets angry sometimes, but for most of us, it's mild anger a couple of times a week. Mild anger often emerges if a loved one or a friend performs what we perceive to be a misdeed, whether it is being late, promising one thing and doing another, or neglecting a duty, for example. Anger disorders, on the other hand, are characterized as enraged, uncontrollable, and frequent.

In this chapter, we present the ratings and descriptions of anger self-help books and Internet resources, respectively.

SELF-HELP BOOKS

Strongly Recommended

★★★★★ *The Anger Control Workbook* (2000) by Matthew McKay and Peter Rogers. Oakland, CA: New Harbinger.

Psychologists McKay and Rogers provide a step-by-step, cognitive-behavioral approach for individuals seeking to control their anger. In 19 chapters, they describe how to identify, understand, respond to, and cope with hostile feelings. Especially recommended is learning how to relax in the face of physical tension in provocative situations; the authors state that it is almost impossible to get angry when you are able to relax your body. Numerous helpful exercises and worksheets are provided. This book is an excellent choice for those seeking to control their anger. Along with the *Dance of Anger* (reviewed below), *The Anger Control Workbook* was judged to be the best self-help book for anger.

RECOMMENDATION HIGHLIGHTS

Self-Help Books

- For advice and methods based on cognitive-behavioral therapy:

  ★★★★★ *The Anger Control Workbook* by Matthew McKay and Peter Rogers

  ★★★★ *The Anger Workbook* by Lorrainne Bilodeau

  ★★★★ *How to Control Your Anger before It Controls You* by Albert Ellis and Raymond Chip Tafrate

  ★★★★ *Letting Go of Anger* by Ron Potter-Efron and Pat Potter-Efron

- For women who want to understand and moderate their anger:

  ★★★★★ *The Dance of Anger* by Harriet Lerner

- For learning to control anger through cognitive therapy:

  ★★★ *Prisoners of Hate* by Aaron Beck

- For coping with anger in many different facets of life:

  ★★★★ *Anger: The Misunderstood Emotion* by Carol Tavris

- For helping children control their anger:

  ◆ *A Volcano in My Tummy* by Elaine Whitehouse and Warwick Pudney

Internet Resources

- For understanding how anger works and how it is treated:

  ★★★★★ *Controlling Anger—Before It Controls You*
  http://www.apa.org/pubinfo/anger.html

  ★★★★★ *Anger—Part I: Identifying Anger* http://www.heart7.net/anger1.html

- For articles offering guidelines on anger management:

  ★★★★ *Get Your Angries Out*
  http://members.aol.com/AngriesOut/index.htm

★★★★★ *The Dance of Anger: A Woman's Guide to Changing the Patterns of Intimate Relationships* (reissued ed., 1997) by Harriet Lerner. New York: Harper Perennial.

This popular and prized book was written mainly for women about the anger in their lives, both their own anger and that of the people they live with, especially men. It has sold more than a million copies and deservedly has been on the *New York Times* bestseller list. Lerner maintains that expressions of anger are not only encouraged more in boys and men than in girls and women but also may be glorified to maladaptive extremes. By contrast, girls and women have been denied even a healthy and realistic expression of anger. Lerner argues that to express anger—especially openly, directly, or loudly—traditionally is considered to make a woman appear unladylike, unfeminine, and sexually unattractive. Lerner explains the difficulties women have in showing anger and describes how they can use their anger to gain a stronger, more independent sense of self. Rooted in both family systems and psychoanalytic theory, *The Dance of Anger* has nine chapters and an epilogue. Lerner describes the circular dances of couples, such as the all-too-familiar situation of the nagging wife and the withdrawing husband. The more she nags, the more he withdraws, and the more he withdraws, the more she nags. Lerner goes on to provide valuable advice about how to deal with anger when interacting with "impossible" mothers, with children, and in family triangles. This excellent guide is a compassionate exploration of women's anger and an insightful guide for turning anger into a constructive force that can reshape women's lives.

★★★★　*Anger: The Misunderstood Emotion* (revised and updated, 1989) by Carol Tavris. New York: Touchstone.

This excellent self-help book covers the wider terrain of anger and its manifestations. Indeed, it is hard to come up with any facet of anger—from wrecked friendships to wars—that Tavris does not address. The revised and updated edition includes new coverage of highway anger, violence in sports, young women's anger, and family anger, and it suggests strategies for getting through specific anger problems. The book consists of 10 entertaining chapters. In the first several chapters, Tavris debunks a number of myths about anger and highlights anger's cultural rules. She persuasively argues that "letting it all out" is not the best solution for defusing anger and effectively coping with stress. She dislikes pop-psychology approaches that tell people that anger is buried within them, and she argues that such notions are dangerous to the mental health of participants and to the social health of the community. She also sharply criticizes psychotherapy approaches that are based on the belief that inside every tranquil soul is a furious person screaming to get out. Later chapters present helpful ideas about anger in marital relationships and situations involving justice. In the final two chapters, Tavris tells readers how to rethink anger and make more adaptive choices. The book is well-researched, and Tavris's delivery is witty and eloquent. Anyone wanting to cope more effectively with the anger in their lives will find this book a welcome tonic.

★★★★　*The Anger Workbook* (1992) by Lorrainne Bilodeau. Minneapolis: CompCare.

This information manual and workbook explains how to understand anger, see its usefulness, and have healthier anger. A cognitive-behavioral approach to anger is taken. The book presents a self-assessment questionnaire, followed by recommended changes in thought patterns and behaviors. The chapters are structured effectively for instruction; the several questionnaires are followed by chapters that address the potential clusters of answers the reader could have given and responds to them in a decision-making format. Concepts include taking a new perspective on anger, acknowledging the complexities of anger, understanding how anger goes awry, changing the experience of anger, and responding to another person's anger. This valuable and practical book clearly explains how to understand anger problems and how to move toward their resolution.

★★★★　*How to Control Your Anger before It Controls You* (1997) by Albert Ellis and Raymond Chip Tafrate. Secaucus, NJ: Birch Lane.

The treatment model of Rational–Emotive Behavior Therapy (REBT) developed by Albert Ellis has evolved over the years into many applications, all with the same underlying goal of controlling thoughts in order to control feelings. Ellis and his coauthor have adapted the REBT model to reducing or eliminating anger. They consider myths about dealing with anger, rational and irrational aspects of anger, and identifying self-anger-ing beliefs. Multiple techniques are taught for thinking ways out of anger, as are well-described relaxation exercises and self-help forms that allow the reader to record experiences and self-guide through the cognitive-behavioral treatment of anger reduction. This practical volume is easy to read, understand, and apply. The REBT principles are presented with clarity in an inviting manner.

★★★★ *Letting Go of Anger: The Ten Most Common Anger Styles and What to Do about Them* (1995) by Ron Potter-Efron and Pat Potter-Efron. Oakland, CA: New Harbinger.

The authors take a systematic approach to identifying and treating types of anger, often using cognitive-behavioral strategies. A questionnaire allows readers to categorize themselves into anger styles: masked anger, explosive anger, or chronic anger. Each chapter further describes several ways of manifesting anger within each of the three primary styles. Clarity and conciseness are strengths of this self-help resource. Each chapter outlines the characteristics of the anger style, typical examples of how the anger plays out, and remedies for counteracting anger. The suggested treatments are understandable and easily conducted by nonprofessionals.

Recommended

★★★ *Prisoners of Hate: The Cognitive Basis of Anger, Hostility, and Violence* (1999) by Aaron Beck. New York: Harper Perennial.

Psychiatrist Beck applies his cognitive therapy to helping individuals learn how to control their anger. Beck describes recognizable examples from everyday life of how people turn anger into hatred. He also tackles the history of hostility and violence on the part of societies and governments. His historical analysis of anger is somewhat tedious though, especially for a self-help book. Beck argues that cognitive distortions involving hostile framing can lock the mind in a "prison of hate." He believes that hostility, anger, and violence can be greatly reduced when rational thinking overrides cognitive distortions. This valuable book was very highly rated by psychologists in our national studies and likely would have been given five stars if it had been rated more frequently.

★★★ *When Anger Hurts* (1997) by Matthew McKay, Peter Rogers, and Judith McKay. Oakland, CA: Fine Communications.

This book presents a cognitive-behavioral approach to coping with anger. Subtitled *Quieting the Storm Within*, it is divided into three main sections that focus on understanding anger, building skills to cope with anger, and dealing with anger at home. The section on building skills to cope with anger contains a number of helpful strategies, including how to control stress step-by-step, how to keep anger from escalating, how to use healthy self-talk to deal with angry feelings, and how to engage in problem-solving communication when anger is harming relationships. The authors instruct readers in the specifics of keeping an anger journal.

★★★ *Angry All the Time: An Emergency Guide to Anger Control* (1994) by Ron Potter-Efron. Oakland, CA: New Harbinger.

This book was written for and about people who regularly function at a high level of anger. The author provides candid descriptions of the angry lifestyle, myths, and excuses for anger, along with a road map for breaking the cycle. Validating checklists enable the reader to clearly understand how to change, and include The Six Main Reasons People Stay Angry, The Violence Ladder, and a chapter for partners of angry people. This book hits anger behavior head on with a no-nonsense but understanding approach. The mental health experts in our study preferred Potter-Efron's later work, *Letting Go of Anger*, slightly more than this book. Refer to its earlier review in the Strongly Recommended listing.

★★★ *Anger: How to Live with and without It* (1986) by Albert Ellis. New York: Lyle Stuart.

This is one of pioneering cognitive therapist Albert Ellis's many books on how to cope more effectively. Here, Ellis applies his Rational–Emotive Therapy to help people deal with anger. He provides step-by-step instructions for how to cognitively and behaviorally rearrange anger. Readers are given a number of homework assignments to help them rethink how they deal with anger. This book is a bit dated, and our mental health experts preferred Ellis's (and Tafrate's) newer book on the same topic, *How to Control Your Anger before it Controls You*, reviewed earlier in the Strongly Recommended category.

★★★ *The Angry Book* (1969, reissued 1998) by Theodore Rubin. New York: Macmillan.

This early, psychoanalytically oriented book advocates the "let it all out" catharsis approach to anger. Rubin warns readers about the dangers that await them if they bottle up their anger and "twist" or "pervert" it. He says that a "slush fund" of accumulated, unexpressed anger builds up in the body, waiting for the opportunity to produce high blood pressure, depression, alcoholism, sexual problems, and other diseases. At the end of *The Angry Book*, Rubin asks readers 103 questions that are intended to give them therapeutic guidance. One of these questions is whether readers have ever experienced the good, clean feeling that comes after expressing anger, as well as the increased self-esteem and feeling of peace that such expression brings. The "let it all out" approach was widely accepted by many clinicians in the past, but it is less accepted today. Rubin's recommendations directly contradict the approaches advocated by cognitive-behaviorists in multiple books reviewed earlier. This book barely makes it into the three-star category, and many experts see it as seriously dated.

Diamonds in the Rough

◆ *A Volcano in My Tummy—Helping Children to Handle Anger* (1996) by Elaine White-house and Warwick Pudney. Gabriola Island, BC: New Society.

This valuable workbook is written in a lesson-plan format that structures key anger concepts into activities for children age six through teens. The book is written for parents and teachers, with emphasis on use by teachers. The activities are well designed for the targeted age groups, and demonstrate creativity and variety that hold the attention of children, whether in school or at home. The purpose of the book is to help children become aware of their anger and learn safe, alternative responses to anger. It is listed as a Diamond in the Rough because the few ratings it received in two of our studies were consistently high.

♦ *The Angry Self: A Comprehensive Approach to Anger Management* (1999) by M. M. Gottlieb. Phoenix: Zeig, Tucker, & Theisen.

Practical, step-by-step cognitive-behavioral, Ericksonian, and relaxation strategies are outlined to help control anger more effectively. This workbook includes extensive exercises and assignments that can be used effectively in anger control. It is placed in the Diamond in the Rough category for positive evaluations but a low number of raters.

♦ *Anger Kills: Seventeen Strategies for Controlling the Hostility That Can Harm Your Health* (1994) by Redford Williams and Virginia Williams. New York: Harper Perennial.

The health costs to a person who experiences ongoing anger is the focus of *Anger Kills*, cited as a Diamond in the Rough for its modest number of raters but very high ratings. Hostility and its effect on individuals and those around them are outlined in factual terms and through scientific study. This area of study was pioneered by coauthor Redford Williams. A self-administered hostility questionnaire is followed by a road map of strategies to overcome hostility. Chapters are grouped by recommendations to alter thinking patterns, cope with volatile situations, react to others' hostility, improve relationships, and adopt positive attitudes. Cognitive-behavioral strategies are suggested and demonstrated through decision-making diagrams, making this book a good companion to cognitive-behavioral therapy on anger.

Not Recommended

★★ *Anger: Deal with It, Heal with It, Stop It from Killing You* (1991) by Bill Defoore. Deerfield Beach, FL: Health Communications.

INTERNET RESOURCES

Metasite

★★★★★ *Anger* http://www.angelfire.com/hi/TheSeer/anger.html

After a two-page introduction, there are perhaps 50 links to all aspects of anger, including treatment, dynamics, self-therapy, relating your spouse and kids, and so on.

Psychoeducational Materials for Clients and Families

★★★★★ *Controlling Anger—Before It Controls You*
　　　　http://www.apa.org/pubinfo/anger.html

A five-page overview from the American Psychological Association that offers several approaches.

★★★★★   *Anger—Part I: Identifying Anger*   http://www.heart7.net/anger1.html

★★★★   *Anger—Part II: Using Anger's Power Safely*
http://www.heart7.net/anger2.html

These sites present an excellent overview with many quotations and guidelines from books. No great psychological sophistication is required; material is accessible to the average reader.

★★★★   *Get Your Angries Out* http://members.aol.com/AngriesOut/index.htm

The 40 or 50 articles by Lynn Namaka offer guidelines and directions for adults, kids, parents, and teachers. They are comprehensive and speak directly and productively.

★★★   *When Anger Hurts* by Mathew McKay, Peter D. Rogers, and Judith McKay http://www.alzwell.com/Clues.html

A three-page list of the verbal, gestural, facial, and other behaviors that trigger anger. It could be useful for clients who do not recognize their triggers.

★★★   *Anger and Aggression* http://mentalhelp.net/psyhelp/chap7

This chapter of an online book offers a wide-ranging presentation (for example, marriage, prejudice, distrust, and gender) and cites a dozen therapeutic approaches and techniques.

★★★   *Temper Tantrums: What Causes Them and How Can You Respond?* by Dawn Ramsburg http://npin.org/pnews/1997/pnew997/pnew997g.html

Two useful pages from *Parent News.*

★★★   *Time Out* http://www.noah-health.org/english/illness/mentalhealth/cornell/recovery/timeout.html

A short but very good list of self-talk to use when enraged.

★★★   *Why Am I So Angry?* http://arthritis.about.com/library/weekly/aa022498.htm?COB=home&terms=anger&PM=113_300_T

Anger is a major component in flare-ups of rheumatoid arthritis. These four pages are a good introduction to the topic of anger for patients.

★★   *Plain Talk About . . . Dealing with the Angry Child*
http://npin.org/library/pre1998/n00216/n00216.html

About three pages from the U.S. Department of Health and Human Services.

See also Stress Management and Relaxation (Chapter 32) and Violent Youth (Chapter 37).

CHAPTER 7

Anxiety Disorders

Anxiety is a highly unpleasant feeling that comes in different forms. Sometimes it is a diffuse, vague feeling; at other times, it is a fear of something specific. People who have an anxiety disorder often feel motor tension (jumpy, trembling, or can't relax), are hyperactive (dizzy, their heart races, or they perspire), and are apprehensive.

All these anxiety symptoms exist to a lesser or greater degree in the spectrum of anxiety disorders: generalized anxiety disorder (GAD), phobias, panic disorders, hypochondriasis, obsessive–compulsive disorder (OCD), and posttraumatic stress disorder (PTSD). The latter two disorders are covered in separate chapters: PTSD in Chapter 26, and OCD in Chapter 25. Also falling into the anxiety category is the controversial and rare diagnosis of dissociative identity disorder (DID), previously known as multiple personality disorder.

Controversy swirls around the causes of anxiety disorders. Some mental health experts, especially in the medical field, believe that anxiety is biologically determined and should be treated with medications. Other mental health experts, including many psychologists, argue that anxiety is primarily caused by what we experience and how we think. They maintain that anxiety reduction involves rearranging the environment and cognitively reinterpreting the world. The following self-help resources include both schools of thought.

As with the other chapters, we begin with a synopsis of our primary recommendations and proceed through the ratings and descriptions of the respective self-help books, autobiographies, films, Internet resources, and national support groups.

SELF-HELP BOOKS

Strongly Recommended

★★★★★ *The Anxiety and Phobia Workbook* (3rd ed., 2001) by Edmund J. Bourne. Oakland, CA: New Harbinger.

In the third edition of his workbook, psychologist Bourne describes specific skills needed to overcome problems with panic, anxiety, and phobias, and provides step-by-

RECOMMENDATION HIGHLIGHTS

Self-Help Books

- For cognitive, behavioral, and social tools to reduce anxiety:

  ★★★★★ *The Anxiety and Phobia Workbook* by Edmund J. Bourne

  ★★★★★ *Mastery of Your Anxiety and Panic III* by Michelle G. Craske and David H. Barlow

- For helping the shy and socially anxious:

  ★★★★ *The Shyness and Social Anxiety Workbook* by Martin Anthony and Richard Swinson

- For holistic and integrative approaches to anxiety:

  ★★★★ *Beyond Anxiety and Phobia* by Edmund J. Bourne

  ★★★★ *Feel the Fear and Do It Anyway* by Susan Jeffers

- For those with a sophisticated knowledge of psychological problems:

  ★★★★ *Anxiety Disorders and Phobias* by Aaron Beck and Gary Emery

- For reducing or eliminating panic attacks:

  ★★★★ *Don't Panic* by Reid Wilson

- For treating phobias, panic, and obsessive–compulsive behaviors:

  ◆ *The Sky Is Falling* by Raeann Dumont

Autobiographies

- For recovering from dissociative identity disorder:

  ★★★★ *A Mind of My Own* by Chris Costner Sizemore

- For a treatment program for panic attacks and agoraphobia:

  ★★★ *The Panic Attack Recovery Book* by Shirley Swede and Seymour S. Jaffe

- For recovering from hypochondria:

  ★★★ *Phantom Illness* by Carla Cantor

Films

- For the (controversial) treatment of dissociative identity disorder:

  ★★★ *Sybil*

Internet Resources

- For a comprehensive site on cognitive-behavioral therapy:

  ★★★★★ *Panic Anxiety Education Management Services*
  http://www.healthyplace.com/communities/anxiety/paems/index.html

- For a site with humor and knowledge about specific anxiety disorders:
  ★★★★★ *the Anxiety Panic internet resource (tAPir)*
  http://www.algy.com/anxiety/index.shtml

- For superb information on shyness:
  ★★★★ *The Shyness Home Page: An Index to Resources for Shyness*
  http://www.shyness.com

- For a great overview written by experts for their clients:
  ★★★★ *The Causes of Anxiety and Panic Attacks*
  http://www.algy.com/anxiety/files/barlow.html

- For explicit detail on the development of panic:
  ★★★★ *Understanding Panic Disorder*
  http://www.nimh.nih.gov/anxiety/panicmenu.cfm

step procedures for mastering these skills. The book contains a fair amount of descriptive material but emphasizes cognitive-behavioral skills, strategies, and exercises to foster recovery. Its approach is strongly holistic, focusing on multiple dimensions (e.g., body, behavior, feelings, mind, interpersonal relations, self-esteem, and spirituality). The latest edition offers additional information on medications, herbal supplements, and the patient's support persons. For the layperson, this is a concise, practical, and comprehensive directory on how to reduce anxiety. A highly regarded and widely known resource.

★★★★★ *Mastery of Your Anxiety and Panic III* (2000) by Michelle G. Craske and David H. Barlow. Albany, NY: Graywind Publications. (Also distributed by the Psychological Corporation.)

Barlow and Craske, nationally known researchers in the treatment of anxiety disorders, have updated their original self-help offering. The book is based on empirically supported and clinically proven treatments that cover the cognitive, behavioral, physical, and social aspects of anxiety. This third edition is easier to read, includes new methods for providing exposure to feared sensations, and offers a series of separate manuals (Therapist Guide, Client Workbook, Client Monitoring Forms, and Client Workbook for Agoraphobia). Record forms, case vignettes, and self-assessments are both numerous and useful. Questions and answers about medications are reviewed. An excellent and scientifically based self-help approach for anxiety-ridden patients, either as an independent self-help book or as an adjunct to psychotherapy.

★★★★ *Beyond Anxiety and Phobia* (2001) by Edmund J. Bourne. Oakland, CA: New Harbinger.

Another excellent self-help resource by Edmund Bourne, who authored the *The Anxiety and Phobia Workbook* (reviewed above). This book covers the spectrum of mainstream and complementary approaches to self-enhancement and includes using cognitive-behavioral methods, rearranging the environment, helping to define life purposes, embracing spirituality, using herbs, modifying diet, and incorporating yoga, massage, acupuncture, and meditation. This down-to-earth, easy-to-read workbook includes appendices listing a variety of organizational and treatment resources. A useful self-help book for those interested in a mixture of traditional and alternative methods.

★★★★ *The Shyness and Social Anxiety Workbook* (2002) by Martin Anthony and Richard Swinson. Oakland, CA: New Harbinger.

This highly rated resource was written to help people be more comfortable around other people. The book provides worksheets and exercises that can be easily incorporated into their daily lives. Cognitive-behavioral, empirically supported techniques to combat social anxiety are presented in a step-by-step manner for the lay public. It is an excellent book: well organized, easy to read, and useful for those in or out of psychotherapy. The highest rated self-help book specifically on social anxiety in our national studies.

★★★★ *Anxiety Disorders and Phobias: A Cognitive Perspective* (1985) by Aaron Beck and Gary Emery. New York: Basic Books.

This sophisticated book provides information about different types of anxiety and how sufferers can rearrange their thoughts to overcome crippling anxiety. Author Aaron Beck is an internationally acclaimed expert on anxiety disorders and depression, and is one of the founders of cognitive therapy. Beck and Emery describe the nature of anxiety and how it is distinguished from fear, phobia, and panic. They believe that the core problem for anxiety sufferers is their sense of vulnerability and their ineffective cognitive strategies. The latter portion of the book contains a treatment program based on cognitive therapy that can help individuals cope effectively with anxiety and phobias. Separate chapters tell readers how to change the way they develop images of themselves and their world, how to change feelings, and how to modify behavior. This highly rated volume received rave reviews in the academic community, but it is not primarily a self-help book. It is written at a very high level that is appropriate for psychotherapists or for graduate students. Only lay readers who are already fairly sophisticated about the nature of psychological problems and how they can be treated, or who seek an intellectual challenge, will want to tackle this volume.

★★★★ *Feel the Fear and Do It Anyway* (reissued ed., 1992) by Susan Jeffers. New York: Fawcett.

This book offers positive and concrete techniques for turning fear, indecision, and anger into power, action, and love. The author helps people reach, understand, and convert negative paths of thinking that feed fear and inactivity. Jeffers uses a 10-step program to help convert negative thinking. Visualization techniques are one of the cognitive exercises that help people rid themselves of destructive fear. Other methods entail power vocabulary, turning decisions into no-lose situations, and adoption of an optimistic perspective about life. The author's belief is that fear can be dealt with through reeducation. For those who struggle with their feelings of fear and indecision, this is a useful book.

★★★★ *Don't Panic: Taking Control of Anxiety Attacks* (revised ed., 1996) by Reid Wilson. New York: Harper & Row.

This book covers the diagnosis and treatment of panic, an anxiety disorder in which the main feature is recurrent panic attacks marked by the sudden onset of intense apprehension or terror. People who suffer from panic disorder may have feelings of impending doom but aren't necessarily anxious all the time. Wilson describes a self-help program for coping with panic attacks. In Part I, readers learn what panic attacks are like, how it feels to undergo one, and what type of people are prone to panic attacks. Advice is given on how to sort through the physical and psychological aspects of panic attacks. In Part II, readers learn how to conquer panic attacks, especially by use of self-monitoring, breathing exercises, focused thinking, mental imagery, and deep muscle relaxation.

Recommended

★★★ *Overcoming Shyness and Social Phobia: A Step-by-Step Guide* (1998) by Ronald M. Rapee. Northvale, NJ: Jason Aronson.

Rapee educates, coaches, and guides those who struggle with social anxiety toward a more comfortable lifestyle. The nine thoughtful lessons are grounded in a systems perspective. The reader will learn ways to think and act differently, and will be able to challenge and defeat the negative assumptions that limit personal growth. The author emphasizes learning and practice, and the case studies illuminate the path to change. A valuable self-help book for the general public and psychotherapy clients. In fact, had the book been more widely known by the mental health experts in our studies, it would have probably received a four- or five-star rating.

★★★ *Worry: Controlling It and Using It Wisely* (1997) by Edward Hallowell. New York: Pantheon.

Worry is uniquely human. The author focuses on the many forms of worry (both destructive and productive), their underlying causes, and how these patterns can be changed. Illustrating his theories with case histories and therapy dialogues, Hallowell emphasizes the physical, not the psychological aspect of worrying, which helps reduce the self-blame to which many worriers are prone. The treatment and preventive steps are holistic, eclectic, and straightforward. First comes awareness, which, over time, sets the stage for new pattern making in the brain. Then, treatment consists of medication and psychotherapy, as well as exercise, diet, and sufficient sleep. Another key to not fretting excessively is "connectedness"—to other people, to ideas, and to spirituality. The experts in our national studies were very positively disposed toward this integrated self-help resource; indeed, if more had rated it, it would have been a four- or five-star self-help book. A valuable aid to understanding and modifying one of the most common maladies.

★★★ *Panic Disorder: The Facts* (1996) by Stanley Rachman and Padmal de Silva. New York: Oxford University Press.

This self-help resource book covers the experience, assessment, and treatment of panic attacks. The authors provide sound, practical advice to family members about choosing a therapist and self-help. Some of the common questions asked by people with panic disorder are reviewed. This book is a valuable scientific resource for both sufferers of this disorder and their families. It can be integrated into a patient's treatment and is easy to read.

★★★ *An End to Panic* (1995, reissued 2000) by Elke Zuercher-White. Oakland, CA: New Harbinger.

The author's goal is to teach the cognitive-behavioral methods that have proven effective for panic disorders. In other words, changing one's style of thinking, believing, and behaving can reduce anxiety. Medication is also discussed, as is a combination of medication and cognitive-behavioral therapy. Part I explains panic disorder and agoraphobia, and sets the stage for the work ahead. Parts II and III review theory and practical methods to overcome panic. Part IV works on mastery of the techniques taught. This book is for people with panic disorders, with or without agoraphobia, who want to prevent further panic attacks. It was highly regarded by the psychologists in our national studies but not well known, leading to the three-star rating.

★★★ *Life without Fear: Anxiety and Its Cure* (1988) by Joseph Wolpe with David Wolpe. Oakland, CA: New Harbinger.

Joseph Wolpe, an international expert in the field of behavior therapy, provides a clear and authoritative account of the essential features of behavior therapy and its application to anxiety. With the help of his son David, a playwright, the two translate into nontechnical language information about behavior therapy and anxiety. Topics include useful and useless fears, how useless fears are developed, how thoughts and feelings are controlled by habit, how habits are formed and extinguished, coping in real-life situations, special behavior techniques for anxiety, getting help for behavior analysis, and the advantages and limits of behavior therapy. This book can be a useful self-help manual for adults engaged in behavior therapy for anxiety.

★★★ *How to Control Your Anxiety before It Controls You* (1998) by Albert Ellis. Secaucus, NJ: Carol.

Ellis, one of the world's most influential psychologists, bases this book on his particular brand of cognitive-behavioral therapy known as Rational–Emotive Behavior Therapy. Ellis talks about how anxious feelings and behaviors go with specific kinds of anxiety-provoking thinking. You think, act, and feel together. That's the way, as a human, you behave. In the final three chapters, he emphasizes rational maxims and beliefs that can help change anxiety-provoking thinking, emotions, and actions. This book can be valuable for the average reader or used as a self-help resource during psychotherapy.

★★★ *Peace from Nervous Suffering* (1972, reissued 1990) by Claire Weekes. New York: Hawthorn.

This book concerns itself with one type of phobia—agoraphobia, the fear of entering unfamiliar situations, especially open or public spaces. It is the most common type of phobic disorder. Weekes maintains that the cure for agoraphobia involves four simple rules: Face the phobia, don't run away from it; accept it, don't fight it; float past it, don't stop and listen in; and let time pass, don't be impatient. Weekes includes extensive case studies from around the world in which agoraphobics have successfully overcome their fear of leaving the safety of their homes. *Peace from Nervous Suffering* was given three stars: On the positive side, Weekes's book was one of the first to deal with agora-phobia, and it helped many people recognize their problem; on the negative side, it is dated and misses many of the advances in cognitive and medical treatments.

★★★ *Anxiety and Panic Attacks: Their Cause and Cure* (1985) by Robert Handly. New York: Fawcett Crest.

This text, about both panic attacks and agoraphobia, begins with the author's description of his own struggle with agoraphobia and the successful strategies he used to overcome it. Handly believes that five basic methods are involved in coping with anxiety and panic at-tacks: (1) Use the creative powers of your unconscious mind to help yourself; (2) use visual-izations and affirmations to improve your self-image; (3) engage in rational and positive thinking; (4) act as if you are already who you want to be; and (5) set goals to be the person you want to be. Handly also stresses the importance of physical health, fitness, and good nutrition in overcoming anxiety. This book has an easy-to-read writing style and provides in-depth analysis of one person's experience. However, it suffers from inattention to cur-rent developments in treating panic disorder and agoraphobia, and from the rather loose inclusion of many different ideas that have not been well tested.

★★★ *The Anxiety Disease* (1983) by David Sheehan. New York: Scribner.

This book astutely reviews the biological factors involved in anxiety and the effective treatment of anxiety disorders by appropriate drugs and behavior therapy. Sheehan de-scribes a number of case studies from his psychiatric practice to illustrate how to recog-nize anxiety problems and successfully treat them. He believes that anxiety disorders progress through seven stages—spells, panic, hypochondriacal symptoms, limited pho-bias, social phobias, agoraphobia/extensive public avoidance, and finally depression—and that recovery from an anxiety disorder occurs in four phases—doubt, mastery, in-dependence, and readjustment. Individuals go through the phases as their medications eliminate chemically induced panic attacks and psychotherapy overcomes their avoid-ance tendencies.

★★★ *The Good News about Panic, Anxiety, and Phobias* (1990) by Mark Gold. New York: Bantam.

This text, like that above, stresses the biological basis of anxiety disorders and their treatment with medications. Gold asserts that if a person has an anxiety disorder, it is not the person's fault. Instead, the disorder is the fault of inherited dysfunctions in the biochemistry of the person's body. Gold recommends variations in drug therapy for dif-ferent types of anxiety disorders. At the end of the book, he provides a state-by-state list-ing of resources and medical experts on anxiety disorders.

Diamonds in the Rough

♦ *The Sky Is Falling* (1996) by Raeann Dumont. New York: Norton.

This author provides information that will help the reader understand and cope with phobias, panic, and obsessive-compulsive behavior. Using case vignettes, Dumont alerts the reader to the danger of forming conclusions that increase anxiety without the bene-fit of rational thought. She explains how magic thinking evolves out of faulty cause-and-effect understanding. The book provides directions on planning treatment programs. Clients, family members, and professionals will find this book to be informative and practical. It was highly but infrequently rated in our national studies, leading to its placement in the Diamonds in the Rough category.

♦ *Overcoming Generalized Anxiety Disorder* (1999) by John White. Oakland, CA: New Harbinger.

Psychologist White has written separate client and therapist manuals to overcome GAD by means of relaxation, cognitive restructuring, and exposure. The client manual is a user-friendly workbook divided into 10 sessions/chapters, each addressed to a particular treatment method. Self-assessments, skill buildings, homework assignments, and cute illustrations fill each session/chapter. A valuable and evidence-based self-help resource that is not yet widely known among mental health professionals.

AUTOBIOGRAPHIES

Strongly Recommended

★★★★ *A Mind of My Own* (1989) by Chris Costner Sizemore. New York: William Morrow.

The protagonist of *Three Faces of Eve* describes her successful battle with multiple personality disorder. Now married with two children, the author has become a lecturer on mental health topics. A tale of hope and the success of psychotherapy, it has become a perennial favorite of those fascinated by—or suffering from—dissociative identity disorder. The book helps explain some of the puzzling aspects of the film and take the reader further along in the author's life.

Recommended

★★★ *The Panic Attack Recovery Book* (revised ed., 2000) by Shirley Swede and Seymour S. Jaffe. New York: New American Library/Dutton.

Jointly written by a former agoraphobic and her psychiatrist, this updated edition outlines a treatment program that does not depend on medication. The PASS program is based on seven steps to recovery from panic attacks: a healthy balanced diet; relaxation; exercise; a positive attitude; imagination (pretending to feel confident); social support; and spiritual values (faith, hope, and forgiveness). The book is clearly written, an easy read, and includes many helpful recommendations based on the personal experiences of an agoraphobic (Swede) and the medical knowledge of a psychiatrist (Jaffe).

★★★ *Memoirs of an Amnesiac* (1990) by Oscar Levant. Hollywood, CA: Samuel French.

A famed pianist recounts a life with many mental and physical disorders. In a humorous and acerbic style, Levant describes his obsessive–compulsive disorder, phobias, and addiction to barbiturates. Chapter titles include "Total Recoil," "My Bed of Nails," and "Stand Up and Faint." Levant was treated with an enormous number of different drugs and had psychotherapy, several hospitalizations, and electroconvulsive therapy. Through it all, he appeared to lack the motivation to get well. The book might best be received by someone with a multiplicity of disorders. Also reviewed in Chapter 25 on obsessive–compulsive disorder.

★★★ *Phantom Illness: Recognizing, Understanding, and Overcoming Hypochondria* (1997) by Carla Cantor with Brian Fallon. New York: Houghton Mifflin.

Cantor's serious problems began when she crashed her car, killing a passenger. She became depressed and was briefly hospitalized. In the hospital, her diagnosis was changed to hypochondria. The book describes her intense struggle with bodily preoccupations and the lessons she learned on the road to recovery. The author has collected a tremendous amount of material, which she shares with the readers. There are not many autobiographies on this disorder, which often goes undiagnosed and untreated.

★★★ *Afraid of Everything: A Personal History of Agoraphobia* (1984) by Daryl M. Woods. Saratoga, CA: R&E.

A first-person account by a young woman with agoraphobia, the book includes information on what is known about causes and treatment of the disorder. It is a helpful memoir in the self-help tradition, though dated with respect to treatments. Out-of-print and not easy to obtain.

Not Recommended

★★ *Sybil* (1995) by Flora Rheta Schreiber. New York: Warner Books.

A reissue of a book that has become a classic in the multiple personality literature, now more accurately known as dissociative identity disorder (DID). Sybil Dorsett had 16 separate personalities before her recovery. The dissociation is attributed to childhood abuse by her schizophrenic mother, which also produced unusual blackouts. With intensive psychotherapy, Sybil's personalities merged in 1965 when she was 42. It is difficult to sort out fact from fiction in the actions of Sybil's various personalities; indeed, some professionals believe that several of the personalities were created by hypnosis. Our mental health experts give the television movie higher marks than the book.

★★ *When Rabbit Howls: The Troops for Truddi Chase* (1987) by Truddi Chase. New York: Dutton.

The troops are the numerous personalities of the author. She did not know they existed until adulthood. Troop members speak of their empathy for Chase, who was abused from ages 2 to 16 by her stepfather. The troops, all 92 of them, speak in disjointed voices, and it is often difficult to keep them straight, leading many readers to find the book confusing.

FILMS

Recommended

★★★ *Sybil* (1976) directed by Daniel Petrie. Not rated. 198 minutes.

The horrific physical and psychological abuse Sybil experienced as a child led to multiple personalities that served as protection, comfort, and survival through her tormented years. She commits herself to the journey of therapy and healing with a caring and courageous therapist who essentially reparents Sybil and gives her the healthier relationship that she never had. This 1970s film was made for television, featuring Sally Field as Sybil and Joanne Woodward as Dr. Wibur. A moving and complex movie about the human spirit, the extraordinary ways in which people survive, and the miraculous healing power of human connection.

Not Recommended

★ *What about Bob?* (1992) directed by Frank Oz. PG rating. 99 minutes.

Strongly Not Recommended

† *High Anxiety* (1977) directed by Mel Brooks. PG rating. 94 minutes.

INTERNET RESOURCES

Metasites

★★★★★ *Panic Anxiety Education Management Services*
        http://www.healthyplace.com/communities/anxiety/paems/index.html

This site is enormously comprehensive, with sections on treatment, chat, resources, support, and so on. Especially strong on cognitive-behavioral therapy—including cost comparisons, outcomes, methods, questions, and answers. See *The Politics of Anxiety Disorder Treatments* for support of cognitive-behavioral therapy.

★★★★★ *The Anxiety Panic Internet Resource*
        http://www.algy.com/anxiety/index.shtml

A dry sense of humor underlies a rich site with chat, listserve, and loads of good-quality links. Each of the anxiety disorders has section with a brief but meaningful description and authoritative materials and handouts. The URL http://www.algy.com/anxiety/links/websearch2.pl?category=an will bring you to a annotated list of links addressing many questions about the anxiety disorders.

★★★★ *Mental Health Articles: General Anxiety Disorder*
        http://www.queendom.com/articles/mentalhealth/gad.html

An overview in about 10 pages, with solid information on cognitive therapy, relaxation approaches, and hyperventilation control methods.

★★★★ *The Shyness Home Page: An Index to Resources for Shyness*
        http://www.shyness.com/

The site contains the most complete resources, with hundreds of links to all aspects of shyness (and social anxiety) by an expert, Lynne Henderson, PhD. It offers brochures, questionnaires, program descriptions, a complete list of readings, and links to local programs.

★★★ *Duke University's Program in Child and Adolescent Anxiety Disorder*
       http://www2.mc.duke.edu/pcaad

A very large site, with materials on every aspect of anxiety disorders in children.

Psychoeducational Materials for Clients and Families

★★★★ *The Causes of Anxiety and Panic Attacks* by Ron Rapee, Michelle J. Craske, and
        David H. Barlow http://www.algy.com/anxiety/files/barlow.html

In probably the best overview written by noted experts for their clients, the aim is to
teach about the physical and mental components of anxiety so that "(1) you realize that
many of the feelings which you now experience are the result of anxiety and (2) you
learn that these feelings are not harmful or dangerous."

★★★★ *National Institute of Mental Health's Library*
        http://www.nimh.nih.gov/anxiety/anxietymenu.cfm

NIMH offers 12 booklets (most about 20 pages long) on anxiety disorders and their
treatment. They can be read online or ordered (call 1-888-8-ANXIETY). Authoritative
and very well done on all anxiety disorders. All are available in Spanish.

★★★★ *Social Phobia/Social Anxiety Association* http://www.socialphobia.org

Several informational brochures, fact sheets, a well-described audiotape series (20
hours, $360) on cognitive-behavior therapy for sales, links, and so on.

★★★★ *Understanding Panic Disorder*
        http://www.nimh.nih.gov/anxiety//panicmenu.cfm

Seven excellent brochures from NIMH.

★★★★ *FAQ: Panic Disorder* http://www.algy.com/anxiety/panicfaq.html

An excellent overview with many resources in just 12 pages.

★★★★ *Panic Disorder, Separation, Anxiety Disorder, and Agoraphobia in Children and Ado-
        lescents* by Jim Chandler, MD
        http://www.klis.com/chandler/pamphlet/panic/panicpamphlet.htm

About 15 pages from a medical perspective, filled with vignettes. The site can also provide a basis for educational materials.

★★★★ *Madison Institute of Medicine*
        http://socialanxiety.factsforhealth.org/index.html

Their "Facts for Health" is a perfect 15-page introductory brochure on social anxiety,
with links, readings, and referrals. Emphasizes both medications and behavior therapy.

★★★★ *Anxiety Disorders—The Caregiver* http://www.pacificcoast.net/~kstrong

A site offering advice, support, and information.

★★★ *Social Phobia* http://www.rcpsych.ac.uk/info/help/socphob/index.htm

A six-page brochure in a friendly style suitable for an introduction.

★★★ *Coping With Performance Anxiety*
       http://www.engr.unl.edu/eeshop/anxiety.html

Focusing on musicians, these three pages are quite thorough.

★★★ *Answers to Your Questions about Panic Disorder*
       http://www.apa.org/pubinfo/panic.html

A good, four-page overview from the American Psychological Association.

★★★ *Social Anxiety Test*
       http://www.queendom.com/tests/health/social_anxiety_r_access.html

A 25-item interactive test for social anxiety. Probably most useful for organizing and understanding symptoms.

★★★ *Agoraphobia: For Friends and Family*
       http://panicdisorder.about.com/msubagora05.htm?pid=2791&cob=home

Seven articles with guidance for those assisting people with agoraphobia.

★★★ *For the Support Person: Helping Your Partner Do In-Vivo Exposure* by
       Edmund J. Bourne, PhD
       http://www.Open-Mind.org/SP/Articles/3a.htm

Brief and clear guidelines.

★★★ *Anxiety and Phobias* http://www.rcpsych.ac.uk/info/help/anxiety/index.htm

A five-page introductory brochure with good information in a friendly presentation.

★★ *Anxiety Disorders* http://www.psych.org/public_info/anxiety.cfm

About eight pages from the American Psychiatric Association, with an emphasis on diagnostic criteria. The treatment suggested at this site is combined behavior therapy and medication.

Treatment

★★★★ *The Systematic Desensitization Procedure* by R. Richmond, PhD
       http://members.aol.com/avpsyrich/sysden.htm

An excellent eight-page presentation of the logic and methods of systematic desensitization.

★★★★ *Relaxation* http://www.algy.com/anxiety/relax.html

A dozen good lists of tips and suggestions for coping with anxiety, including tools, tips, advice, and wisdom.

★★★★ *Panic Attack Treatment*
       http://www.psycheducation.org/anxiety/panic/introduction.htm

A brief guide to weighing medications and/or therapy and siding with therapy, which would make a fine handout for ambivalent clients.

★★★ *Getting Treatment for Panic Disorder*
       http://www.nimh.nih.gov/anxiety/getpd.cfm

Eight pages with an emphasis on cognitive-behavioral therapy and medications.

★★★ *Basics of Cognitive Therapy* http://mindstreet.com

Click on About Cognitive Therapy on the left. An overview with references in a couple of pages. This is part of a cognitive-based treatment program.

★★ *Diaphragmatic Breathing* http://www.algy.com/anxiety/A2Z/diaph.html

See also http://www.angelfire.com/id2/cafe/Mentaldiphram.html

★★ *Anxiety and the Workplace* http://www.pacificcoast.net/~kstrong/work.html

This is a discussion and list of suggestions for modifying the workplace for the anxious worker.

Other Resources

★★★★ *Self-Help Brochures* http://www.couns.uiuc.edu/brochures/brochure.htm

These may be relevant to people with an anxiety disorder: Dissertation Success Strategies, Overcoming Procrastination, Perfectionism, Stress Management, Test Anxiety, and Time Management.

★★★ *Panic Disorder Treatment and Referral: Information for Health Care Professionals* http://www.algy.com/anxiety/files/treatref.html

If you need to educate referral sources, this eight-pager will do it. It includes How to Recognize Panic Disorder, Biological and Psychological Causes, Treatment and Referral, and Sources of Further Information.

★★ *Anxiety: Theoretical Views and Therapeutic Techniques* by David W. Ayer
       http://www.algy.com/anxiety/files/outline.html

If you need notes for a lecture or presentation, this is a useful site.

NATIONAL SUPPORT GROUPS

Agoraphobics Building Independent Lives (ABIL)
400 West 32nd Street
Richmond, VA 23225
Phone: 804-353-3964
E-mail: answers@anxietysupport.org
http://www.anxietysupport.org/
b001menu.htm

Agoraphobics in Motion (AIM)
1719 Crooks
Royal Oak, MI 48067
Phone: 248-547-0400
E-mail: anny@ameritech.net
http://www.aim-hq.org

Anxiety Disorders Association of America (ADAA)
8730 Georgia Avenue, Suite 600
Silver Spring, MD 20910
Phone: 240-485-10001
http://www.adaa.org

A nonprofit organization "whose mission is to promote the prevention and cure of anxiety disorders." Their bookstore is excellent for its prices and the wide range of books.

Emotions Anonymous
PO Box 4245
St. Paul, MN 55104-0245
Phone: 651-647-9712
E-mail: info@emotionsanonymous.org
http://www.emotionsanonymous.org

Twelve-step program of recovery from emotional difficulties.

Recovery
802 North Dearborn Street
Chicago, IL 60610
Phone: 312-337-5661
E-mail: inquiries@recovery-inc.org
http://www.recovery-inc.com

"Self-help method of will training; a system of techniques for controlling temperamental behavior and changing attitudes toward nervous symptoms, anxiety, depression, anger and fears."

tAPir Registry
E-mail: tapir@algy.com
http://www.algy.com/anxiety

This is a search engine for support groups. Although new, it is a wonderful idea and helps locate many people and organizations.

See also Obsessive–Compulsive Disorder (Chapter 25), Posttraumatic Stress Disorder (Chapter 26), and Stress Management and Relaxation (Chapter 32).

CHAPTER 8

Assertiveness

The famous behavior therapist Joseph Wolpe said that there are essentially three ways to relate to others. The first is to be aggressive, considering only ourselves and riding roughshod over others. You count, but others don't. The second is to be nonassertive, always putting others before ourselves and letting others run roughshod over us. Others count, but you don't. The third approach is the golden mean—to be assertive, placing ourselves first, but taking others into account. That is, you count *and* other people count.

In most cultures, women have traditionally been socialized to be passive and men to be aggressive. In today's world, an increasing number of women have stepped up their efforts to reduce their passivity and be more assertive, and more men are choosing to be less aggressive. Many mental health professionals believe that our society would benefit from increased assertiveness by women and decreased aggression by men. Breaking out of traditional patterns, though, can be difficult and stressful. In the case of working hard to become more assertive, it's clearly worth the effort.

In this chapter, we present evaluative ratings and brief descriptions of self-help books and Internet resources on assertiveness.

SELF-HELP BOOKS

Strongly Recommended

★★★★★ *Your Perfect Right: A Guide to Assertive Living* (7th ed., 1995) by Robert Alberti and Michael Emmons. San Luis Obispo, CA: Impact.

This national best-seller, periodically updated, emphasizes the importance of developing better communication skills in becoming more assertive. Initially published in 1970, *Your Perfect Right* is divided into two main parts: Part I speaks to the self-help reader

RECOMMENDATION HIGHLIGHTS

Self-Help Books

- For practical and comprehensive training in assertion skills:

    ★★★★★ *Your Perfect Right* by Robert Alberti and Michael Emmons

    ★★★★ *Asserting Yourself* by Sharon Anthony Bower and Gordon H. Bower

    ★★★★ *Stand Up, Speak Out, Talk Back* by Robert Alberti and Michael Emmons

    ★★★★ *When I Say No, I Feel Guilty* by Manuel Smith

    ★★★ *The Assertiveness Workbook* by Randy Peterson

- For women who want to become more assertive:

    ★★★★★ *The Assertive Woman* by Stanlee Phelps and Nancy Austin

- For assertion and communication skills for children:

    ◆ *Stick Up for Yourself* by Gershen Kaufman and Lev Raphael

Internet Resources

- For quality information on assertion from a rights perspective:

    ★★★★ *Assertiveness* http://www.couns.uiuc.edu/brochures/assertiv.htm

- For a simple way to understand assertion:

    ★★★ *Learn to Be Assertive* http://www.utexas.edu/student/cmhc/booklets/assert/assertive.html

who wants to learn how to become more assertive; Part II, a guide for assertiveness training leaders, teaches techniques to help others become more assertive. In Part I, the reader learns how to distinguish assertive, nonassertive, and aggressive behavior, and why assertive behavior is the best choice. Among the key components of assertive behavior are self-expression, honesty, directness, self-enhancement, not harming others, being socially responsible, and learned skills. Readers complete a questionnaire to evaluate their own level of assertiveness, and they learn about the obstacles they will face in trying to be more assertive. Step-by-step procedures are presented for getting started and for gaining the confidence to stand up for their own rights. An excellent chapter on soft assertions gives information about how to be more assertive with friends and family members. Interactions in school, work, and community are also covered, with tips on how to be assertive in those contexts. Readers learn how anger needs to be expressed in assertive, nonaggressive ways. An extensive annotated list of readings about assertiveness is provided toward the end of the book. *Your Perfect Right* received the highest rating in the Assertiveness category and is widely respected; almost 300 respondents rated it. Indeed, some mental health professionals call it the assertiveness bible, they think so highly of it.

★★★★★   *The Assertive Woman* (3rd ed., 1997) by Stanlee Phelps and Nancy Austin. San Luis Obispo, CA: Impact.

This book is about how women can become more assertive. The third edition addresses the challenge for women to be assertive in the workplace, socially, at home, and with various sets of people with whom they come into contact. The topics of body image, attitude, power, compliments, saying no, and anger, among others, are approached with illustrative scenarios, checklists, and exercises that readers may use to learn the concepts presented. A strength of the book is that the authors adapt assertion principles to relevant contemporary contexts rather than to conventional scenarios. An effective question-and-answer section at the end of the book presents questions that the authors have found women ask most frequently. A fine, five-star resource specifically for women.

★★★★   *Asserting Yourself: A Practical Guide for Positive Change* (1991) by Sharon Anthony Bower and Gordon H. Bower. Reading, MA: Addison-Wesley.

The authors maintain that individuals lack communication and coping strategies for everyday living and that these deficits are often the root of interpersonal conflict and general unhappiness. The purpose of their program is to help individuals learn to change behavior in positive ways and to relate to others more effectively. Several self-tests help the reader identify desired areas of change and goals. Then, the text focuses on success exercises that the reader can do initially, followed by sample scripts for common situations that can be practiced and, finally, ways to handle situations when people react negatively to new assertive behaviors. In addition to the major focus of assertiveness training, the authors address the often-accompanying problem of self-esteem and conclude with a chapter on how to develop friendships.

★★★★   *Stand Up, Speak Out, Talk Back* (1975, reissued 1982) by Robert Alberti and Michael Emmons. New York: Pocket Books.

This book tackles the same problem as its sister publication, *Your Perfect Right*: how to become more assertive by improving communication skills. The authors discuss developing self-confidence and specific strategies that will help readers become more assertive. Alberti and Emmons give artful advice on how to become assertive without stepping on others. Their 13-step assertiveness training program is based on the premise that it is easier to change people's behavior than to change their attitudes. The steps are clearly described and easy to understand. Readers learn some fascinating strategies for using nonverbal behavior—eye contact, body posture, gestures, facial expressions, voice, and timing—to present themselves more assertively. Readers are also taught how to handle potential adverse reactions to their assertiveness, and situations are presented in which they might not want to assert themselves (such as when interacting with overly sensitive people). Not as well-known or as highly regarded by our mental health experts as the authors' *Your Perfect Right*, this book nonetheless is a solid, practical text on assertiveness training.

★★★★   *When I Say No, I Feel Guilty* (1975) by Manuel Smith. New York: Bantam.

This volume was especially written for people who feel that they are always being talked into doing something they don't want to do. It falls into the category of assertiveness books that emphasize the importance of learning better communication skills to become more assertive. Its 11 chapters cover such important topics as how other people violate our rights, an assertiveness bill of rights, the importance of persistence in becoming assertive, how to assertively cope with supervisors and experts, how to work out compromises and say no, and how to be assertive in sexual encounters. Interspersed through the book are 34 annotated dialogues that illustrate key skills, such as using calm persistence to get what we want, disclosing our worries to others, agreeing with critical truths and still doing what we want, asserting our negative points, prompting criticism, and keeping our self-respect. Many mental health professionals praise the book, commenting about the down-to-earth advice and the many examples of timid people who gained assertive skills.

Recommended

★★★   *The Assertiveness Workbook* (2000) by Randy Peterson. Oakland, CA: New Harbinger.

This book seeks to help people build their confidence, express their ideas, and say "no" without feeling guilty. Step-by-step methods assist individuals in standing up for their rights in work, love, and many other aspects of their lives. Cognitive-behavioral techniques help individuals to set and maintain personal boundaries, to be more open in relationships without getting hurt, and to defend themselves when they are criticized or asked to submit to unreasonable requests. This fine self-help book likely would have received a higher rating if it had been better known by more psychologists in our national studies.

★★★   *Don't Say Yes When You Want to Say No* (1975) by Herbert Fensterheim and Jean Baer. New York: Dell.

This behaviorally oriented book contains 13 chapters, 7 of which are devoted to the behavioral approach to assertiveness training. In the early chapters, the reader learns how to target assertiveness difficulties, use behavioral rehearsal and other strategies to learn to say no, call on assertiveness training techniques to develop a social network of friends and acquaintances, and learn assertiveness skills that help at work. Other chapters explore a wide range of topics, some of which are not found in other assertiveness self-help books, including using assertiveness to combat depression, reduce eating disorders, and improve sexual relationships. The book was published some 25 years ago and has become dated in many ways; for example, in discussing mental disorders, the outmoded category of neurosis is used.

★★★   *Good-Bye to Guilt* (1985) by Gerald Jampolsky. New York: Bantam.

This self-help book presents an emotionally and spiritually based approach to becoming more assertive. Jampolsky uses the term *good-bye* for the process of letting go of guilt, fear, and condemning judgments. In Part I, the reader learns about the spiritual transformations involved in moving from fearfulness to forgiveness to unconditional love. In Part II, the majority of the book, 14 lessons apply the knowledge in Part I to real-life situations. Among the chapters are "Only My Condemnation Injures Me" and "In My Defenselessness My Safety Lies." Exercises, such as becoming one with a flower introduce vivid images of the spiritual healing process.

★★★ *The Gentle Art of Verbal Self-Defense* (1980) by Suzette Elgin. Englewood Cliffs, NJ: Prentice-Hall.

This self-help book presents a communication skills approach to becoming more assertive. The 18 chapters train readers in verbal judo, which involves using an opponent's strength and momentum as tools for self-defense. Elgin describes four basic principles of verbal self-defense: (1) know that you are under attack; (2) know what kind of attack you are facing; (3) know how to make your defense fit the attack; and (4) know how to follow through. A number of examples and exercises help readers learn to use these principles. On the positive side, the book includes effective verbal strategies for seizing control of a situation, and the extensive exercises are good learning devices. However, the consensus of the mental health experts in the national studies was that the four- and five-star books listed earlier do a better job of teaching assertion skills.

Diamond in the Rough

♦ *Stick Up for Yourself: Every Kid's Guide to Personal Power and Positive Self-Esteem* (1990) by Gershen Kaufman and Lev Raphael. Minneapolis: Free Spirit.

Written for children ages 8 to 12, this book begins with the elusive concept of sticking up for yourself. The authors effectively use cognitive techniques in walking the child through definitions, explanations, and numerous scenarios with which he or she can identify. Getting to know yourself is a central idea of the book, and the breadth and intensity of human feelings are discussed using short narratives, illustrations, writing exercises, and questions to generate thinking (e.g., Write about a time when you felt angry; tell what happened and what you did). A strength of *Stick Up for Yourself* is its section on learning to like yourself, which includes a self-esteem self-quiz, do's and don'ts, and good things to do for yourself. This book is cited as a Diamond in the Rough because few of our mental health experts were familiar with it, but it is particularly well presented and appropriate for the young.

Not Recommended

★★ *Creative Aggression: The Art of Assertive Living* (1974) by George Bach and Herb Goldberg. Garden City, NY: Doubleday.

★ *Pulling Your Own Strings* (1977) by Wayne Dyer. New York: Crowell.

★ *Control Freaks: Who Are They and How to Stop Them from Running Your Life* (1991) by Gerald Piaget. New York: Doubleday.

Strongly Not Recommended

† *Looking Out for Number One* (1977) by Robert Ringer. Beverly Hills, CA: Los Angeles Book Company.

† *Winning through Intimidation* (1973) by Robert Ringer. Beverly Hills, CA: Los Angeles Book Company.

INTERNET RESOURCES

Psychoeducational Materials for Clients and Families

★★★★ *Assertiveness* http://www.couns.uiuc.edu/brochures/assertiv.htm
A three-page brochure with many specific self-statements from a rights perspective.

★★★ *Learn to Be Assertive—In a Positive Way*
    http://www.utexas.edu/student/cmhc/booklets/assert/assertive.html
Three brief pages, including Four Types of Assertion and What Is Being Assertive?

★★ *Assertive Behavior: An Outline* http://www.upenn.edu/fsap/assert.htm
A list of 10 well written and thought provoking points.

★★ *Basic Strategies for Behaving More Assertively*
    http://www.unc.edu/depts/unc_caps/assert.html
A one-page listing.

See also Communication and People Skills (Chapter 14).

CHAPTER 9

Attention-Deficit/ Hyperactivity Disorder

The diagnosis of attention-deficit/hyperactivity disorder (ADHD) has proliferated over the past decade, with some experts asserting that this neurobehavioral disorder is finally being effectively diagnosed and other experts claiming that we are unduly labeling fidgety or misbehaving children. The attention deficit part of the disorder is characterized by an inability to pay attention to details, a failure to sustain attention, easy distractibility, and forgetfulness in daily activities. Hyperactivity is characterized by fidgeting, squirming, talking excessively, moving around during sedentary activity, and impulsiveness, such as interrupting and displaying impatience. Adolescents and adults report restlessness and inability to engage in quiet activities. ADHD is estimated to affect 3–5% of school-age children and occurs between four and nine times more frequently in males than in females.

ADHD can dramatically impact children's lives and, correspondingly, parents find their lives and families in turmoil. The symptoms become evident during early school years. Academic achievement often declines, and behavioral problems in school develop. The child's inability to apply him- or herself to concentrated work often has the appearance of disinterest, lack of discipline, and contrary behavior. The symptoms of ADHD can shift in intensity and frequency, resulting in the parents' and teachers' perception of willfulness and deliberateness in oppositional behavior. The understandable fallouts from ADHD include family discord, discipline problems, and educational frustrations, while the child feels isolated, misunderstood, and sometimes rejected.

The self-help books, autobiographies, websites, and support groups described in this chapter target parents of children with ADHD and the children–adolescents themselves. An increasing number of self-help resources also address adults grappling with lifelong ADHD.

RECOMMENDATION HIGHLIGHTS

Self-Help Books

- For parents of ADHD children:

  ★★★★★ *Taking Charge of ADHD* by Russell Barkley

- For adults with ADHD:

  ★★★★★ *Driven to Distraction* by Edward M. Hallowell and John J. Ratey

  ◆ *Adventures in Fast Forward* by Kathleen G. Nadeau

- For teens with ADHD:

  ★★★ *ADHD and Teens* by Colleen Alexander-Roberts

- For children with ADHD:

  ★★★★ *Putting on the Brakes* by Patricia O. Quinn and Judith M. Stern

  ★★★ *Learning to Slow Down and Pay Attention* by Kathleen G. Nadeau and Ellen B. Dixon

- For parents, teachers, and family members with questions about ADD:

  ★★★ *Answers to Distraction* by Edward M. Hallowell and John J. Ratey

Autobiographies

- For coping strategies from two parents of ADHD children:

  ★★★★ *Parenting a Child with Attention Deficit/Hyperactivity Disorder* by Nancy S. Boyles and Darlene Contadino

- For advice from a psychotherapist who has ADHD:

  ★★★ *ADHD Handbook for Families* by Paul L. Weingartner

Internet Resources

- For excellent general information about ADHD:

  ★★★★ *National Attention Deficit Disorder Association* http://www.add.org

  ★★★★ *Attention Deficit Hyperactivity Disorder* http://www.nimh.nih.gov/publicat/adhd.cfm

- For common questions and authoritative answers:

  ★★★★ *What Is ADHD? A General Overview* http://www.helpforadd.com/over.htm

- For materials for diagnosis, outcomes, and medications:

  ★★★★ *CHADD* http://CHADD.org

SELF-HELP BOOKS

Strongly Recommended

★★★★★ *Taking Charge of ADHD* (revised ed., 2000) by Russell A. Barkley. New York: Guilford Press.

Psychologist Barkley adopts an empathic stance toward parents of children with ADHD, offering illustrations of how parents and children are misunderstood and misinformed. The purpose of this popular self-help resource is to describe how ADHD impairs the lives of parents and children and to empower parents to take a proactively executive role in decisions about their children. The theme of the book is upbeat in that the author offers parents many practical and effective methods for managing their children, taking care of themselves as parents, becoming effective as advocates for their children, and implementing techniques to help ADHD children succeed at school and feel better about themselves. This stellar book, which received a ringing endorsement from our mental health experts, is written for beleaguered parents who have not given up hope.

★★★★★ *Driven to Distraction: Recognizing and Coping with Attention Deficit Disorder from Childhood through Adulthood* (1994) by Edward M. Hallowell and John J. Ratey. New York: Simon & Schuster.

This superb book is written for all people with ADHD, family members, and others in their lives, with special focus on adults suffering from ADHD. The experience of ADHD is realistically portrayed through case studies that illustrate specific problems, such as secondary symptoms of depression, low self-esteem, fear of learning new things, and the fear of diagnosis as an educational death sentence. The reader is taught how to obtain a diagnosis, what one can do when the diagnosis is suspected, how to explain the diagnosis to a child, and how to structure the child's daily life. There is a thorough description of treatment possibilities. The experience of ADHD and its effects on the relationships of adults, couples, the family, and schoolchildren are addressed. *Driven to Distraction* also presents an informative description of ADHD effects when coupled with anxiety, depression, learning disabilities, substance abuse, conduct disorders, and other conditions. An early and influential self-help book on ADHD throughout the lifespan.

★★★★ *Putting on the Brakes: Young People's Guide to Understanding Attention Deficit Hyperactivity Disorder (ADHD)* by Patricia O. Quinn and Judith M. Stern. New York: Magination.

This book speaks directly to children between the ages of 8 and 13 from a pediatric and educative perspective about their ADHD. The purpose is to give children a sense of control and encouragement that they can, in fact, achieve. Chapters on understanding ADHD ask questions such as What is ADHD? How Do You Know If You Have ADHD? Are You the Only One? Then the chapter explains in bullet formats, graphics, and symptom listings what the child is likely experiencing and what it means. The second half of the book addresses ways children can gain a sense of control of their lives, including getting support, making friends, understanding medications, and becoming more organized. A letter of encouragement written to children concludes the book. An excellent activity book, *The Best of Brakes: An Activity Book for Kids with ADD* (2000), accompanies this book. Probably the best book on the market that speaks directly to children about their ADHD.

Recommended

★★★ *Answers to Distraction* (1994) by Edward M. Hallowell and John J. Ratey. New York: Pantheon.

Answers To Distraction, written by Hallowell and Ratey shortly after they wrote *Driven To Distraction*, is a compilation of the questions they were asked about ADHD since the publication of the first book (reviewed above). This highly readable text focuses on ADHD's impact on children, teachers, women, work, couples, and families. The chapter on ADHD and children clusters questions from parents, young children (ages 4–10), and adolescents (ages 11–18), and answers them in an age-appropriate manner. Questions are effectively organized into topics of medication, creativity, diagnosis, addiction, and anger. The questions are clear and crisp, and the answers are informative. The authors take on the myths and stereotypes of ADHD and in the last section of the book offer 100 tips on managing adult ADHD, ADHD in families, and ADHD in couples. The recommendations are doable and practical.

★★★ *ADHD and Teens* (1995, reissued 2002) by Colleen Alexander-Roberts. Dallas, TX: Taylor.

This volume is written for parents and, secondarily, for those working with teens with ADHD. The roller-coaster ride of adolescent ADHD is described by identifying problem areas, offering warning signs, suggesting coping techniques, and explaining improved parenting skills. The approach assumes a partnering of behavioral and educational models with medication (for moderate to severe cases). The author also addresses the larger context of ADHD effects on family dynamics, school and peer interactions, and stages of development. This book includes helpful chapters on coexisting special problems, such as substance abuse, sexuality, suicide risk, and oppositional defiant/conduct disorder.

★★★ *Learning to Slow Down and Pay Attention: A Book for Kids about ADD* (2nd ed., 1997) by Kathleen G. Nadeau and Ellen B. Dixon. Washington, DC: Magination.

This second edition of *Learning to Slow Down and Pay Attention* retains the fundamental elements of the first but adds several strong areas, including many more "things I can do to help myself," increased focus on attentional problems without hyperactivity, and a greater emphasis on problems experienced by girls. The writing style, page layout, and funny cartoons lend themselves effectively to the interests of children. A checklist about the child at home, at school, and with friends, and about the child him- or herself allows youth to identify specific concerns and frustrations on which they can work with parents and teachers. "Things I can do for myself," an excellent activity list, includes getting ready for school, paying attention, completing homework, controlling anger, solving problems, and making friends. A section on special projects that children can do with parents adds positive experiences.

★★★ *Living with ADHD Children: A Handbook for Parents* (1998) by Peter H. Buntman. Los Alamitos, CA: Center for Family Life.

This handbook written in a workbook format presents the major topics concisely but thoroughly. The focus areas start with how it feels to be a parent and to be a child coping with ADHD, moves into symptoms, other causes of hyperactivity that need to be ruled out, and then targets behavioral change. The instructional chapters teach the parent how to change the child's behavior, how to get the child to listen, how to work with self-esteem and school problems, and about medication. The last chapter, a compendium of questions from parents, is quite comprehensive.

Diamonds in the Rough

♦ *Adventures in Fast Forward* (1996) by Kathleen G. Nadeau. New York: Brunner/Mazel.

Adults with symptoms of attention deficit disorder (ADD) are often anxious and confused. This highly readable and informative book is written for them. The early chapters are devoted to defining ADD and to explaining the scope of diagnosis and assessment; the latter chapters enumerate the treatment choices, including medication and psychotherapy. Two chapters on life management skills and social skills are very instructive in teaching individuals how to counteract ADD-related difficulties. Time management techniques, stress management, money management, coping with hyperactivity and impulsivity, and memory techniques are among the life management skills recommended. Interpersonal behaviors, including interrupting, distractibility, bluntness, hypersensitivity, poor listening skills, and missed social cues, are among the problems described. Coping techniques for each problem behavior are suggested. Examples of ADD difficulties in the workplace are described, and modifications of behavioral patterns are recommended. This book was highly but infrequently rated in our studies, thus receiving the Diamond in the Rough designation.

♦ *Teenagers with ADD: A Parents' Guide* (1995) by Chris A. Zeigler Dendy. Bethesda, MD: Woodbine House.

The agony of being the parent of a child with undiagnosed ADD motivated the author to write this book for parents of adolescents who may not have been diagnosed as children. The distinctive contributions of this self-help resource, unlike many others, are the specific focus on teen years (ages 13–20) and the real-life vignettes of teenagers and parents who have experienced success, as well as challenges. Neglected topics are discussed, including sports participation, driving privileges, speeding tickets, sleep disturbances, drug and alcohol use, and college attendance. Chapters include excellent "easy reference guides" that summarize the full content of the chapter and provide categorized listings of recommendations. These include a list of common learning problems and adaptations for home and school, guiding principles for parent–teen interpersonal interaction, and a warning list about problem behaviors that have potential for greater concerns. This text is an effective compendium for parents who want tools to help teens.

AUTOBIOGRAPHIES

Strongly Recommended

★★★★ *Parenting a Child with Attention Deficit/Hyperactivity Disorder* (1999) by Nancy S. Boyles and Darlene Contadino. Los Angeles: Lowell House.

The two authors, both parents of children with ADHD and professionals in the field, have also collaborated on *The Learning Differences Sourcebook*. Here, they present management, coping, and advocacy strategies for parents based on their own experiences and those of other parents. A self-help source as well as personal account, the book discusses test interpretation, diagnosis, and intervention strategies. It is a highly valued and practical volume with a strong insider's voice.

Recommended

★★★ *ADHD Handbook for Families: A Guide to Communicating with Professionals* (1999) by Paul L. Weingartner. Washington, DC: Child Welfare League of America.

An experienced therapist who works with children with ADHD, Weingartner brings a personal perspective in that he has ADHD himself. He describes his coping mechanisms and the methods he uses to work with children and educate parents about the disorder. A central theme of the book, encapsulated in its subtitle, is enhancing the family's ability to communicate and lobby effectively with health care professionals. The thrust of the book is family empowerment through behavior management, realistic goals, and effective reinforcement. Sample behavior contracts are presented. A very good and scientifically based approach that can benefit many parents of ADHD children.

Diamond in the Rough

♦ *Maybe You Know My Kid: A Parents' Guide to Helping Your Child with Attention Deficit Hyperactivity Disorder* (3rd ed., 1999) by Mary Fowler. Secaucus, NJ: Birch Lane.

Faced with the challenge of raising a son with ADHD, Mary Fowler researched the topic. Her book describes theories in the field, available treatments, educational programs, and advocacy techniques related to the Americans with Disabilities Act. The new edition features recent material on treatments and on sources of assistance for families. It was named a Diamond in the Rough because of its high rating but low number of ratings; our experts may have not been familiar with the revised edition.

INTERNET RESOURCES

Metasites

★★★★ *CHADD: Children and Adults with Attention Deficit/Hyperactivity Disorder*
http://CHADD.org

CHADD is both an educational and advocacy organization. Their Fact Sheets of 3 to 10 pages are a solid starting place. Particularly useful is a discussion of treatments that do *not* work and how to evaluate "alternative" treatments (Fact Sheet 6). The FAQ of about eight pages covers legal, social, and other aspects.

★★★ *The National Attention Deficit Disorder Association*
       http://www.add.org/content/menu1.html

This site offers dozens of articles under the first three headings of Information. None are very recent, but many could be offered as general educational handouts. There is much material for support and guidance of parents and children relative to school, family, career, coaching, and treatment.

Psychoeducational Materials for Clients and Families

★★★★ *Attention Deficit-Hyperactivity Disorder (ADHD)* by Jim Chandler, MD
        http://www.klis.com/chandler/home.htm

About 40 pages of solid information with lots of cases. It is an excellent educational product because it offers more than medications for treatment.

★★★★ *Attention Deficit Hyperactivity Disorder*
        http://www.nimh.nih.gov/publicat/adhd.cfm

This 30-page booklet from the federal government is packed with factual information. A good start for many who want to know all the science as of 1996. Also available in Spanish at http://www.nimh.nih.gov/publicat/spadhd.cfm.

★★★★ *110 Diagnosis and Treatment of Attention Deficit Hyperactivity Disorder*
        http://odp.od.nih.gov/consensus/cons/110/110_intro.htm

This is a Consensus Conference Statement from November 1998 on the scientific data on diagnosis, effects, effective treatments, risks of treatments, and so forth. For those who need this level of professional evidence, this is the best and latest source available.

★★★★ *What Is ADHD? A General Overview* http://www.helpforadd.com/over.htm
Nine pages of well-written and accurate questions and answers.

★★★★ *ADDvance Magazine* http://www.addvance.com
Because considerably fewer females have ADHD, this site may be of special value. Some of the articles and resources are specific to females—girls, students, and mothers—and the site also has chat, links, and support groups.

★★★★ *Attention Deficit Disorder without Hyperactivity* by Jennifer Wheeler, MA, and
        Caryn L. Carlson, PhD http://www.kidsource.com/lda-ca/add_wo.html

A solidly research-based, seven-page article on this subtype.

★★★★ *Attention Deficit Disorder* http://add.miningco.com

This website's dozens of headings lead the reader to hundreds of sites. The breadth is amazing, and almost any need can be met here—from medications to allopathy, from doing homework to college work, from using Ritalin to saying no to Ritalin. Quite worthwhile.

★★★ *Learning Disabilities* http://www.nimh.nih.gov/publicat/learndis.htm

This is a professionally written, comprehensive, 24-page pamphlet from the National Institute of Mental Health.

★★★ *Attention-Deficit/Hyperactivity Disorder in Children and Adolescents*
        http://www.mentalhealth.org/publications/allpubs/ca-0008/default.asp

A three-page fact sheet perhaps useful as a handout because it lists the symptoms very fully.

★★★ *Special Education Rights and Responsibilities* http://adhdnews.com/sped.htm

Here, a child advocate will find all the federal rules, policies, and advice for writing IEPs and TIEPs needed to pursue special educational services. See also the section on *Advocating for Your Child* at http://adhdnews.com/advocate.htm, which provides guidance and encouragement.

★★★ *Born to Explore! The Other Side of ADD* http://borntoexplore.org/sitemap.htm

"ADD is a difference not a defect" is the theme here. Creativity, Positive Quotes, and The Other Side are highlights. Lots of loose hypotheses about causation and treatments, so please be cautious.

★★★ *Social Security* http://adhdnews.com/ssi.htm

Advice is given here on applying for Social Security disability benefits for a child with ADHD.

Other Resources

★★★★ *Forms* http://www.add-plus.com/

Devised by John F. Taylor, PhD, these five data collection forms can enhance communication with teachers and physicians. They are not available online but can be ordered at no cost. Titles include Academic Problem Identification Checklist, Classroom Daily Report Form, Hyperactivity Screening Checklist, Medication Effectiveness Report Form (Parents' and Teachers' versions), and Social/Emotional/Academic Adjustment Checklist. Also consider ordering Preventing Misbehavior from Boredom: The Fun Idea List, which is also free.

★★★★ *Amen Clinic ADD Subtype Test*
http://www.amenclinic.com/ac/addtests/default.asp

An interactive test to diagnose five subtypes of ADD and a checklist for adult ADD.

★★★ *ADDitude: The Happy Healthy Lifestyle Magazine for People with ADD*
http://www.additudemag.com

Articles, information, and encouragement.

NATIONAL SUPPORT GROUPS

Attention Deficit Disorder Association (ADDA)
1788 Second Street, Suite 200
Highland Park, IL 60035
Phone: 847-432-ADDA
E-mail: mail@add.org
http://www.add.org

Also an online support group at http://www.add.org/content/group1.htm.

Attention Deficit Information Network (AD-IN)
58 Prince Street
Needham, MA 02492
Phone: 781-455-9895
http://www.addinfonetwork.com/
E-mail: adin@gis.net

CHADD: Children and Adults with Attention Deficit/Hyperactivity Disorder
8181 Professional Place, Suite 201
Landover, MD 20785
Phone: 800-233-4050
E-mail: national@chadd.org
http://www.chadd.org/index.htm

Council for Exceptional Children
1110 North Glebe Road
Arlington, VA 22201-5704
Phone: 888-CEC-SPED
http://www.cec.sped.org/

Federation of Families for Children's Mental Health
1101 King Street, Suite 420
Alexandria, VA 22314
Phone: 703-684-7710
E-mail: ffcmh@ffcmh.org
http://www.ffcmh.org

HEATH Resource Center
2121 K Street, NW Suite 220
Washington, DC 20037
Phone: 800-544-3284
E-mail: askheath@heat.gwu.edu
http://www.heath.gwu.edu

National Association of Private Schools for Exceptional Children
1522 K Street, NW, Suite 1032
Washington, DC 20005
Phone: 202-408-3338

Provides referrals to private special education programs.

National Information Center for Children and Youth with Disabilities
PO Box 1492
Washington, DC 20013-1492
Phone: 800-695-0285
E-mail: nichcy@aed.org
http://www.nichcy.org

Learning Disabilities Association of America
4156 Library Road
Pittsburgh, PA 15234-1349
Phone: 412-341-1515 and 888-300-6710
E-mail: info@ldaamerica.org
http://www.ldanatl.org/

For people with learning disabilities and their families.

See also Child Development and Parenting (Chapter 13) and Violent Youth (Chapter 37).

CHAPTER 10

Bipolar Disorder (Manic–Depression)

We all experience the routine ups and downs of life, but some people suffer from extreme and pathological mood swings. Bipolar disorder, previously called manic–depression, is characterized by extreme mood swings between depression and mania. In the manic phase, people are exuberant, have tireless stamina, and tend toward excess. The manic symptoms—decreased sleep, racing thoughts, intense distractibility—may be so severe that people appear to be temporarily psychotic. In the depressed phase, people are fatigued, sad, indecisive, and generally feel hopeless. (Chapter 17 is devoted entirely to depression.)

As with most clinical conditions, there are multiple forms of bipolar disorder. Bipolar I disorder is diagnosed when the person has experienced one or more manic episodes along with depression. Bipolar II disorder, by contrast, is diagnosed when the depression has been accompanied by at least one hypomanic episode. The term *hypomanic* refers to a less severe or "below" manic condition. In this respect, a person may receive a diagnosis of bipolar (II) disorder without having suffered through full-blown mania.

Bipolar disorder is increasingly seen as a brain or biological disease, but all experts acknowledge the reciprocal interaction of psychology and biology. Experts also increasingly see this volatile disorder showing up in older children and adolescents. And virtually all experts recommend a combination of medication, psychotherapy, family support, and self-help.

In this chapter, we critically review the self-help books, autobiographies, and Internet resources dedicated to bipolar disorder.

RECOMMENDATION HIGHLIGHTS

Self-Help Books

- For individual and families coping with bipolar disorder:
    - ★★★ *The Bipolar Disorder Survival Guide* by David J. Miklowitz
    - ★★★ *The Depression Workbook* by Mary Ellen Copeland

- For parents and children:
    - ★★★ *The Bipolar Child* by Demitri F. Papolos and Janice Papolos

Autobiographies

- For moving accounts of bipolar disorder:
    - ★★★★★ *An Unquiet Mind* by Kay R. Jamison
    - ★★★★ *A Brilliant Madness* by Patty Duke and Gloria Hochman

- For understanding the treatment of bipolar disorder:
    - ★★★ *Breakdown* by Stuart Sutherland

- For appreciating life with a bipolar parent:
    - ◆ *Daughter of the Queen of Sheba* by Jacki Lyden

Internet Resources

- For well-organized information on all aspects of bipolar disorder:
    - ★★★★ *Internet Mental Health* http://www.mentalhealth.com/fr20.html

- For an excellent starting place with links to everything:.
    - ★★★★ *Bipolar Planet*
      http://mywebpages.comcast.net/bipolarplanet/MHLinks.html

- For bipolar disorder in kids:
    - ★★★★ *Bipolar Affective Disorder in Children and Adolescents*
      http://www.klis.com/chandler/pamphlet/bipolar/
      bipolarpamphlet.html

SELF-HELP BOOKS

Recommended

★★★ *The Bipolar Disorder Survival Guide: What You and Your Family Need to Know* (2002) by David J. Miklowitz. New York: Guilford Press.

This self-help book was designed to help readers recognize the early warning signs of mania or depression and to secure the right medication and treatment. The author's research shows that education about bipolar disorder and its treatment can actually alter the course of the illness, even though it stems from biological causes. Miklowitz offers much wise advice on preventing mood swings from dominating life and on remaining on track at home and at work. The most highly rated book on bipolar disorder in our national studies; it offers the right tools for both patients and families.

★★★ *The Depression Workbook: A Guide for Living with Depression and Manic Depression* (1996) by Mary Ellen Copeland. Oakland, CA: New Harbinger.

A useful and comprehensive self-help book for unipolar and bipolar depression. Part I provides symptom outlines of depression and mania, along with help in understanding the emotional context of these mood disorders. Part II offers information on how to secure family, professional, and social support systems. In Part III, Copeland reviews lifestyle and counseling techniques to build one's self-esteem. Part IV addresses suicide and prevention strategies. Part V provides a resource list on career planning, psychotherapy, diet, health, medications, sleep, substance abuse, self-esteem, and the like. This is a balanced and practical workbook for living with mood disorders.

★★★ *The Bipolar Child: The Definitive and Reassuring Guide to Childhood's Most Misunderstood Disorder* (1999) by Demitri F. Papolos and Janice Papolos. New York: Broadway.

This book provides a balance of scientific knowledge, clinical experience, and family tales about children suffering from bipolar disorder. Papolos and Papolos walk the reader through the diagnostic dilemma, helping one to select treatments and to monitor the course of the disorder. Also helpfully discussed are the multiple causes of the disorder, the impact on the family, school concerns, dealing with adolescence, the timing of hospitalizations, and the insurance maze. The authors include clearly written and sensitive accounts of families who have lived with a bipolar child. There are few books dedicated to this child–adolescent problem, and *The Bipolar Child* is quite useful for those living with and caring for such children.

Not Recommended

★★ *Bipolar Disorder: A Guide for Patients and Families* (1999) by Francis M. Mondimore. Baltimore: Johns Hopkins University Press.

AUTOBIOGRAPHIES

Strongly Recommended

★★★★★ *An Unquiet Mind* (1997) by Kay R. Jamison. New York: Random House.

A psychologist known for her research on the relationship between bipolar disorder and creativity, Jamison discusses in this frank autobiography her own history of bipolar disorder. It started in adolescence and is now controlled by lithium. Although the author had studied psychopathology, she did not connect the lectures with her own life. Jamison acknowledges the risks of going public with her disorder while still working professionally in a medical school. She presents bipolar disorder as having been a mixed blessing: It complicated her life but also contributed to her creativity, productivity, and empathy. A sensitive and compelling autobiography and deservedly rated with five stars.

★★★★   *A Brilliant Madness* (1993) by Patty Duke and Gloria Hochman. New York: Bantam.

Cowritten by actress Duke and medical writer Hochman, the book details the disastrous effects of untreated bipolar disorder on the young actress's life and career. Duke suffered through periods of wild euphoria and crippling depression for almost 20 years before being properly diagnosed and treated with lithium, to which she attributes her recovery. Duke's work in the mental health field and collaboration with a respected medical writer increase the book's credibility beyond that of the usual celebrity story. Hochman describes the different forms of affective disorder, treatments, and support groups available.

Recommended

★★★   *Pain: The Essence of Mental Illness* (1980) by Anna Eisenhart Anderson. Hicksville, NY: Exposition.

This repetitive, rambling book describes the author's life in and out of mental hospitals with a diagnosis of bipolar disorder. There were numerous separate admissions. Anderson describes herself as "a highly cultivated intellectual somewhat frail of body and very frail of mind." A recurring theme is that she viewed the hospital as her refuge and was most happy when she was there; as such, this book might be most useful for people who are apprehensive about hospitalization.

★★★   *Call Me Anna: The Autobiography of Patty Duke* (1988) by Patty Duke with Kenneth Turan. New York: Bantam.

Patty Duke was a successful child actress, but at the cost of normal contact with her family and with other children. She became a show-business legend but was an unfulfilled, disturbed individual still searching for her lost childhood. She won three Emmy Awards, divorced three husbands, and became notorious for tantrums, spending sprees, and promiscuous behavior. When her bipolar disorder was diagnosed, she began receiving treatment with lithium that enabled her to become a successful wife, mother, and political activist. This book serves as a sequel to her *A Brilliant Madness*, reviewed earlier in this chapter, and contains more information on bipolar disorder and Duke's work in the mental health movement. An inspiring and brutally honest story.

★★★   *Breakdown: A Personal Crisis and a Medical Dilemma* (revised ed., 1987) by Stuart Sutherland. New York: Oxford University Press.

In this update of a 1976 account, psychology professor Sutherland describes his bipolar episodes (including a description of hypomania), experiences with psychodynamic and behavioral therapy, drug treatments, yoga, and two hospitalizations. This edition also presents the author's views on the way society treats the mentally ill, including ethical aspects of treatment. Simon Gray's book and play were based on *Breakdown*. It is a good description of the full range of available treatments. Drawing upon his background as a psychologist, the author discusses the history and rationale of the various treatments.

Diamond in the Rough

♦ *Daughter of the Queen of Sheba* (1998) by Jacki Lyden. New York: Viking Penguin.

Foreign correspondent Jacki Lyden describes her childhood in a dysfunctional family with a manic–depressive mother and a controlling stepfather who committed her mother and beat his stepdaughter. As a child, Lyden would find her mother wrapped in bedsheets, with hieroglyphics drawn on her arms, convinced that she was the Queen of Sheba. Lyden and her sisters attempted to find treatment for their mother, who now functions on lithium. This book, though positively rated, was recently published at the time of the national study and is thus designated a Diamond in the Rough.

Not Recommended

★ *The Loony-Bin Trip* (1990) by Kate Millett. New York: Simon & Schuster.

INTERNET RESOURCES

Metasites

★★★★★ *Bipolar (Manic Depressive) Disorder*
        http://www.psycom.net/depression.central.bipolar.html

About a hundred unorganized articles on absolutely every aspect from an acknowledged expert, Dr. Ivan Goldberg. Use the Find function of your browser.

★★★★ *Internet Mental Health* http://www.mentalhealth.com/fr20.html

Click on Bipolar Disorder in the left column for a varied but quality collection of linked articles. They are organized under many headings, but include medical, legal, children, violence, deinstitutionalization, personal stories, patient education booklets, and so forth. There are hundreds of magazine articles and journal abstracts on each of the medications. The site is weak on nonmedical treatments, but for those who are already informed, this is encyclopedic. Thank you, Dr. Long.

★★★★ *BPSO-Bipolar Significant Others* http://www.bpso.org/

The focus is on supporting the "significant others" of persons with bipolar disorder, and to do so the authors offer hundreds of current, high-quality articles, sites, and readings. There is much here to offer to clients.

Psychoeducational Materials for Clients and Families

★★★★★ *Manic–Depressive Illness: An Information Book for Patients, Their Families and Friends* by Erika Bukkfalvi Hillard, MSW
        http://www.mentalhealth.com/book/fr40.html

Click on Mood Disorders in the left column and, under Bipolar Disorders, this is the first booklet listed. In 35 pages, Hilliard covers the theory, treatments (with short shrift given to psychotherapy), hospitalization, and especially family considerations that might make a good family support handout, especially after a hospitalization.

★★★★ *Bipolar Planet* http://mywebpages.comcast.net/bipolarplanet/MHLinks.html

Hundreds of links to both formal and personal sites on mood disorders, support, search engines, researchers, and humor.

★★★★ *McMan's Depression and Bipolar Web*
        http://www.mcmanweb.com

A vast collection, with links, of articles, FAQs, essays, scientific publications, and much more. It has great depth as well as breadth and will reward your exploring. Thank you, John McManamy.

★★★★ *Bipolar Affective Disorder in Children and Adolescents* by James Chandler, MD
        http://www.klis.com/chandler/pamphlet/bipolar/bipolarpamphlet.html

About 20 pages of solid information and three cases written for the public and teens. Although nonmedical treatments are only briefly addressed, the rest is a very good introduction for families.

★★★★ *Expert Consensus Treatment Guidelines for Bipolar Disorder: A Guide for Patients and Families* http://www.psychguides.com/bphe.html

A large (16-page) overview of bipolar disorder, with almost no attention paid to psychotherapy.

★★★★ *Bipolar Kids Homepage* http://www.geocities.com/EnchantedForest/1068

A large set of links, but the Articles for Families of Bipolar Kids and the School Issues sections contain much of use to families. Written for an educated audience.

★★★★ *How to Explain Bipolar Disorder to Others*
        http://bipolar.about.com/library/howto/ht-explain.htm

A one-page how-to that authors suggest might take an hour to do with a friend. Full of excellent ideas on detecting and managing, as well as explaining, one's disorder to trusted others.

★★★ *Questions I Had, Answers I Got* http://bipolar.about.com/cs/faqs/

For the impatient (manic? depressed? frightened?), here are about 30 questions and answers that are direct and relevant for correcting misunderstandings and teaching needed information.

★★★ *Tempering the Mania of Manic Depression* by Stephen L. Bernhardt
        http://www.have-a-heart.com/bipolar-depression.html

Five pages of very solid advice from Bernhardt's book.

★★★   *Understanding Bipolar Disorder*
        http://www.nami.org/helpline/UnderstandingBipolarDisorder.pdf

A 30-page discussion of all aspects of bipolar disorder, well suited as an introduction, although very heavy on the "brain disorder" perspective.

★★★   *Alternative Approaches to the Treatment of Manic–Depression*
        http://www.pendulum.org/articles/articles_misc_lisaalt.html

A nine-page overview suitable as an introduction to the use of nutrients and the like.

Other Resources

★★★★   *Bipolar Disorders Information Center*
         http://www.mhsource.com/bipolar/treat.html

For the medically sophisticated, there are two dozen articles. This is a good source of updated information on medications, odd issues, and guidelines.

★★★★   *Mood Charting* by Gary Sachs, MD
         http://www.manicdepressive.org/tools.html

Here are three charting forms: information on progress, symptom data, and mood charting. These could be useful for assessment and treatment purposes.

★★★   *Creativity and Depression and Manic-Depression*
        http://www.drada.org/OurPrograms/creativity_keats.html
        http://www.drada.org/OurPrograms/creativity_fitzgerald.html

Talks by Dr. Kay Redfield Jamison on four famous writers with mood disorders. They are not linked, so you have to use the site's Search function.

Online Support Groups

Pendulum

"The Pendulum mailing list is a support group for people who have a cyclical affective disorder (either bipolar or unipolar depression)." To subscribe to Pendulum, send a message to majordomo@ucar.edu containing this command: "subscribe pendulum [your e-mail address]."

Walkers-in-Darkness

"Walkers-in-Darkness is a list for people diagnosed with various depressive disorders (unipolar, atypical, and bipolar depression, seasonal affective disorder, related disorders). To subscribe to Walkers or Walkers-Digest, send a message to majordomo@world.std.com containing one of the following lines: "subscribe walkers [your e-mail address]" for the mailing list, or "subscribe walkers-digest [your e-mail address]" for the digest.

Madness

"An electronic action and information letter for people who experience moods swings, fright, voices, and visions." To subscribe, send a message to listserv@sjuvm.stjohns.edu with this command in the body of the message: "subscribe madness [first name] [last name]."

BiPolar Children and Teens Homepage
http://hometown.aol.com/DrgnKpr1/BPCAT.html
A site with links to perhaps hundreds of home pages of families with a bipolar child.

NATIONAL SUPPORT GROUPS

Depression and Related Affective Disorders Association
Johns Hopkins Hospital
600 North Wolfe Street
Baltimore, MD 21287-4647
Phone: 410-955-4647
Email: drada@jhmi.edu
http://www.drada.org

National Alliance for the Mentally Ill
Colonial Place Three
2107 Wilson Boulevard, Suite 300
Arlington, VA 2201
Phone: 703-524-7600 or 800-950-NAMI
   (Hotline)
http://www.nami.org

Manic Depressives Anonymous
PO Box 212
Collingswood, NJ 08107
Phone: 856-869-5508
E-mail: mda@manicdepressivesanon.org
http://www.manicdepressivesanon.org

National Depressive and Manic Depressive Association
730 North Franklin, Suite 501
Chicago, IL 60610
Phone: 800-826-3632
E-mail: questions@ndmda.org
http://www.ndmda.org

Recovery
802 North Dearborn Street
Chicago, IL 60610
Phone: 312-337-5661
http://www.recovery-inc.org

   An organization that offers a self-help method of will training: a system of techniques for controlling temperamental behavior and changing attitudes toward nervous symptoms, anxiety, anger, and fears.

See also Depression (Chapter 17) and Suicide (Chapter 33).

CHAPTER 11

Borderline
and Narcissistic
Personality Disorders

Personality disorders are recurrent interpersonal patterns that exasperate other people and ultimately harm the afflicted person. It is frequently said that neurotics make themselves miserable, but those with personality disorders make everyone else miserable. Many types of personality disorders are recognized by mental health professionals, but we cover only two in this chapter: borderline personality disorder and narcissistic personality disorder.

Individuals suffering from Borderline Personality Disorder (BPD) typically exhibit mood swings, inappropriate anger, impulsivity, chronic feelings of emptiness, unstable relationships, identity disturbances, frenzied attempts to avoid abandonment, and risky behaviors (such as promiscuous sex, substance abuse, and shoplifting). People with BPD also frequently engage in self-destructive acts, such as suicide attempts and cutting themselves. Borderlines are described as impulsive, unpredictable, angry, and empty; their only stable feature seems to be instability. Approximately 2% of the general population suffers from this disorder. Of those diagnosed with BPD, nearly 75% are women.

The term *narcissistic* is derived from Narcissus, a handsome character in Greek mythology who could only love himself. One day, Narcissus bent down to drink from a stream and saw his reflection in the water. He became so captivated with his own beauty that he stared at his reflection until he grew weak and died.

Individuals diagnosed with narcissistic personality disorder (NPD) suffer from a grandiose sense of self-importance, an unlimited need for admiration, and a lack of empathy for others. Their entitlement, arrogance, and interpersonal exploitation result in disrupted relationships with friends and family. However, most clinicians believe that

RECOMMENDATION HIGHLIGHTS

Self-Help Books

- For cognitive-behavioral skills training for BPD:

  ★★★★★ *Skills Training Manual for Treating Borderline Personality Disorder* by Marsha Linehan

- For the adult children of narcissistic families:

  ★★★★★ *The Drama of the Gifted Child* by Alice Miller

  ◆ *Trapped in the Mirror* by Elan Golomb

- For managing relationships with people afflicted with BPD:

  ★★★ *I Hate You, Don't Leave Me* by Jerold Kriesman.

Autobiographies

- For a best-selling story of an adolescent with borderline personality disorder:

  ★★★★ *Girl, Interrupted* by Susanna Kaysen

Films

- For narcissistic personality disorder:

  ★★★★ *The Great Santini*

  ★★★★ *Sunset Boulevard*

  ★★★★ *Like Water for Chocolate*

- For borderline personality disorder:

  ★★★★ *Girl, Interrupted*

  ★★★ *Fatal Attraction*

Internet Resources

- For just about anything you might want to know about BPD:

  ★★★★ *BPD Central* http://www.bpdcentral.com

- For overcoming the isolation of those who self-injure:

  ★★★★★ *Self-Injury: You Are NOT the Only One* http://www.palace.net/~llama/psych/injury.html

- For many short pieces on narcissism:

  ★★★★ *Narcissistic Personality Disorder* http://www.suite101.com/articles.cfm/npd

narcissists are actually plagued by low and fragile self-esteem; they feel so bad about themselves that they behave in an opposite manner by acting so important. Up to 1% of the population displays NPD; approximately 75% of these individuals are men.

In this chapter, we review self-help books, autobiographies, films, and Internet sites addressing BPD and NPD. Some of the self-help resources are written for the afflicted individuals, and others are written for their suffering families.

SELF-HELP BOOKS

Strongly Recommended

★★★★★ *Skills Training Manual for Treating Borderline Personality Disorder* (1993) by Marsha M. Linehan. New York: Guilford Press.

This skills manual accompanies Linehan's professional text on cognitive-behavioral therapy for BPD. The manual presents lecture notes, discussion questions, exercises, and practical advice. Especially helpful are the reproducible client handouts and home-work sheets on many of the skills borderline patients are learning. The manual is a step-by-step guide to teaching clients four broad sets of skills: interpersonal effectiveness, emotion regulation, distress tolerance, and mindfulness. An extremely practical and re-search-based guide for clinicians implementing skills training and for clients hoping to master these skills. Indeed, this self-help resource was one of the highest rated books in all of our national studies.

★★★★★ *Drama of the Gifted Child: The Search for the True Self* (1994) by Alice Miller. New York: Basic Books.

Originally published in German as *Prisoners of Childhood,* this book demonstrates how disturbed parent–child relationships negatively affect children's development. Miller tries to get parents to recognize the dangers of misusing their power. The title of the book is somewhat misleading in that *gifted* does not mean talented in ability or intellect; rather, it means sensitive and alert to the needs of others, especially to the feelings and needs of parents. As a result of parents' unintentional or unconscious manipulation of them, gifted children's feelings are stifled. While gifted children become reliable, empathic, and understanding in order to keep their parents happy, they end up never having experienced childhood at all. Miller believes that gifted children's sensitivity, empathy, and unusually powerful emotional antennae predispose them to be used by people with intense narcissistic needs. Miller argues that narcissistic individuals do not experience genuine feelings, and ultimately they destroy the authentic experiencing of genuine feelings in their children. *Drama of the Gifted Child* is beautifully written and can help gifted readers gain insight into their own feelings.

Recommended

★★★ *The Culture of Narcissism: American Life in an Age of Diminishing Expectations* (1974) by Christopher Lasch. New York: Norton.

Lasch provides a cultural assessment on how the concept of self has invaded contempo-rary society. It is a study of narcissism that takes a developmental look from birth to college, mixing sociology and individuality. Now somewhat dated, *The Culture of Narcissism* was a best-seller in the mid-1970s. The book is far more a cultural critique than a self-help book, but its general point is well taken.

★★★ *I Hate You—Don't Leave Me* (1991) by Jerold Kriesman and Hal Straus. New York: Avon.

Psychiatrist Kriesman and writer Straus offer a diagnostic picture and treatment plan for borderline personality disorder. The book title aptly captures the highly charged, hate–love relationship experienced by many of those living with people suffering from BPD. The authors describe how the person with BPD creates chaos or adds to existing chaos within a family unit, and address comorbid disorders, seeking therapy, communicating with the afflicted individual, and coping with BPD. A helpful resource for families and individuals wishing to better understand and live with BPD.

★★★ *Stop Walking on Eggshells: Taking Your Life Back When Someone You Care about Has Borderline Personality Disorder* (1998) by Paul T. Mason and Randi Kreger. Oakland, CA: New Harbinger.

This self-help book was explicitly written for family members and individuals in a relationship with someone diagnosed with BPD. *Stop Walking on Eggshells* begins by helping people understand the character of a person with this diagnosis; feeling out of control is one of the most common emotions in such a relationship. The book offers advice on how to make the necessary changes within yourself and within your relationship. Establishing clear boundaries, developing coping skills, and instituting a safety plan are among the strategies discussed. The appendices contain reading lists and additional resources. A useful, easy-to-read book on a neglected topic.

Diamond in the Rough

♦ *Trapped in the Mirror* (1992) by Elan Golomb. New York: William Morrow.

This book is intended to help adult children of narcissists in the struggle for self. As the author writes in the epilogue, "Because children of narcissists are raised to follow parental dictates, to believe that what the parent thinks is right and to defer to authority, it is important for these individuals to break the habit of allowing other people to set their path." The author presents various examples and offers methods to discover and maintain true identity. Golomb, a clinical psychologist, shares her own childhood development influenced by narcissism. She knowingly demonstrates how narcissistic parents project onto their child negative emotions and self-images. A fine book for laypersons and therapists alike, this book was highly but infrequently rated in one of our studies, meriting the Diamond in the Rough designation.

AUTOBIOGRAPHIES

Strongly Recommended

★★★★ *Girl, Interrupted* (1993) by Susanna Kaysen. New York: Random House.

Written 25 years after her hospitalization with probable diagnoses of BPD and depression, the author describes her self-mutilation and suicide attempts; problems at school and work, where she was chronically afflicted with boredom and ennui; and her 18-month hospital stay. A perennial favorite of our college students, this popular book became a film showing how a rebellious and self-destructive teenager can end up in a psychiatric hospital. Trenchant observations of ward life, it is a great read but probably less valuable as a self-help resource.

Diamonds in the Rough

♦ *Welcome to My Country* (1997) by Lauren Slater. New York: Anchor Books/Doubleday.

This unusual book is a combination of case studies, memoir, and literature bordering on poetry. Psychotherapist and former client Lauren Slater has experienced life on both sides of the desk. Now a psychologist, she spent much of her adolescence and young adulthood in a psychiatric hospital diagnosed with BPD. Sessions with her clients awaken memories of her own time in treatment. Like the work of Oliver Sacks, the book can be read as literature and will be most useful to individuals already in a helping profession or clients who want to understand the complexity, subjectivity, and uncertainties of treatment for serious mental disorder. *Welcome to My Country* received the designation Diamond in the Rough because it was infrequently but positively evaluated in one of our studies.

♦ *Skin Game* (2000) by Caroline Kettlewell. New York: St. Martin's Press/Griffin.

Why would a young person, almost always female, repeatedly cut herself with a razor? Writer Caroline Kettlewell, a former cutter now married and a mother, tries to answer this question. As a child, she was insecure, apprehensive, and unconnected. Self-injury, the feeling of a sharp steel blade against soft skin, brought her into contact with a physical reality absent in her inner life. This is a solid book for understanding that self-mutilation is not necessarily attention seeking. It is not clear that the account will benefit someone presently engaged in self-mutilation, although it can provide insight to parents and others close to such individuals. Too new to be widely known in professional circles, this book carries a Diamond in the Rough designation.

FILMS

Strongly Recommended

★★★★ *The Great Santini* (1979) directed by Lewis Carlino. PG rating. 115 minutes.

A Marine pilot, the self-described "great Santini," is devoted to his family and troops but is an unpredictable and alcoholic narcissist. He must be in charge and victorious at home, as well as at work. He subjects his codependent wife and resentful kids to white-glove inspections, verbal rants, and violent retributions in order to bolster his own self-esteem. He will not tolerate soft feelings or failures. One of his sons eventually takes a courageous stand and assertively defies his father's direct orders. *The Great Santini* is, at once, a harrowing film and an inspiring film. It is harrowing in its realistically dark portrayal of abuse and narcissism. Viewers will learn how families survive a domineering narcissist, perennially walking on eggshells and maneuvering around his abuse. However, the film is also an inspiring demonstration of the resilience of children and the possibility of escape. In both respects, it is a deeply emotional experience.

★★★★   *Sunset Boulevard* (1950) directed by Billy Wilder. Not rated. 110 minutes.

An aging star of silent movies, Norma Desmond (Gloria Swanson), harbors the narcissistic delusion that millions of fans still adore her, and she plans a comeback playing the lead in her own screenplay. William Holden plays a young screenwriter who exchanges admiration and sexual favors for the security she affords. In the end, though, the silent screen star's pathological possessiveness, jealousy, and entitlement get the best of both of them. A sad but accurate film about elderly narcissists, left only with their grandiosity.

★★★★   *Girl, Interrupted* (1999) directed by James Mangold. R rating. 127 minutes.

Based on Susanna Kaysen's memoir of the same title (reviewed above), the film traces her 18-month stay at a mental hospital in the 1960s. Susanna (Winona Ryder) is admitted following a probable suicide attempt, feeling depressed, directionless, and interpersonally alienated. She befriends the band of troubled women in her ward, addresses her borderline personality features in psychotherapy and in her relationships, and gradually pulls herself together. The ensemble cast is marvelous, especially Angelina Jolie as the resident antisocial. As a self-help resource, the film explores the hazy line between Susanna as confused adolescent and as sufferer from BPD. It is a film (and autobiography) especially popular among young women.

★★★★   *Like Water for Chocolate* (1993) directed by Alfonso Arau. R rating. 123 minutes. In Spanish with English subtitles

Family tradition dictates that Tita, the youngest daughter, remain unmarried and take care of her aging, self-absorbed Mama. But Tita falls in love with Pedro, who, bowing to the Mexican culture and Mama's wishes, marries Tita's older sister. Living in the same house, their love changes everything. Tita ultimately confronts the spirit of her narcissistic Mama and gains her autonomy despite the oppressive tradition. *Like Water for Chocolate* is a love story overflowing with romantic grandeur, but for self-help purposes, it also realistically portrays the suffering of children of narcissistic or tyrannical parents. The film vividly, if symbolically, displays Tita's liberation in wrenching free from her mother's oppression.

Recommended

★★★   *Misery* (1990) directed by Rob Reiner. R rating. 107 minutes.

In a horror and thriller flick based on a Stephen King novel, Kathy Bates stars as an obsessed and delusional fan who imprisons her favorite novelist and forces him to rewrite his latest novel to suit her tastes. He is bound, crippled, and drugged at her mercy. Bates displays classic borderline behaviors and deservedly won an Oscar for her role alternating between the extremes of a sweet nurse and a wicked torturer.

★★★   *Fatal Attraction* (1987) directed by Adrian Lyne. R rating. 119 minutes.

In probably the most eerily accurate portrayal of borderline personality disorder in cinematic history, Glenn Close plays Alex, who has an affair with her married colleague and will not let go of him. She engages in impulsive sex, intense anger, suicidal gestures, and disturbed interpersonal relationships alternating between idealization and devaluation. Her classic examples of borderline rage include throwing acid on her ex-lover's car, stalking his family, and cutting herself, all of it ending with violence. If you can ignore the contrived ending, the film brilliantly captures the psychological manifestations of borderline pathology (even though it never explains or treats it).

Not Recommended

★★ *In the Company of Men* (1997) directed by Neil Labute. R rating. 97 minutes.

★ *Groundhog Day* (1993) directed by Harold Ramis. PG rating. 101 minutes.

★ *After Hours* (1985) directed by Martin Scorcese. R rating. 96 minutes.

Strongly Not Recommended

† *Murder by Numbers* (2002) directed by Barbet Schroeder. R rating. 120 minutes.

INTERNET RESOURCES

Metasites

★★★★ *BPD Central* http://www.BPDCentral.com/

Lots of information, support, and stories for those who care about someone with BPD. The Basics of BPD (on the left) is about 10 pages of well-balanced information—an excellent starting place. It starts with DSM-IV criteria but goes on to much more familiar indicators, myths, and a discussion of games. Books are for sale, and there are support, legal and medical links, treatment and research. Something for everyone.

★★★★ *Helen's World of BPD Resources* http://www.bpdresources.com/

Hundreds of links, annotated by Helen, for the friends, family, and loved ones of those with BPD. The site is comprehensive and searchable, with authoritative materials collected by a sophisticated woman. Use the list of pages on the left to explore the site. The Recommended Books page describes perhaps 200 books on the important aspects of BPD, and most are linked to Amazon.com, so you can see details and others' reviews. This site is all anyone needs.

★★★★ *Narcissistic Personality Disorder*
        http://www.halcyon.com/jmashmun/npd/index.html

Joanna M. Ashmun's dozen or so essays here can extend one's understanding enormously. In the first, she translates the DSM-IV criteria into the familiar language of living with a narcissist. The second and third essays discuss how to recognize a narcissist by the traits displayed and provide an excellent discussions of the traits. All presentations are well written, thoughtful, and sensitive.

★★★★ *Narcissistic Personality Disorder* http://www.suite101.com/articles.cfm/npd

Sam Vaknin is still a narcissist. His 60 short essays here could be useful for getting a person with NPD to recognize his or her narcissism, if in denial. Vaknin explores multiple aspects of society, history, and psychology through the lens of narcissism. More of his essays are available as FAQs at http://www.healthyplace.com/communities/personality_disorders/narcissism/faq_index.html and as articles at http://www.healthyplace.com/communities/personality_disorders/narcissism/articles.html.

Psychoeducational Materials for Clients and Families

★★★★★   *Self-Injury: You Are NOT the Only One*
                http://www.palace.net/~llama/psych/injury.html

By the author of a book with the same name, the site offers support, links, and much practical information in 50 or more pages. Excellent for self-harmers who need to know they are not alone as well as those who need guidance and help now.

★★★★   *An Overview of Dialectical Behavior Therapy in the Treatment of Borderline Personality Disorder* by Barry Kiehn and Michaela Swales
                http://www.mentalhelp.net/poc/view_doc.php?type=doc&id=1020

In about 15 pages, the authors cover just about everything of importance on the treatment of BPD. An excellent handout for patients.

★★★★   *Kathi's Mental Health: Toddler Time*
                http://www.toddlertime.com/menu_borderline_personality_diso.htm

There are about 40 articles (about half by Ms. Stringer) for clients, relatives, and professionals on this page. The six professional articles by Ms. Stringer are highly recommended. Every client will find much stimulation and hope on this site.

★★★★   *A Primer on Narcissism*
                http://www.mentalhelp.net/poc/view_doc.php/type/doc/id/419

About a dozen tightly written pages of description covering definitions, dynamics, major theories, family dysfunction, and trauma. If you need a history of views on the topic, this is solid.

★★★★   *Voicelessness: Narcissism*   http://voicelessness.com/narcissism.html

"Many people spend a lifetime aggressively trying to protect an injured or vulnerable self. Traditionally, psychologists have termed such people "narcissists," but this is a misnomer. To the outside world, it appears that these people love themselves. Yet at their core, they don't love themselves—in fact, their self barely exists, and what part does exist is deemed worthless."

★★★   *The Other Side of Power* by Claude M. Steiner, PhD
                http://www.igc.org/emlit/osp.htm

This is a free, full-length online book using transactional analysis to deal with manipulation and power plays. Steiner suggests not responding in kind, no matter how good it might feel or how socially supported. Especially useful for those in relationships with narcissists or BPD people.

★★★ *BPD Recovery.com* http://pub69.ezboard.com/bashrisen40890

Although it has resources and links, the best part of this site is the well-organized links to bulletin boards and chat for support, clarification, and other communal activities.

★★★ *Were You Raised by a Narcissistic Father?* by Kathleen Brizendine, MA
     http://www.toddlertime.com/were_you_raised_by_a_narcissisti.htm

A short but telling essay.

★★★ *Dual Diagnosis: Resources for Co-Occuring Addiction and Personality Disorders* http://
     /www.toad.net/%7earcturus/dd/ddhome.htm

The links to Online Docs (on the left) take the reader to many professional resources.

★★★ *Dual Diagnosis—Online Library*
     http://www.dualdiagnosis.org/library/library.html

Although most of the 30 articles here are for professionals, some are for clients, and others can be adapted for sophisticated clients.

★★★ *You Owe Me! Children of Entitlement* by Lynne Namka, EdD
     http://members.aol.com/AngriesOut/teach9.htm

About 10 pages on understanding children's selfish (narcissistic) behavior—its causes, dynamics, and management. It may be helpful to parents in understanding normal and abnormal behaviors or to adults in recalling their pasts.

★★★ *Self-Confident Personality Type*
     http://www.geocities.com/ptypes/narcissistic.html

After a list of nine characteristics of this type, there is much material on noteworthy people who have this type of personality. Useful to help distinguish high self-confidence from narcissism for family, friends, and perhaps the person with NPD.

★★★ *Narcissism: A Nine Headed Hydra? Exploring Types of Narcissism* by Bruce
     Stevens http://www.psychotherapy.com.au/august00/featart1.html

In about 15 pages, Stevens describes in ordinary language the types of presentation, interactions, and relationships that are, for him, variants on NPD. This site is quite useful as an introduction to the topic of abusive relationships and recognizing the dynamics of relationships for those who do not see what is happening.

★★★ *So, You're in Love with a Narcissist* by Alexandra Nouri
     http://www.angelfire.com/indie/aanouri/

In 11 short essays, the author presents pleasures, benefits, and problems of living with a NPD in clear and ordinary terms. Rather bitter, but probably useful for partners who do not understand what is wrong with their relationship.

CHAPTER 12

Career Development

Too often, we perceive developing a career plan as a one-time event, as making a single major commitment. But each of us probably experiences life changes that require modifications in employment, adjustments in career goals, and sometimes a change of careers. In fact, the average worker now makes five to six job transitions in a lifetime.

Careers occupy a crucial role in our life satisfaction and our family relationships. Cost reduction and downsizing by businesses have translated into displacement and job loss. The workforce is rapidly becoming diverse, international, and service-oriented. Many jobs are more complex and technically demanding. Workers are increasingly perceiving the workplace as a means of enhancing their health and well-being, not simply as a place for earning a living. Dual-career couples predominate. And now, more than ever, people are concerned about the role of work in their lives, wanting to strike the best balance between work and other life tasks.

Self-help resources on career development traverse a number of topics, including career choice, job hunting, interviewing, career changes, dual-career families, and effective communication in the workplace. A large number of self-help books on specific components of work have been written—how to become a better salesperson, how to be an effective manager, how to improve the corporate workplace—but such books are not included here.

What follows are national ratings and evaluative descriptions of self-help books and Internet resources devoted to career development.

SELF-HELP BOOKS

Strongly Recommended

★★★★★ *What Color Is Your Parachute?* (2002 edition) by Richard Bolles. Berkeley, CA: Ten Speed.

This extremely popular book about job hunting was first published in 1970. Since 1975, an updated edition has appeared annually. This is an enormously successful self-help

RECOMMENDATION HIGHLIGHTS

Self-Help Books

- On career choice, job hunting, and interviewing:

  ★★★★★   *What Color Is Your Parachute?* by Richard Bolles

  ★★★   *Knock 'Em Dead* by Martin Yate

- On the meaning of work for traditional males and traditional females:

  ★★★★   *Staying the Course* by Robert Weiss

- On turning conflict into career and interpersonal advancement:

  ★★★★   *Win–Win Negotiating* by Fred Jandt

- On the meaning of work:

  ◆   *Lives without Balance* by Steven Carter and Julia Sokol

Internet Resources

- On everything you want to know about college and graduate school:

  ★★★★★   *Petersons.com*   http://www.petersons.com

- On great suggestions for a career:

  ★★★★   *Career Interests Game!*
  http://web.missouri.edu/~cppcwww/holland.shtml

- On accessing a workbook for moving your career forward:

  ★★★★★   *Career Development Manual*   http://www.cdm.uwaterloo.ca/

book that has become the career seeker's bible. Bolles tries to answer readers' concerns about the job-hunting process and gives many sources that can provide further information. Unlike many books on job hunting, *What Color Is Your Parachute?* does not assume that readers are recent college graduates seeking their first jobs. He spends considerable time discussing job hunting for people seeking to change careers. Bolles describes a number of myths about job hunting and successfully debunks them. He also provides invaluable advice about where jobs are, what to do to get hired, and how to cut through the red tape and confusing hierarchies of the business world to meet the key people who make hiring decisions. The book has remained appreciably the same over the years, with updates as appropriate. Recent editions have added material on job hunting for handicapped workers, on the effective use of career counselors, and on finding a mission in life. This five-star book was one of the most frequently rated books in our national studies—more than 300 mental health professionals evaluated it. It is indeed an excellent self-help book about job hunting and career change. Bolles writes in a warm, engaging, personal tone. His chatty comments are often witty and entertaining, and the book is attractively packaged with cartoons, drawings, and many self-administered exercises.

★★★★ *Staying the Course: The Emotional and Social Lives of Men Who Do Well at Work* (1990) by Robert Weiss. New York: Free Press.

This book is based on Weiss's interviews with 80 men, ages 35 to 55, in upper-middle-class occupations. He explores the nature of the men's work and nonwork lives—their activities, relationships, goals, and stresses. He also delves into their psychological lives to discover what has motivated them to meet their obligations year after year after year. Weiss found that men who stayed the course had established social status and self-worth at work, had experienced emotional and social support from their marriages and families, and had benefited from loyal friendships. He says that, all too often in our society, successful men are portrayed as exploiters. He found this not to be the case. Successful men had made compromises with their youthful dreams and had developed respectful and caring relationships both in and out of the workplace. Their lives revolved around steady career advancement instead of ruthless ambition, and they cared more about family stability than sexual conquest. *Staying the Course* contains high-quality research, careful interpretation, and useful insights. However, there is something of an old-fashioned cast to Weiss's men and his interpretation of their lives. Feminists, especially, do not appreciate some of the conclusions that can be drawn from Weiss's work (e.g., if wives work, their jobs are secondary in terms of economics and status).

★★★★ *Win–Win Negotiating: Turning Conflict into Agreement* (1987) by Fred Jandt. New York: Wiley.

The main themes of this book are that conflict is inevitable but not always bad, and that if everyone involved makes an honest effort, the conflict can be resolved. In the first four chapters, Jandt describes the basic nature of conflict and includes a self-assessment so that readers can determine how they deal with conflict and identify sources of conflict. He shows readers how to keep minor disagreements from turning into major battles. Jandt makes the important point that when one party is the "winner" in a conflict, in the long run, both parties often lose when the losing party avoids future contact or tries to get even. Ultimately, the relationship dies. Thus, the goal is to develop a solution that will satisfy both parties and let the relationship continue in much the same way as in the past. *Win–Win Negotiating* is a good introduction to learning how opponents or adversaries think and how they negotiate their positions. Anyone who wants to learn about negotiating techniques and resolving conflict in the workplace can benefit from reading it.

Recommended

★★★ *Shifting Gears* (1990) by Carole Hyatt. New York: Simon & Schuster.

Hyatt calls attention to research that indicates that most people go through several career changes. She uses the results of interviews with 300 individuals who succeeded in career transitions to develop a framework for self-guidance in making career transitions. She advises how to:

- Adapt to today's marketplace.
- Determine your work style.
- Identify trigger points that require change.

- Explore the psychological barriers to change and overcome them.
- Learn strategies to define a career path and repackage yourself.

This addition to the self-help literature was not well-known among the mental health professionals; only 20 rated it, but they accorded it moderately positive value.

★★★ *Knock 'Em Dead* (10th ed., 2002) by Martin Yate. Holbrook, MA: Bob Adams.

This regularly updated guide to job interviewing is subtitled *With Great Answers to Tough Interview Questions*. Yate gives the best answers to a number of key questions likely to be asked in a job interview:

- Why do you want to work here?
- How much money do you want?
- What can you do that someone else can't?
- What decisions are the most difficult for you?
- What is your greatest weakness?
- Why were you fired (if you lost your last job)?

According to Yate, the best jobs go to the best-prepared rather than to the best-qualified candidates. Yate prepares the potential interviewee with the inside scoop on stress interviews, salary negotiations, executive search firms, and drug testing. He also provides advice about how to respond to illegal questions and other hardball tactics. In the most recent editions, Yate has added sections on dress and body language. This three-star book was not well known among the mental health professionals, but the experts who did rate it thought it gives sound advice for job interviewing, especially on handling tough interviews.

★★★ *Do What You Love, the Money Will Follow* (1987) by Marsha Sinetar. New York: Dell.

This book is subtitled *Discovering Your Right Livelihood*, and that is what Sinetar tries to encourage readers to do. Sinetar strongly believes that people should try to find jobs that fulfill their needs, talents, and passions. She provides a step-by-step guide to doing this and includes dozens of real-life examples of how people have overcome their fears and found work that allows them to grow. Readers learn how to get in touch with their inner selves and true talents, evaluate and build their self-esteem, get rid of their "shoulds," overcome resistance, and get out of unfulfilling jobs and into fulfilling ones. *Do What You Love, the Money Will Follow* barely received a three-star rating; that is, it was given mixed reviews. Some of the mental health professionals felt that Sinetar does a good job of helping people stuck in jobs they don't like to break free and find jobs they truly enjoy doing. Others said that Sinetar's approach borders on naiveté and might encourage people to leave jobs they probably shouldn't in search of the ultimate, perfect job.

Diamonds in the Rough

♦ *Lives without Balance* (1992) by Steven Carter and Julia Sokol. New York: Villard.

The authors describe the problem of unbalanced living because of outdated values and false premises. Among the modern destructive myths highlighted are the limitless credit card; you are the master of your own fate; think and grow rich; you can have it all; and you can do it all. Using catchy phrases, the authors evaluate four types of unbalanced lives: the downward slide, the never-ending treadmill, the uncontrollable escalator, and the roller coaster. Carter and Sokol also analyze image fixes, power fixes, glamour fixes, buying and selling fixes, job perks fixes, and status fixes—along with the problems entangled in the fixes. *Lives without Balance* was published between our national studies and, unfortunately, we neglected to secure experts' ratings on it. But the book raises important issues and stimulates thought about work, careers, and meaning in life.

♦ *Career Mastery* (1992) by Harry Levinson. San Francisco: Berrett-Koehler.

This introspective exploration of career choices is not a how-to book, nor does it give advice on practical aspects of a job search. Rather, it is a psychological self-assessment and a values clarification that enables readers to decide how to direct themselves through a lifetime of careers. Topics involve the larger context of decision making, not about a specific job but about the direction in which the individual wants to go in shaping a professional future. Some of these topics include how to cope with change in an organization, how to avoid self-blame, how to make sense of a defeat or failure, how to cultivate good work relationships, and how to relate to good and problem bosses. This book falls into the Diamonds in the Rough category because it received positive but infrequent ratings and because it reflects on the psychological aspects of work.

Not Recommended

★★ *The Portable MBA* (1990) by Eliza Collins and Mary Devanna. New York: Wiley.

★★ *The 100 Best Companies to Work for in America* (revised ed., 1994) by Robert Levering and Milton Moskowitz. New York: Signet.

INTERNET RESOURCES

There are numerous sites to post resumes, search for openings, locate recruiters, and apply for specialized jobs. None of these have been included here, because they are not direct self-help resources and they do not assist in psychotherapy.

Metasites

★★★★★ *Petersons.com* http://www.petersons.com

If someone needs college, this is the place to start. Just about anything and everything about college and graduate school are here: selecting a college, studying abroad, financing school, job searching, admission tests, adult students, executive education programs, and so on.

★★★★★ *Yahoo—Careers* http://www.yahoo.com

Searching Yahoo under Careers produces about 60 sections, including information about each of 100 careers (at http://dir.yahoo.com/Business_and_Economy/Companies/Corporate_Services/Human_Resources/Recruiting_and_Placement/Career_Fields).

★★★★   *Career Interests Game!*   http://web.missouri.edu/~cppcwww/holland.shtml
Using Holland's six types of personality, this site will suggest careers. Neat.

★★★   *Graduate and Professional School Guides*
     http://www.jobweb.org/career_development/gguides.htm
Links to sites about applying to and financing graduate school and about making the transition to graduate school.

★★★   *Monster.com*   http://www.monster.com
If you are seeking a job, this is the largest list of job openings. The readings can be very helpful.

Psychoeducational Materials for Clients and Families

★★★★★   *Career Development Manual*   http://www.cdm.uwaterloo.ca/
This small, book-size site covers all the steps in detail: self-assessment, researching occupations, making decisions, contacting employers, working, and life planning. From the University of Waterloo.

★★★★★   *The Princeton Review*   http://www.review.com/
The authors' specialty is coaching for the standardized admission tests to college and graduate schools, and the site offers a great deal of support, direction, and information. The site also offer lots of good introductory advice on choosing a college and an advanced search engine.

★★★★★   *How to Conduct an Effective Job Search*
     http://www2.jobtrak.com/help_manuals/jobmanual/
This is actually a small book on how to find a job, aimed at college students but of value to anyone. It covers areas such as networking, business letters, resumes, and interviewing.

★★★★★   *Developing A Career Transition Strategy*
     http://www.doi.gov/octc/strategy.html
An interactive guidebook with 10 sections on career transitions, this site offers assessment tools, areas of occupational growth, interviewing tips, resumes, and retirement information.

★★★★★   *The Student Guide*   http://www.ed.gov/prog_info/SFA/StudentGuide
This online book is the most comprehensive resource on student financial aid. From the U.S. Department of Education.

★★★★   *Career Adviser: Your Channel Guide to Career Resources*
     http://www.careeradviser.com
If you know what you want to explore but don't know where to start, this site will take you to just about all the online information about the job.

★★★★ *Your Self-Assessment* http://www.cats.ohiou.edu/careers/students.html

Download this worksheet to assess interests, skills, and values. This may help clarify issues in an open-ended way.

★★★★ *Feminist Career Center* http://www.feminist.org/911/jobs/911jobs.asp

Listings of available positions with about 200 feminist and progressive organizations.

★★★★ *Job Hunters Bible* http://www.jobhuntersbible.com

This site is designed to supplement the valuable book *What Color Is Your Parachute?* Best if the client is familiar with the book, but the 25 articles in the Parachute Library are of value by themselves.

★★★★ *Conference Calls in Your Pajamas: The Pros and Cons of Working from Home*
          by Bradley Richardson
          http://editorial.careers.msn.com/articles/workfromhome/

A two-page summary to help a person decide. The other articles here are also useful.

★★★ *iVillage Work* http://www.ivillage.com/work

Many practical articles on confidence and persisting, balancing work and home, self-employment, job finding, and other aspects of being employed.

★★★ *Interviewing for a Job Assembled* by Carter McNamara, PhD
          http://www.mapnp.org/library/career/ntrvwing.htm

About a dozen links to solid advice on handling tough or illegal questions, salary negotiations, and lots more.

★★★ *Career Goals* http://www.careernet.state.md.us./goalsetting.htm

For those who cannot decide on goals, this essay and worksheet will help them focus.

★★★ *Major to Career Converter*
          http://www.content.monstertrak.monster.com/tools/careerconverter/

If one has already declared a major but doesn't know what kind of careers one can enter with that major, it may help to search Monster.com's gigantic list of jobs.

★★★ *The Riley Guide: Research for Career and Work Options*
          http://www.rileyguide.com/

This site is eight links to the best sites for job and career research. If you need the facts, here is how to find them on employers, education, salary, the future of different careers, career counselors, and so on.

★★★ *iVillage Work at Home* http://www.ivillage.com/topics/work/0,,165441,00.html

Support and information for those who work at home, especially women.

★★★   *ACCESS: Networking in the Public Interest* http://www.accessjobs.org

This site includes some articles and a large listing of jobs in the nonprofit area. "An excellent resource for anyone seeking jobs, internships, volunteer positions, and career development in nonprofit organizations." See also *Opportunity NOCs: Nonprofit Organization Classifieds* at http://www.opportunityknocks.org where jobs can be searched by region, state, or keyword.

★★★   *The Red Guide to Temp Agencies: Tips for Temps; Strategies for Successful Temping*
          http://www.panix.com/~grvsmth/redguide/tips.html

Lots of guidance for seeking and using temporary employment agencies.

CHAPTER 13

Child Development and Parenting

Playwright George Bernard Shaw once commented that although parenting is a very important occupation, no test of fitness for it is ever imposed. If a test were imposed, some parents would turn out to be more fit than others. Most parents hope that their children will grow into socially mature individuals, but they often are not sure how to help their children reach this goal.

Child development and parenting are probably the largest categories of self-help resources. If parents are not confused about what to do before they visit a bookstore or surf the Internet to obtain information on parenting, they may well become confused when they see the bewildering array of advice. The ratings of the mental health experts in our national studies provide valuable advice about how to navigate the maze of parenting self-help books.

In this chapter we evaluate self-help resources that focus on parenting children. Other chapters consider closely related topics, notably Infants (Chapter 21), Pregnancy (Chapter 27), Families and Stepfamilies (Chapter 20), and Teenagers and Parenting (Chapter 34). Entire chapters are also devoted to attention-deficit/hyperactivity disorder (9) and violent youth (37).

Because there are so many resources, we had to decide which to include and exclude. We primarily included resources that deal with parenting in general rather than parenting strategies for specific problems. For example, we evaluate parenting books on discipline but for the most part do not rate books that exclusively cover topics such as learning disabilities or mental retardation. Of course, some of the general parenting books include the specific topics in their overview of parenting and child development.

Even with these exclusions, be forewarned: This is one of the lengthiest chapters in the book. It is also, rewardingly, the chapter with the largest number of strongly recommended self-help resources.

RECOMMENDATION HIGHLIGHTS

Self-Help Books

- On the normal course of child development and coping with problems:

  ★★★★★ *To Listen to a Child* by T. Berry Brazelton

  ★★★★★ *Your Baby and Child* by Penelope Leach

- On parenting toddlers:

  ★★★★★ *Toddlers and Parents* by T. Berry Brazelton

- On parenting 3- to 6-year-olds:

  ★★★ *Touchpoints* by T. Berry Brazelton and Joshua Sparrow

- On general parenting and communication skills:

  ★★★★★ *Between Parent and Child* by Haim Ginott

  ★★★★★ *How to Talk So Kids Will Listen and Listen So Kids Will Talk* by Adele Faber and Elaine Mazlish

  ★★★★ *Parent Effectiveness Training* by Thomas Gordon

  ★★★ *Raising Resilient Children* by Robert Brooks and Sam Goldstein

- On effective discipline for children:

  ★★★★★ *Children: The Challenge* by Rudolph Dreikurs

  ★★★★★ *1-2-3 Magic* by Thomas W. Phelan

  ★★★★ *Parenting the Strong-Willed Child* by Rex Forehand and Nicholas Long

  ★★★ *Living with Children* by Gerald Patterson

- On parenting defiant and difficult children:

  ★★★★★ *Your Defiant Child* by Russell Barkley and Christine Benton

  ★★★★ *The Difficult Child* by Stanley Turecki

- On the problem of children growing up too soon:

  ★★★★ *The Hurried Child* by David Elkind

- On parenting African American children:

  ◆ *Raising Black Children* by James P. Comer and Alvin E. Poussaint

- On understanding motherhood at different points in life:

  ★★★ *The Mother Dance* by Harriet Lerner

Films

- On pushing children and on children trying to please their parents:

  ★★★★ *Searching for Bobby Fischer*

- On discovering what is in a child's best interest:
    - ★★★★ *Little Man Tate*
    - ★★★★ *I Am Sam*

Internet Resources

- On parenting information in general:
    - ★★★★★ *Parenthood.com* http://www.parenthood.com/links.html
    - ★★★★★ *Tufts University Child and Family Webguide* http://www.cft.tufts.edu
    - ★★★★★ *NPIN: National Parent Information Network*
      http://ericps.crc.uiuc.edu/npin/index.html

- On what to expect by the child's age:
    - ★★★★★ *Today's Parent Online* http://www.todaysparent.com

- On substance abuse concerns:
    - ★★★★★ *Common Sense* http://www.pta.org/commonsense

SELF-HELP BOOKS

Strongly Recommended

★★★★★ *Your Defiant Child: Eight Steps to Better Behavior* (1998) by Russell A. Barkley and Christine Benton. New York: Guilford Press.

This excellent self-help book, one of the most highly rated in all of our studies, is written for parents who have a child who is unyielding or combative. The book examines what causes children to become defiant, when the defiance reaches problem proportions, and how to deal with the defiance. The authors' eight-step program emphasizes consistency and cooperation, as well as instituting changes through a system of praise, reward, and mild punishment. Parents learn how to establish effective discipline, communicate with children at a level they can understand, and reduce family stress. An exceptional resource (also reviewed in Chapter 37 on violent youth).

★★★★★ *To Listen to a Child* (1984) by T. Berry Brazelton. Reading, MA: Addison-Wesley.

Brazelton's focus here is primarily on problematic events that arise in the lives of children. Fears, feeding difficulties, sleep problems, stomachaches, and asthma are among the problems that Brazelton evaluates. He assures parents that only when they let their own anxieties interfere do problems such as bedwetting become chronic and guilt-laden. Each chapter closes with practical guidelines for parents. This five-star book is easy to read, includes well-chosen and clearly explained examples, and is warm and entertaining. Its descriptions are not as detailed as those in some other books that focus on specific periods of development—for example, Brazelton's own *Toddlers and Par-*

ents—but it is a very good resource for parents to refer to throughout the childhood years when normal problems emerge.

★★★★★ *Toddlers and Parents* (2nd ed., 1989) by T. Berry Brazelton. New York: Delacorte.

This Brazelton contribution traces normal child development and advises parents on how to handle typical problems and issues that arise during the toddler years. Each of the 11 chapters interweaves the narrative of an individual child's experiences (e.g., the birth of a sibling or a typical day at a day care center) with Brazelton's moment-by-moment descriptions of what the child may be feeling, explanations of the child's behavior, and supportive suggestions for parents that help them cope with their own feelings, as well as their child's behavior. Among the topics addressed by Brazelton are the following:

- The toddler's declaration of independence at about one year of age, a time when the toddler becomes alternately demanding and dismissing.
- The nature of working parents' family life and their toddler's development at 18 and 30 months.
- Life with a toddler of different ages in nontraditional families (divorced, stepfamily).
- Special considerations for withdrawn, demanding, and unusually active toddlers.
- Coping with the 18-month-old's frequent no's.
- The 30-month-old's developing self-control and self-awareness.

All told, this is an excellent self-help book for the parents of toddlers. The writing is clear, and Brazelton's tone is warm and personal. He not only provides parents with a guide to survival but also helps them develop a sense of delight in the struggles and triumphs of their toddlers.

★★★★★ *Between Parent and Child* (1965) by Haim Ginott. New York: Avon.

This aging classic provides parents with a guide to improving communication with their children and understanding their feelings. Ginott's aim is to help parents understand the importance of listening to the feelings behind their child's communication. Ginott says that children who feel understood by their parents do not feel lonely, and they develop a deep love for their parents. Toward this end, he describes a communication technique he calls "childrenese," which is based on parents' respect for the child and statements of understanding preceding statements of advice or instruction. Since its publication in 1965, millions of copies of the book have been sold. *Between Parent and Child* has been praised for being simple and clear. Although almost four decades old, *Between Parent and Child* continues to be one of the books that many mental health professionals recommend for parents. The age of the book is a problem: For example, the material on sex education and sex roles is severely outdated; mothers are always at home, and fathers are off at work. The book was never revised; however, we were recently informed that Alice Ginott (Haim's widow and a psychologist herself) and H. Wallace Goddard will be updating the book for a late 2003 release.

★★★★★ *Children: The Challenge* (1964, reissued 1991) by Rudolph Dreikurs. New
York: Hawthorn.

This aging classic's central concern is effective and loving discipline. Dreikurs believes
that parents have to learn how to become a match for their children by becoming wise
to their children's ways and capable of guiding them without letting them run wild or
stifling them. Unfortunately, says Dreikurs, most parents don't know what to do with
their children. Dreikurs teaches parents how to understand their children and meet
their needs. He stresses that the main reason for children's misbehavior is discourage-
ment. Discouraged children often demand undue attention. Parents usually respond to
this negative attention-getting behavior by trying to impose their will on the children,
who in turn keep misbehaving. Dreikurs says that parents who get caught up in this cycle are actually rewarding their children's misbehavior. He tells parents instead to remain calm and pleasant when disciplining the child. Each of the 39 brief chapters involves a different type of discipline problem in which children misbehave and parents
respond inappropriately. Dreikurs clearly spells out effective ways to handle each of
these situations. He also recommends a "family council" for solving family problems.
This book remains an excellent guide for parents to use in learning how to discipline
their children more effectively. It is easy to read; the examples are clear and plentiful;
the strategies for discipline are good ones. Although written over four decades ago,
Children: The Challenge still is a widely recommended book on parental discipline.

★★★★★ *How to Talk So Kids Will Listen and Listen So Kids Will Talk* (20th ed., 1999) by
Adele Faber and Elaine Mazlish. New York: Avon.

This is a how-to book written with the goal of teaching methods that affirm the dignity
and humanity of parents and children. After years of conducting workshops on communication skills for parents, the authors assembled the many ideas, activities, and lessons
learned into this book. Each chapter presents ways to put the principles into action and
addresses topics such as dealing with children's feelings, cooperation, alternatives to
punishment, autonomy and praise, and putting it all together. In their regularly revised
editions, Faber and Mazlish include open-ended answers for reader response, cartoons
that teach key principles, feeling and context exercises, parent–child role plays, and
questions and answers. This is a good book for parent–child interaction in that it is both
understandable and practical.

★★★★★ *1-2-3 Magic: Effective Discipline for Children 2–12* (2nd revised ed., 1996) by
Thomas W. Phelan.

This humorous book takes the reader through the 1-2-3 disciplinary approach with colorful and applicable illustrations. How to successfully start behaviors (e.g., cleaning
room) and stop them (e.g., tantrums) are clearly described. The false assumption that
the child is a little adult and the big mistakes parents make of showing too much emotion and explaining too much are played out in lighthearted but all too familiar scenarios. Phelan demonstrates established behavioral and Adlerian principles in novel and
interesting ways. The book is written not only to instruct parents in accomplishing the
program but also to demonstrate empathic support of the discipline challenges confronted by contemporary families.

★★★★ *The Difficult Child* (2nd revised ed., 2000) by Stanley Turecki. New York: Bantam.

This book tells parents how to deal more effectively with a child who has a difficult temperament. Turecki's book is based on his experience with thousands of families in the Difficult Children Program he created at Beth Israel Medical Center in New York City. He guides parents in identifying whether they have a difficult child; managing conflicts with their child; disciplining more effectively; obtaining support from schools, doctors, professionals, and support groups; and ensuring that they acknowledge and reward the difficult child's strengths. The revised second edition also addresses ADHD.

★★★★ *Parent Effectiveness Training: The Tested New Way to Raise Responsible Children* (1975) by Thomas Gordon. New York: Peter Wyden.

First published in 1970, this book, revised in 1975, is designed to educate parents about the nature of children's development and to help parents communicate more effectively with them. The book opens with a discussion of how parents are blamed but not trained (which underscores the rationale for Gordon's Parent Effectiveness Training program). Gordon advocates an authoritative parenting strategy that involves being neither permissive nor punitive but, rather, emphasizes nurturing and setting clear limitations. Gordon provides especially good advice about how to communicate more effectively with children. Included in his recommendations are how to engage in active listening, how to make frank statements of feeling without placing blame, and how to deal with children's problems. Gordon's approach enables parents to show children how to solve their own problems rather than inappropriately accusing or blaming children. The widespread popularity of this four-star book was reflected in the large number of respondents who rated the book—more than 250. The book and the Parent Effectiveness Training course, taught through numerous parenting groups and classes across the country, have helped millions of parents gain a better understanding of their children and learn to communicate more effectively with them. Despite its age, it remains one of the best books available for improving parent–child communication.

★★★★ *Parenting the Strong-Willed Child* (1996) by Rex Forehand and Nicholas Long. Chicago: Contemporary.

Parents of strong-willed children will learn a system of techniques and interactive skills that have been shown by research to be effective in significantly improving child behavior. Well-accepted behavioral techniques are taught in very clear and understandable terms. A five-week program is outlined, with step-by-step instructions that teach attending to the child, rewards, when to ignore the behavior, how to give directions, and how to implement an effective time-out. The program is then integrated with a focus on improved relationship, communication, and dealing with specific problem behaviors (e.g., tantrums, aggression, lying). This book will capture the interest of frustrated parents and effectively lead them through steps to improve their children's behavior.

★★★★ *The Hurried Child: Growing Up Too Fast Too Soon* (3rd ed., 2001) by David Elkind. Reading, MA: Addison-Wesley.

This book describes a pervasive and harmful condition that many children experience—growing up too fast and too soon. Elkind believes that many parents place excessive pressure on children to grow up quickly. He says that parents too often push children to be superkids, competent to deal with all of life's ups and downs. He believes that parents have invented the superkid to alleviate their own anxiety and guilt. But he doesn't just blame parents; he also faults schools and the media. Elkind argues that many parents expect their children to excel intellectually and demand achievement early in their lives. Excessive expectations are both academic and athletic: Parental pressures let children know that to be fully loved they have to win. In response, Elkin recommends respecting children's own developmental time tables, encouraging children to play and fantasize, making sure that expectations and support are in reasonable balance, and being polite. This four-star book highlights an important theme and provides insightful analysis: Parents want children to be stars but don't give them the necessary time and support.

★★★★   *Dr. Spock on Parenting* (1988) by Benjamin Spock. New York: Simon & Schuster.

This book is primarily a collection of articles that Dr. Spock wrote for *Redbook* magazine in the 1970s and 1980s. Topics include anxieties in our lives, being a father today, divorce and its consequences, the new baby, sleep problems, discipline, stages of childhood, difficult relationships, behavior problems, influencing personality and attitudes, and health and nutrition. In a chapter on discipline, Spock rebuts the criticism leveled at *Dr. Spock's Baby and Child Care* that he encourages parents to be too permissive. Spock says that he never promulgated such a philosophy and believes that parents should deal with their children in firm, clear ways. This four-star book is easy to read and generally dispenses sound parenting advice. The consensus of our experts in the national studies, however, was that several of the preceding books would be better choices on general approaches to parenting.

Recommended

★★★   *Touchpoints: Three to Six* (2001) by T. Berry Brazelton and Joshua Sparrow. Cambridge, MA: Perseus.

This book describes effective parenting techniques for parents with children who are 3–6 years of age. Teaming with child psychiatrist Joshua Sparrow, leading pediatrician T. Berry Brazelton addresses key issues in this developmental time frame, such as sibling rivalry, bed wetting, tantrums, and lying. Especially helpful are strategies for staying emotionally calm when children engage in these behaviors. The second half of the book provides approximately 200 pages of advice for parents on topics such as ADHD, divorce, computers, bad habits, and sadness. Brazelton's other self-help books are rated as four- and five-star books, and this recent book would have also reached five-star status if it had been known by more psychologists.

★★★   *Raising Resilient Children* (2001) by Robert Brooks and Sam Goldstein. New York: McGraw-Hill.

This book seeks to help parents focus on their children's strengths rather than spending too much time on improving their weaknesses. The authors argue that children's resilience has its most important roots in the home, nurtured by parents who provide their children with healthy doses of empathy, optimism, respect, unconditional love, listening skills, and patience. Detailed steps are given for rewriting negative parenting scripts, teaching and modeling empathy, and creating opportunities for children to be-have in responsible ways. This excellent self-help book likely would have been desig-nated a four- or five-star resource had been it more frequently rated in our national studies.

★★★ *The Mother Dance: How Your Children Change Your Life* (1999) by Harriet Lerner. New York: Harper Perennial.

Psychologist Lerner writes about the experience of being a mother and all of the changes that it entails, beginning with pregnancy and continuing through birth, power struggles, guilt, anxiety, relationship challenges, and other aspects of motherhood. The book is especially helpful for mothers-to-be as a guide for what they are likely to experi-ence in the future. Also, women who already are mothers can gain a better understand-ing of their experiences as mothers by reflecting on the experiences that Lerner frames.

★★★ *Positive Discipline A–Z* (1993) by Jane Nelsen, Lynn Lott, and H. Stephen Glenn. Rocklin, CA: Prima.

This book addresses 1,001 solutions to everyday parenting problems. The text covers parenting any age child but focuses on preteen children. Part I consists of helpful par-enting tools that set the stage for use of the positive discipline solutions to everyday problems (Part II). The tools are well-explained and include how to affect your child's behavior using concepts such as natural consequences, honesty, saying no, and using your sense of humor. The book also covers beliefs behind behavior. The text is guided by Adlerian principles and implements the approach effectively.

★★★ *Living with Children* (3rd ed., 1987) by Gerald Patterson. Champaign, IL: Research Press.

This behavior modification approach to disciplining children has an unusual style for a self-help book. It is written in a programmed instruction format that makes the material easy to learn. In this approach, main ideas are broken down into small units or items. Parents are asked to respond to the items actively, rather than just read them. Four sec-tions tell parents how learning takes place, how to change undesirable behavior, how normal children have normal problems, and what the problems of more seriously dis-turbed children are like. Patterson explains how reinforcement works and the impor-tance of rewarding children immediately. Parents learn to develop a plan for changing their child's undesirable behavior. They begin by observing and recording the child's behaviors, detecting what led to the behaviors and what followed them, as well as how the parents responded when the child behaved in undesirable ways. Parents then learn to respond to the child's behaviors differently than they have in the past. Time-out fig-ures prominently in replacing the child's negative behaviors with positive ones. This simple but powerful book helps parents replace a child's undesirable behaviors with de-sirable ones by rearranging the way they respond to the child. Its three-star rating is somewhat misleading: The book secured very positive ratings but was not rated fre-quently enough to reach the four- or five-star categories.

★★★ *How to Discipline Your Six- to Twelve-Year-Old without Losing Your Mind* (1991) by Jerry Wyckoff and Barbara Unell. New York: Doubleday.

As its title suggests, this book falls into the category of discipline techniques for parents. The authors define discipline as a teaching system that leads to orderliness and control. Chapters focus on topics such as social problems, school problems, noise, children wanting their own way, irresponsibility and disorganization, sleeping and eating, hygiene problems, self-image problems, and activities. Each chapter begins with the statement of a problem followed by a brief description of how the problem can be prevented. Then, the authors tell parents how to solve the problem. A "what not to do" section is also included. Although the book's title indicates that it is about discipline, in reality the book is a general parenting guide that provides suggestions for preventing and solving typical childhood problems. The experts' three-star rating conveys the impression that the book does a good job of providing parents with concrete advice in an easy-to-read format.

Diamonds in the Rough

◆ *Helping the Child Who Doesn't Fit In* (1992) by Stephen Nowicki and Marshall Duke. Atlanta, GA: Peachtree.

Nonverbal communication deficits are described as the most common reason for social rejection and alienation suffered by children. The authors present skills and accompanying exercises for the parents and children to practice together. Receptive or expressive deficits in the areas of facial gestures, body gestures, voice tone, use of timing, and style of dress are identified through assessment exercises conducted by the parents. Once the problem is targeted, remedial exercises are recommended and explained. This book registers as a Diamond in the Rough for its favorable but few ratings and its effective materials in helping children build interpersonal skills.

◆ *Common Sense Parenting* (1996) by Ray Burke and Ron Herron. Boys Town, NB: Boys Town.

Many parents doubt their effectiveness as parents. This book is written for those parents who wish to improve their parenting skills with what the authors call a blueprint for parenting: practical, down-to-earth teaching and unconditional love coupled with spending time together. The skills material is systematically presented in an understandable manner in the following format: presentation of a skill, examples and illustrations of how to use it, how not to use it, and a variety of typical situations. The book is applicable to children of any age and includes skills development topics such as positive and negative consequences, praise, clear expectations, making decisions, and teaching self-control. This book is included as a Diamond in the Rough because it received very high ratings, albeit from a small number of psychologists.

◆ *Raising Black Children* (1992) by James P. Comer and Alvin E. Poussaint. New York: Plume.

Written by a pair of highly respected experts on black children, this book argues that African American parents face additional difficulties in raising emotionally healthy children because of problems related to minority status and income. Comer and

Poussaint's guide contains almost 1,000 child-rearing questions they have repeatedly heard from black parents across the income spectrum. Among the issues on which they offer advice are how to improve the child's self-esteem and identity; how to confront racism; how to teach children to handle anger, conflict, and frustration; and how to deal with the mainstream culture and still retain a black identity. This excellent self-help book includes pertinent suggestions that are not found in most child-rearing books. Virtually all other child-rearing books are written for white, middle-class parents and do not deal with many of the problems faced by black parents, especially those from low-income backgrounds.

♦ *Parenting Young Children: Systematic Training for Effective Parenting (STEP) of Children Under Six* (1997) by Don C. Dinkmeyer and Gary D. McKay. Circle Pines, MN: American Guidance Service.

This is the accompanying text for the STEP (Systematic Training for Effective Parenting) program that has trained thousands of parents across the country to become more effective communicators with their children. Dinkmeyer and McKay believe that democratic child rearing is the best strategy for parents. In democratic child rearing, both parent and child are socially equal in the family and mutually respect each other. The authors explain why children misbehave (to get attention, achieve power, mete out revenge, or display inadequacy). They suggest family activities and encourage parents to develop parenting goals. Parents are told how to get in touch with their own emotions and understand their children better. Encouragement, communication skills, and discipline methods that develop responsibility are advocated. One chapter is exclusively devoted to the family meeting, in which all members of the family have an equal opportunity to discuss issues of concern. *Systematic Training for Effective Parenting* received a very high positive rating but was evaluated by only eight respondents. The book is brief (less than 100 pages) and somewhat sketchy, without the accompanying parenting course that it is designed to supplement. Several mental health professionals mentioned that its exercises and goal-setting strategies are especially effective, but that the depth of coverage and extensive examples in other books make them more attractive on their own. The best use of this book is in conjunction with the parent training workshops developed by the authors.

Not Recommended

★★ *Parent Power! A Common Sense Approach to Parenting in the '90s and Beyond* (1990) by John K. Rosemond. Kansas City, MO: Andrews & McMeel.

FILMS

Strongly Recommended

★★★★ *Searching for Bobby Fischer* (1994) directed by Steven Zaillian. PG rating. 110 minutes.

When a seven-year-old boy and his father discover that he has a gift for chess, the boy begins a conflicted journey to become the next Bobby Fischer. His father and coach relentlessly drive him to become ruthless, single-minded, and competitive beyond a level of decency that the boy and his mother value. The boy accommodates the wishes of his father and coach for a while, but when he and his mother realize that his very life is at stake, he returns to playing chess in the local park and makes difficult but confirming choices. This is a compelling morality tale about and for parents who drive their children, children who feel the pressure and desire to please their parents, and families learning to cherish the true value of nurturance.

★★★★ *Little Man Tate* (1991) directed by Jodie Foster. PG rating. 99 minutes.

Young Fred Tate and his single-parent mother are a working-class family. They love each other and find great enjoyment in their lives. Tension and uncertainty arise when the mother realizes that Fred is a genius and, though she can give him the safety and caring, she cannot provide the intellectual stimulation he requires. She sends him to a school for the gifted, where his teacher focuses only on his intellectual abilities. Only when the two women work together for Fred's welfare does he truly grow and learn. The film is about the decision of what is best for one's child and how to balance the many dimensions of a child's growth.

★★★★ *I Am Sam* (2001) directed by Jessie Nelson. PG-13 rating. 132 minutes.

The title character has the mental capacity of a seven-year-old and a daughter with a homeless woman, who abandons father and daughter. Sam raises his daughter, but as she reaches age seven herself, Sam's intellectual limitations begin to impede his daughter's academic performance. The state authorities remove the daughter, and Sam sues for custody. In the process, we learn about genuine parental love and the priority of a child's needs. Despite the predictable plot, a tender parable about parenting.

Recommended

★★★ *Big* (1989) directed by Penny Marshall. PG rating. 104 minutes.

Twelve-year-old Josh yearns to be older, so that he can be taken more seriously, especially by Cynthia, who has stolen his heart. After being rejected by Cynthia at the carnival, he wanders over to the wish machine, where his wish to grow up fast is granted. The next morning, he wakes up as an adult. He remains an imaginative, fun-loving, spontaneous youngster in an adult existence. We are reminded that adults could use a good dose of Josh's qualities in order to enjoy life more and to truly connect with others and with life. Josh's compelling honesty and virtuosity play out in a corporate advertising environment to remind us of the power of basic morality and good deeds.

★★★ *Parenthood* (1990) directed by Ron Howard. PG-13 rating. 124 minutes.

The common yet terribly difficult challenge of raising children is effectively illuminated through the eyes of the main character, Gil (played by Steve Martin). Gil is the son of Frank, whose other three adult children continue to bring their problems home to him. Gil has three children of his own, for whom he wants to be a better dad than his father was. Frank discovers that not rescuing his adult children is in fact the only way to help save them. Gil learns that bringing home the bacon and being home for the family are in a continuing balance. This film lets parents know that they are not alone in their uncertainties, anxieties, and dreams.

Not Recommended

★★ *Baby Boom* (1987) directed by Charles Shyer. PG rating. 110 minutes.

INTERNET RESOURCES

Metasites

★★★★★ *Parenthood.com* http://www.www.parenthood.com/links.html

A comprehensive source of pregnancy, parenting, and child care articles and websites. Categories include child care, education, health, fatherhood, finance, nutrition, organizations, safety issues, product recalls, infertility, and online shopping.

★★★★★ *Tufts University Child and Family Webguide* http://www.cft.tufts.edu

Under five or six headings such as Daycare, Education, and Parenting are links to hundreds of sites. This guide briefly describes and assigns stars to "web sites that contain research-based information about child development . . . [which] have been selected from thousands of sites about children, based primarily on the quality of the information provided. The goal of the WebGuide is to give the public easy access to the best child development information on the Web."

★★★★ *Information for Parents* http://www.childdevelopmentinfo.com

This site offers over a hundred readings in every aspect of development, school, parenting, and disorders. Most are several pages long and well written for handing out. Thank you, Robert Meyers, PhD.

Psychoeducational Materials for Clients and Families

★★★★★ *NPIN: National Parent Information Network*
            http://ericps.crc.uiuc.edu/npin/index.html

This site has endless high-quality information on the education of children for parents, professionals, and researchers. Click for the bimonthly magazine *Parent News*, with first-class articles on a variety of topics, from sexuality and sportsmanship to school safety. One of the best features is that parents can AskERIC and get answers.

★★★★★ *NPIN Resources for Parents: Full Texts of Parenting-Related Materials*
            http://ericps.crc.uiuc.edu/npin/library/texts.html

Full-text electronic versions of pamphlets, brochures, guides, and other materials. Dozens of articles are available under the following headings: Assessment and Testing, Child Care, Children and the Media, Children with Special Needs, Children's Health and Nutrition, Early Childhood–Family/Peer Relationships, Early Childhood—Learning, Gifted Children, Helping Children Learn at Home, Older Children, Pre-Teens and Young Adolescents, Parents and Families in Society, Parents and Schools as Partners, and Teens.

★★★★★   *Today's Parent Online*   http://www.todaysparent.com

For lots of high-quality information on each developmental stage, go to Step and Stages, select an age (from 0 to 12) and use the pop-up menus to choose an article, then click on Go.

★★★★★   *Facts for Families*   http://www.aacap.org/publications/factsfam/index.htm

Almost a hundred "fact sheets" on almost any topic of relevance to adolescents from the American Academy of Child and Adolescent Psychiatry. Ideal for introducing a topic or general public education efforts.

★★★★   *ParenthoodWeb*   http://www.parenthood.com

A magazine with all kinds of information and advice.

★★★★   *KidSource Online*   http://www.kidsource.com

This is basically a magazine with a gigantic collection of good-quality readings. It is perhaps best used by people who need an orientation to the world of children. It is organized by age of children, followed by some general articles.

★★★★   *Parenting: General Parenting Articles*
          http://www.kidsource.com/kidsource/pages/parenting.general.html

About 100 articles are described, rated, and available online. They cover almost everything and will guide parents well.

★★★★   *Family Life Library*
          http://www.oznet.ksu.edu/library/famlf2/#Family%20Living

Page down to Managing Time, Work, and Family for nine articles, suitable as handouts, and brochures from a Kansas State University program. They have to be downloaded and opened in Adobe's Acrobat Reader.

★★★★   *Cambridge Center for Behavioral Studies*   http://www.behavior.org

The Parenting section offers several good essays as well as collections of articles. Solid behavioral approaches.

★★★★   *Children* by Kalman Heller, PhD   http://www.drheller.com/index.html

Here, under Parenting and Marriage, Children, are about 20 short but very well-written and authoritative essays by an obviously experienced psychologist.

★★★   *HealthyKids*   http://www.americanbaby.com/hk/CDA/homepage/

A commercial site with good advice on recipes, activities, illnesses, and the like. This would serve as an ideal introduction to using online resources for guidance and exploration.

★★★   *Family Keys: Self-Care Resources for Children and Their Families*
      http://www.uwex.edu/ces/flp/parenting/keys.html

These 12 brochures cover such topics as family rules, phone skills, first aid, safe at home, nutritious snacks, and the like. They are written at the fifth-grade reading level and were developed by the University of Wisconsin.

Specific Aspects of Parenting

★★★★★   *Project NoSpank* http://www.nospank.net/toc.htm

A superb site for those who wish to campaign against paddling in the schools or to educate parents. Lots of research, cases, links, and logic. For those partial to James Dobson's views, see section 72.

★★★★★   *Common Sense: Strategies for Raising Alcohol- and Drug-Free Children*
      http://www.pta.org/commonsense

A project of the National PTA, the site is simple and pretty. The contents are well-designed for effectiveness. The Parent's Center offers hard-hitting interactive quizzes, drug facts and risk, warning signs, guidance on discipline, being a role model, and getting closer. A nice package of materials that should have an effect on families with drug and alcohol concerns.

★★★★   *People, Places, and Things That Help Me*
      http://www.kidshealth.org/kid/feel_better/index.html

If you need information for children about going to the hospital, dentist, or other medical service, the 20 readings here are excellent.

★★★★   *Contact a Family* http://www.cafamily.org.uk

Information and support for people caring for children with rare disorders. If parents need this kind of material, this is the best place to get it.

★★★★   *Dealing with Feelings* http://www.kidshealth.org/kid/feeling/index.html

There are 50 readings here of about four pages each. They really deal with contexts, not just labeled emotions. Examples are A Kid's Guide to Divorce, Am I Too Fat or Too Thin?, Are You Shy?, and Why Am I So Sad?

★★★★   *National Center for Fathering* http://www.fathers.com

Under Fathering Tips are about 30 practical tips, plus hundreds of brief and sometimes sappy essays on stages, responsibilities, and functions. It is best as a source of beginning ideas or expanding some men's ideas of what it could mean to be a father.

★★★★   *Foster Parent Community* http://www.fosterparents.com

Although the site offers support through chat and boards, the best part is the two-dozen articles under Online Training. They are information-packed and relevant.

★★★   *So What Are Dads Good For?* http://www.io.com/~duanev/family/dads.html

A fine essay, with insight and guidance for the confused.

★★★   *Full Texts of Parenting-Related Materials: Gifted Children*
        http://npin.org/searchvl.html

Type the word *gifted* to find the relevant readings. These readings vary from 3 to about 10 pages and address ADHD and Children Who Are Gifted; College Planning for Gifted and Talented Youth; How Can I Help My Gifted Child Plan for College?; How Parents Can Support Gifted Children; and Should Gifted Students Be Grade Advanced?

See also Infant Development and Parenting (Chapter 21) and Teenagers and Parenting (Chapter 34).

CHAPTER 14

Communication
and People Skills

We get things done by talking with family, friends, colleagues, and neighbors. When someone doesn't quite grasp what we are saying, we often let it go, the talk continues, and nobody pays much attention. But some conversations have critical outcomes that hinge on the effectiveness of the conversation—a job interview, a business meeting, a marriage proposal, a family decision. In these circumstances, ineffective communication can have serious negative consequences: We don't get the job, don't convince our business colleagues, don't get engaged, and don't collaborate as a family.

Sometimes strained conversations reflect genuine differences between people. On many occasions, though, strained conversations develop when people simply are miscommunicating. Their conversations could readily be improved by understanding the nature of interpersonal communication and by acquiring people skills.

Communication and people skills are hot items on self-help lists. Whether it is general interpersonal abilities, female–male communication, or negotiating agreements, humans seem to crave "knowing" one other. In this chapter, we review self-help books, films, and Internet sites devoted to these quintessentially human skills.

SELF-HELP BOOKS

Strongly Recommended

★★★★ *You Just Don't Understand: Women and Men in Conversation* (1990) by Deborah Tannen. New York: Ballantine.

As its title implies, this book is about how women and men communicate—or, all too often, miscommunicate—with each other. *You Just Don't Understand* reached number one

RECOMMENDATION HIGHLIGHTS

Self-Help Books

- On learning a wide range of communication and people skills:
    - ★★★★ *The Dance of Connection* by Harriet Lerner
    - ★★★★ *How to Communicate* by Matthew McKay et al.
    - ★★★★ *People Skills* by Robert Bolton
    - ★★★★ *The New Peoplemaking* by Virginia Satir

- On improving female–male communication:
    - ★★★★ *You Just Don't Understand* by Deborah Tannen
    - ★★★★ *Intimate Strangers* by Lillian Rubin

- On defining boundaries and clarifying responsibilities:
    - ★★★★ *Boundaries* by Henry Cloud and John Townsend

- On negotiating agreements:
    - ★★★★ *Getting to Yes* by Roger Fisher and William Ury

- On the healing power of confiding in others:
    - ★★★ *Opening Up* by James Pennebaker

- On overcoming shyness and being less lonely:
    - ★★★★ *Shyness* by Philip Zimbardo
    - ★★★★ *Intimate Connections* by David Burns

- On friendship and its important roles in our lives:
    - ★★★★ *Just Friends* by Lillian Rubin

Films

- On demonstrating love and triumph over adversity:
    - ★★★★★ *Children of a Lesser God*

- On inspiring creativity and individuality at a cost:
    - ★★★★ *Dead Poets Society*

Internet Resources

- On improving communication skills:
    - ★★★★★ *The Seven Challenges* http://www.coopcomm.org/workbook.htm

- On raising awareness of communication problems:
    - ★★★ *Communication Skills Test–Revised*
      http://queendom.com/tests/relationships/
      communication_skills_r_access.html

- On enhancing public speaking skills:
    - ★★★★ *Virtual Presentation Assistant*
      http://www.ukans.edu/cwis/units/coms2/vpa/vpa.htm

on several best-seller lists. Tannen shows that friction between women and men in conversation often develops because, as girls and boys, they were brought up in two virtually distinct cultures and continue to live in those two different cultures. The two gender cultures are rapport talk (female culture) and report talk (male culture). Rapport talk is the language of conversation and a way of establishing connections and negotiating relationships, with which women feel more comfortable. Report talk is public speaking, with which men feel more comfortable. Tannen illustrates miscommunication in male–female relationships with several cartoons about a husband and wife at the breakfast table. Harmful and unjustified misinterpretations might be avoided by understanding the conversational styles of the other gender. The problem, then, may not be an individual man, or even men's styles, but the difference between women's and men's styles. If so, both women and men need to make adjustments. In the public context, a woman can push herself to speak up without being invited or begin to speak at even the slightest pause in talk. Men can make women feel more comfortable by warmly encouraging and allowing them to speak rather than hogging public talk for themselves. This excellent four-star self-help book has been especially taken up by women who, after reading the book, want their male partner to read it too. Tannen's book is solidly written, well-researched, and entertaining.

★★★★　*Boundaries: When to Say Yes, When to Say No to Take Control of Your Life* (1992) by Henry Cloud and John Townsend. Grand Rapids, MI: Zondervan.

A boundary is a personal line that defines identity and responsibility. In this fine book, Cloud and Townsend define several types of boundaries (e.g., physical, mental, emotional, and spiritual) and help people clarify their boundaries. This is accomplished in various ways, such as setting limits and changing how one feels about setting boundaries. The authors take a biblical and psychological approach to constructing healthy boundaries. Under the Law of Exposure, the authors remind us that the entire concept revolves around the fact that we exist in relationships. An excellent resource for individuals looking to clarify boundaries, especially for those interested in blending psychology and scripture.

★★★　*The Dance of Connection* by Harriet Lerner (2002). New York: Quill.

This book examines the verbal challenges of life's most painful conversations with a special emphasis on women's experiences. Lerner counsels women on how to speak out in stressful circumstances, such as when their husband is having an affair or when friends jeopardize their relationship by becoming roommates. She provides advice on how to complain, how to request, how to apologize, and how to listen and set limits on the extent to which one is willing to listen to others' negativity. It is another excellent resource from psychologist Lerner, who also authored *The Dance of Anger*.

★★★★　*Intimate Strangers* (revised ed., 1990) by Lillian Rubin. New York: Harper & Row.

This book focuses on intimacy and communication difficulties between women and men. Rubin tackles a relationship problem that confronts many women and men—their inability to develop a satisfying intimate relationship with each other. Rubin says that male–female differences in intimacy are related to the fact that it is primarily mothers who raise children and are the emotional managers of the family. Because girls identify with mothers and boys with fathers, females develop a capacity for intimacy and an interest in managing emotional problems, and males do not. Rubin supports her ideas with a number of case studies derived from interviews with approximately 150 couples. She provides detailed insights about the nature of intimacy and communication problems in sexual matters and in raising children. Rubin concludes that the only solution to the intimacy gulf between females and males is for every child to be raised and nurtured by two loving parents, not just the mother, from birth on. That is, Rubin's culprit is the nonnurturant father, who, she says, has to change his ways and serve as a nurturing, intimate role model, committed to managing emotional difficulties. Although this four-star resource is reviewed in this chapter, its contents also apply to several other categories, including marriage, love, and intimacy.

★★★★   *The New Peoplemaking* (1988) by Virginia Satir. Palo Alto, CA: Science & Behavior Books.

This book is aimed at improving communication with a select group of people in your life—family members. Virginia Satir, a pioneer in family therapy, originally published *Peoplemaking* in 1972, then revised it for 1988 publication. Based on her extensive observations as a leading family therapist, Satir describes four areas that can lead to troubles for families: self-worth, communication, family system, and link to society. In her observations, troubled families invariably have low levels of self-worth, communication patterns that are indirect or dishonest, rigid systems of rules, and relate to the rest of society in fearful, placating, and blaming ways. Satir encourages readers to explore their own family dynamics to see how they stack up in regard to the four areas. Although dated in some sections, *The New Peoplemaking* still contains some valuable advice, especially for couples who want to communicate effectively, and for parents who want to communicate with their children.

★★★★   *How to Communicate: The Ultimate Guide to Improving Your Personal and Professional Relationships* (1997) by Matthew McKay, Martha Davis, and Patrick Fanning. New York: Fine.

The premise of this book is that communication makes life work. The authors tell what to do about communicating rather than what to think. The emphasis is on skills (e.g., basic, advanced, conflict, social, family, and public skills). The authors recommend that you read the basic and advanced skills chapters first, then go on to the specific chapters appropriate to your relationships and position in life. Contained in the basic skills section are listening, self-disclosure, and expressing skills. In the advanced skills section is information on body language, paralanguage (vocal component), hidden agendas, and clarifying skills. For adults and older adolescents looking to improve their communication style, this four-star book is worthwhile.

★★★★   *Getting to Yes: Negotiating Agreement without Giving In* (revised ed., 1991) by Roger Fisher and William Ury. New York: Penguin.

This concise book (only about 150 pages) offers a step-by-step method for arriving at mutually acceptable agreements, whether between parents and children, neighbors, bosses and employees, customers and business managers, or tenants and landlords. Fisher and Ury describe how to:

- Separate people from the problem.
- Emphasize interests, not positions.
- Develop precise goals at the outset of negotiations.
- Work together to establish options that will satisfy both parties.
- Negotiate successfully with opponents who are more powerful, refuse to play by the rules, or resort to dirty tricks.

The book is based on the method of principled negotiation developed as part of the Harvard Negotiation Project. This method helps people evaluate issues based on their merits instead of regressing to a haggling process in which each side says what it will and won't do. It teaches negotiators to look for mutual gains whenever possible. The method of principled negotiation is hard on the merits of the issues, soft on the people. It uses no tricks and no posturing. Although written more than a decade ago, this four-star book remains one of the best, easy-to-read resources for learning how to negotiate effectively in a wide range of situations.

★★★★ *Shyness* (1987) by Philip Zimbardo. Reading, MA: Addison-Wesley.

This book is dedicated to helping people overcome social isolation and become more gregarious. What does psychologist Zimbardo say shy people can do about their situation? First, they have to analyze their shyness and figure out how they got this way. Possible reasons include negative evaluations, fear of being rejected, fear of intimacy, and lack of adequate social skills, among others. Second, they need to build their self-esteem. To help with this, Zimbardo spells out 15 steps to becoming more confident. Third, shy people need to improve their social skills. To accomplish this, Zimbardo describes several behavior modification strategies, tells how to set realistic goals, and advocates working hard toward achieving these goals. *Shyness* received a robust four-star rating as a well-known (164 respondents), excellent self-help book for shy people. It gives sound advice, is free of psychobabble, and is easy to read.

★★★★ *Intimate Connections: The New Clinically Tested Program for Overcoming Loneliness* (1985) by David Burns. New York: Morrow.

This book, a program for overcoming loneliness, is authored by David Burns, famous for *Feeling Good*, a book on depression. Burns believes that loneliness is essentially a state of mind that is primarily caused by the faulty assumption that a loving partner is needed before one can feel happy and secure. He says that the first step in breaking free from loneliness is learning to like and love oneself. He also distinguishes between two types of loneliness: situational loneliness, which lasts for only a brief time and can be healthy and motivating; and chronic loneliness, which persists and results from problems that have plagued people for most of their lives. Burns says that to overcome chronic loneliness, a person has to change the patterns of perception that created the loneliness and continue to perpetuate it. Among the topics Burns touches on are how to make social connections, how to get close to others, and how to improve one's sexual life. Checklists, worksheets, daily mood logs, and a number of self-assessments are found throughout the book, which received a four-star rating. This is a good self-help book—full of straightforward advice and helpful examples—for helping people over-come their loneliness.

★★★★ *People Skills* (reissued ed., 1986) by Robert Bolton. New York: Touchstone.

This book, dedicated to improving human communication, is divided into four main parts. Part I, the Introduction, describes a number of skills for bridging gaps in inter-personal communication and barriers to communicating effectively. Part II, Listening Skills, explains how listening is different from merely hearing, how to develop the im-portant skill of reflective listening, and how to read body language. Part III, Assertion Skills, outlines a number of valuable techniques to help a person become more assertive in relationships. Part IV, Conflict Management Skills, discusses how to manage conflict effectively in many different circumstances. *People Skills* received a four-star rating in our studies despite the fact that the book was originally published in 1981. However, a number of the mental health professionals concluded that it remains one of the best general introductions to communication skills.

★★★★ *Just Friends: The Role of Friendship in Our Lives* (1985) by Lillian Rubin. New York: Harper & Row.

Author Rubin, who penned *Intimate Strangers* evaluated earlier in this chapter, examines the nature of intimacy and friendship in this book. She analyzes the nature of the val-ued yet fragile bond of friendship between women, between men, between women and men, between best friends, and in couples. She says that, unlike many other relation-ships, friendship is a private affair, with no rituals, social contracts, shared tasks, role re-quirements, or institutional supports of any kind. Rubin believes friends are central players in our lives—not just in childhood, but in adulthood as well. Friends give us a reference outside of our families against which we can judge and evaluate ourselves; they help us develop an independent sense of self and support our efforts to adapt to new circumstances and stressful situations. This is an insightful analysis of the impor-tant and often overlooked role that friends play in our lives. However, some critics said that Rubin exaggerates sex differences in friendships and fails to provide sufficient practical tools for enhancing friendships.

Recommended

★★★ *That's Not What I Meant! How Conversational Style Makes or Breaks Relationships* (1986, reprinted 1991) by Deborah Tannen. New York: Ballantine.

This book provides a broader understanding of the inner workings of conversation than Tannen's earlier reviewed book, *You Just Don't Understand*. Tannen believes that different conversational styles are at the heart of miscommunication. But conversational confusion between the sexes is only part of the picture. Tannen shows that growing up in different parts of the country, having different ethnic and class backgrounds, being of different ages, and possessing different personality traits all contribute to different conversational styles that can cause disappointment, hurt, and misplaced blame. *That's Not What I Meant!* received a three-star rating in one of our studies, just missing a four-star rating. This is a good self-help book that provides a rich understanding of how conversational styles make or break relationships. Compared to *You Just Don't Understand*, this book includes more basic information about communication skills, which are covered in other books, although Tannen does a better job of describing these skills than most other authors.

★★★   *Opening Up: The Healing Power of Confiding in Others* (1997) by James Pennebaker. New York: Guilford Press.

As its subtitle indicates, this book concerns the healing power of confiding in other people. It deals with the following issues:

- Why suppressing inner turmoil has a devastating effect on health.
- How denial of mental pain can cause physical pain.
- Why talking or writing about troubling thoughts protects us from the internal stresses that cause physical illness.

Psychologist Pennebaker's advice is not based only on his own opinions. For more than a decade, he has studied thousands of people in many different contexts to learn how confessing troubling feelings benefit health. What is surprising about Pennebaker's findings is that the benefits of confession occur whether you tell your secrets to someone else or simply write about them privately. Pennebaker is especially adept at pinpointing how the hard work of inhibiting troublesome thoughts and feelings gradually undermines the body's defenses. *Opening Up* received a three-star rating in our national study, probably because it was not well-known at the time it was rated. One of the rare self-help books that is based on hard science, this contribution deserves to be better known and more frequently read.

★★★   *Coping with Difficult People* (1981) by Robert Bramson. New York: Dell.

In this self-help resource, Bramson describes and presents strategies for coping with the following types of difficult people:

- The Hostile Aggressive, who bullies by bombarding, making cutting remarks, or throwing tantrums.
- The Complainer, who gripes incessantly but never gets any closer to solving the problem.
- The Silent Unresponsive, who is always reasonable, sincere, and supportive to your face but never comes through.
- The Negativist, who responds to any proposal with statements such as "It will never work."
- The Know-It-All, who is confident that he or she knows everything there is to know about anything worth knowing.
- The Indecisive, who delays any important decision until the outcome is certain and refuses to let go of anything until it's perfect—which is never.

Bramson outlines a six-step plan to cope with these people and make life less stressful. This three-star book is entertaining reading, and the author uses a lot of catchy labels to get his points across and grab the reader's attention, such as describing Know-It-Alls as bulldozers and balloons, and Hostile Aggressives as Sherman tanks, snipers, and exploders. Written several decades ago, *Coping with Difficult People* has been successful, with sales of more than 500,000 copies. The mental health experts in our national studies recommended the book for improved understanding of people in work rather than family settings; because the author's background is in managerial consulting, many of the examples come from work settings.

★★★   *Games People Play* (1964) by Eric Berne. New York: Grove.

Psychiatrist Eric Berne was the founder of transactional analysis, an approach to understanding interpersonal relationships that emphasizes communication patterns. He maintained that people live their lives by playing out games in their interpersonal relationships. People play games to manipulate others, avoid reality, and conceal ulterior motives. Berne analyzes 36 different games, which he divides into seven main categories:

- Life games, which pervade every person's behavior.
- Marital games, which partners may use to maintain a frustrating and unrewarding life.
- Sexual games, in which one person provokes sexual reactions in another and then acts like an innocent victim.
- Party games, which are highly social and include perpetual gossip.
- Consulting room games, played by a patient with a doctor to avoid cure (as in psychiatry).
- Underworld games, which are most often played for material gain but can also be played for psychological gain.
- Good games, which involve social contributions that outweigh the complexity of underlying motivation and manipulation.

Games People Play received a three-star rating in one of our national studies. On the positive side, many characterize the book as a self-help classic that has been a huge bestseller. It was one of the most frequently rated books in our studies. People who read it will find numerous examples that apply to their own lives. And Berne connects with readers through catchy, witty writing. You can read about the Sweetheart, the Threadbare, the Schlemiel, the Stocking Game, the Wooden Leg, and the Swymd (see what you made me do). Although the book is now four decades old, some psychotherapists continue to recommend it to clients who are having communication problems and use Berne's transactional analysis in their practice. On the other side, this book has steadily faded in professional popularity, and many will find it dated in content and tone. Some critics opine that Berne overdramatizes the role of game playing in intimate relationships, that the parent–adult–child aspect of Berne's approach is overly simplistic, and that the games reiterate traditional male and female orientations.

★★★   *Difficult People: How to Deal with Impossible Clients, Bosses and Employees* (1990) by Roberta Cava. Toronto: Key Porter.

This book addresses the stress of dealing with rude, impatient, emotional, persistent, and aggressive people. People learn to control their moods by not allowing other people to give them negative feelings, by improving their people skills. The author first helps identify emotional behavior by having readers answer specific questions, examine techniques for specific stressful situations, look at consequences of behavior, and examine approaches to conflict resolution. Reviewed are basic communication skills, communication skills for specific situations, gender influences, and ratings of listening and speaking skills. Three chapters address difficult clients, supervisors, coworkers, and subordinates. For adults who find themselves faced with difficult people, this book could provide some informative advice and practical skills.

★★★ *Stop! You're Driving Me Crazy* (1979) by George Bach and Ronald Deutsch. New York: Berkley.

This book covers a broad array of communication strategies to help, in the authors' words, "keep the people in your life from driving you up the wall." It spells out the authors' catchy concept of "crazymaking." Crazymaking describes a variety of harmful communication patterns that are passive–aggressive in nature. Passive–aggressive individuals consciously like, love, or at least respect each other but unconsciously undermine rather than build up the morale and mental well-being of friends, lovers, or spouses. Some examples of passive–aggressive crazymaking include the following: A husband stirs up a screaming fight and then wants to make passionate love; a boss gives an employee a promotion and then says, "You're worthless"; and a young woman tells her mother that she is on a crash diet, and the mother then bakes her a chocolate cake.

The authors help the reader cope with and eliminate such crazymaking techniques. On the borderline between two and three stars, this book just managed the three-star rating. An early success that achieved best-seller status in the early 1980s, its popularity has waned. Several of our experts criticized the book for being too sensational, gender-biased, and difficult to read in places.

Diamond in the Rough

♦ *The Talk Book: The Intimate Science of Communicating in Close Relationships* (1988) by Gerald Goodman and Glenn Esterly. New York: Ballantine.

Talk is an essential tool for ensuring the success of all close relationships, and *The Talk Book* is about ways to improve face-to-face communication. The authors describe six communication tools that contribute to using talk more effectively: disclosures, reflections, interpretations, advisements, questions, and silences. These talk tools fashion most of the meaning in everyday conversation. Understood well, they can help improve close relationships. Each chapter ends with a section that includes several tested methods for improving mastery of talk and making sense of another person's talk. This resource made the Diamond in the Rough category: It was rated positively but by too few experts. This is a solid book on conversation skills written by a leading expert. *The Talk Book*'s main drawbacks are its length (almost 400 pages of small type) and encyclopedic tendencies.

Not Recommended

★★ *How to Start a Conversation and Make Friends* (2001, revised ed.) by Don Gabor. New York: Simon & Schuster.

★★ *Men Are from Mars, Women Are from Venus* (1992) by John Gray. New York: HarperCollins.

★★ *How to Argue and Win Everytime* (1995) by Gerry Spence. New York: St. Martin's Press.

★ *Body Language* (1970) by Julius Fast. New York: Pocket Books.

★ *How to Win Friends and Influence People* (revised ed., 1981) by Dale Carnegie. New York: Simon & Schuster.

★ *Are You the One for Me?* (1998) by Barbara DeAngelis. London: Thorsons.

Strongly Not Recommended

† *Mars and Venus on a Date* (1997) by John Gray. New York: HarperCollins.

FILMS

Strongly Recommended

★★★★★ *Children of a Lesser God* (1987) directed by Randa Haines. R rating. 119 minutes.

Marlee Matlin, who is hearing impaired, won an Academy Award for her performance as a young hearing-impaired woman who refuses to read lips or try to learn to speak. She encountered a teacher of the deaf who is both attracted to her and single-minded in implementing his ideas that the deaf should read lips and speak. The film, a love story, is more a story of triumph over adversity and the struggle for control between two people. Those who live with physical or emotional obstacles will find spirit and love winning out in this excellent five-star film.

★★★★ *Dead Poets Society* (1990) directed by Peter Weir. PG rating. 129 minutes.

John Keating is a brilliant and inspiring English teacher who returns to the New England private school that he attended as a youth. He brings poetry, literature, and pursuit of life to his students, and in so doing, brings to life their spirit, self-confidence, and independence. The school doesn't approve of his teaching style. When a student is encouraged to confront his parents about his career direction and the parents remove him from the school, the boy commits suicide. The death is subsequently blamed on Keating. The film reminds us that the exhilaration of learning through spontaneity, nurtured curiosity, and creativity is to be cherished; the rebelliousness and individuality that often result from unbridled growth must be handled conscientiously. Also reviewed under Teenagers and Parenting (Chapter 34).

Not Recommended

★★ *He Said, She Said* (1990) directed by Ken Kwapis and Marisa Silver. PG-13 rating. 115 minutes.

INTERNET RESOURCES

Surprisingly little material on the web deals with communication and other people skills. There are many sites about marital and sexual relationships, and those can be found in Marriage (Chapter 23) and Families and Stepfamilies (Chapter 20). The numerous sites about communication in business and in groups are not included here, nor are the commercial sites with little of value to self-changers or psychotherapy clients.

Psychoeducational Materials for Clients and Families

★★★★★ *The Seven Challenges* http://www.coopcomm.org/workbook.htm

Here you will find a seven-chapter workbook in communication skills by Dennis Rivers, MA. Each topic takes only a few pages and is stated as a challenge: listening more attentively and responsively; explaining your conversational intent and inviting consent; expressing yourself more clearly and completely; translating complaints and criticisms into requests; asking more open-ended, creative questions; expressing more appreciation; and making better communication an important part of everyday living. These topics might be assigned as self-help exercises or downloaded and used in therapy.

★★★★ *Arguing and Relationships: Introduction*
        http://www.queendom.com/articles/love/arguing_rules.html

Four pages presenting guidelines for constructive arguing and a list of books on improving communication skills.

★★★★ *Virtual Presentation Assistant*
        http://www.ukans.edu/cwis/units/coms2/vpa/vpa.htm

This is an online tutorial of nine, single-page papers for improving public speaking skills.

★★★ *Communicating When Anger Is Involved*
        http://www.dataguru.org/love/misc/communicate.asp

Only one page, but very clear on how anger is to be expected, and that disagreements are normal and escalation is not. Useful as a starting point.

★★★ *Communication Skills Test–Revised*
        http://queendom.com/tests/relationships/communication_skills_r_access.html

Thirty-four questions with interactive feedback. Most useful for the breadth of the questions in sensitizing a client.

Other Resources

★★ *Toastmasters International* http://www.toastmasters.org

This international voluntary group offers free or low-cost training, feedback, and practice making speeches to business, civic, and other groups. There are chapters everywhere. Click on "Speaking Tips" for 10 tips for successful public speaking.

See also Love and Intimacy (Chapter 22) and Marriage (Chapter 23).

CHAPTER 15

Death and Grieving

The famous psychotherapist Erich Fromm once commented that "Man is the only animal that finds his own existence a problem he has to solve and from which he cannot escape." He went on to say that "in the same sense man is the only animal who knows he must die." Our life does ultimately end, reaching the point when, as Italian playwright Salvadore Quasimodo says, "Each of us stands alone at the heart of the earth pierced through by a ray of sunlight, and suddenly it is evening!" In the end, the years do steal us from ourselves and from our loved ones.

Compared to people in many other cultures around the world, Americans are death avoiders and death deniers. We are rarely prepared to cope with the overwhelming emotions that fear, despair, and grief bring into our lives. Because we are such a death-avoiding and death-denying culture, many people might expect this chapter to be depressing. We think you will not find that to be the case. Self-help writers who dispense advice on coping with the sadness of death balance the sadness with love, support, and spiritual healing.

In this chapter, we review self-help books, autobiographies, films, and Internet sites on the topics of death, loss, and grief. These resources address coping with loss of any kind, including death, impending death (one's own or someone else's), and grieving in general. A listing of pertinent support and self-help groups concludes the chapter.

SELF-HELP BOOKS

Strongly Recommended

★★★★★ *How to Survive the Loss of a Love* (2nd ed., 1991) by Melba Colgrove, Harold Bloomfield, and Peter McWilliams. Los Angeles: Prelude.

This book provides suggestions for coping with the loss of a loved one, through death or otherwise. Since the first edition appeared in 1976, the authors, among them, have experienced the death of a parent, a major stroke, serious car accidents, a bankruptcy, a

RECOMMENDATION HIGHLIGHTS

Self-Help Books

- On coping with loss of any kind, including death:

  ★★★★★ *How to Survive the Loss of a Love* by Melba Colgrove et al.

  ★★★★★ *How to Go on Living When Someone You Love Dies* by Therese Rando

  ★★★★ *The Grief Recovery Handbook* by John W. James and Frank Cherry

  ★★★★ *Recovering from the Loss of a Child* by Katherine Donnelly

- On a spiritual approach to death and grief:

  ★★★★★ *When Bad Things Happen to Good People* by Harold Kushner

- On coping with death (your own or someone else's):

  ★★★★ *Working It Through* by Elisabeth Kübler-Ross

  ★★★ *On Death and Dying* by Elisabeth Kübler-Ross

- On helping children cope with grief:

  ★★★★★ *On Children and Death* by Elisabeth Kübler-Ross

  ★★★★ *Learning to Say Good-By* by Eda LeShan

  ★★★★ *Talking about Death* by Earl Grollman

  ★★★★ *Helping Children Grieve* by Theresa Huntley

  ◆ *When Children Grieve* by John W. James and Russell Friedman

- On sudden infant death syndrome:

  ★★★ *Sudden Infant Death* by John DeFrain et al.

- On life (and death) lessons:

  ★★★★ *Life Lessons* by Elisabeth Kübler-Ross and David Kessler

Autobiographies

- On grieving a spouse's death:

  ★★★★★ *A Grief Observed* by C. S. Lewis

- On grieving a mother's death:

  ★★★★ *Motherless Daughter* by Hope Edelman

- On grieving a child's death:

  ★★★★★ *Death Be Not Proud* by John Gunther

  ★★★ *After the Death of a Child* by Ann Finkbeiner

  ◆ *Hannah's Gift* by Maria Housden

- On living while dying:

  ★★★★★ *Letting Go* by Morrie Schwartz

  ★★★★ *The Wheel of Life* by Elisabeth Kübler-Ross and Todd Gold

Films

- On denial of grief and eventual recovery:

  ★★★★★ *Ordinary People*

  ★★★ *The Accidental Tourist*

- On grieving a loss and choosing life:

  ★★★★★ *Corrina, Corrina*

  ★★★★ *Truly, Madly, Deeply*

- On the death of a child and the desire for revenge:

  ★★★★ *In the Bedroom*

- On women sharing life and grief:

  ★★★★ *Steel Magnolias*

- On choosing how to live one's life:

  ★★★★ *A River Runs through It*

Internet Resources

- On advice on grief and loss:

  ★★★★ *Counseling for Loss and Life Changes*
  http://www.counselingforloss.com

- On information and links on end-of-life care:

  ★★★★★ *Growth House* http://www.growthhouse.org

  ★★★★ *Hospice Net* http://www.hospicenet.org

- On hospice information:

  ★★★★ *National Hospice Foundation* http://www.hospiceinfo.org/
  index.cfm?weburl=/public/articles/index.cfm?cat=2

- On children who are losing a loved one:

  ★★★★ *Safe Crossings* http://www.providence.org/resources/safecrossings

- On an underappreciated source of pain—the death of a pet:

  ★★★★ *Pet Loss* http://www.avma.org/care4pets/losspetl.htm

lawsuit, and an impending divorce. Consequently, the authors view loss broadly. They subdivide loss into four categories: (1) obvious losses, such as death of a loved one, divorce, robbery, and rape; (2) not-so-obvious losses, such as moving, loss of a long-term goal, and success (loss of striving); (3) loss related to age, such as leaving home, loss of youth, loss of hair, and menopause; and (4) limbo losses, such as awaiting medical tests, going through a lawsuit, and having a loved one missing in action. The presentation is unusual for a self-help book. Poetry, common sense, and psychological advice are interwoven throughout more than 100 very brief topics organized according to the categories of understanding loss, surviving, healing, and growing. Topics include it's OK to feel, tomorrow will come, seek the comfort of others, touching and hugging, do the mourning now, when counseling or therapy might be helpful, nutrition, remaining distraught is no proof of love, pray, meditate, contemplate, keep a journal, take stock of the good, and your happiness is up to you. This has been a highly successful book, selling more than 2 million copies. The content is clear, succinct, helpful, and covers a vast range of situations involving loss. It has helped people cope with many types of loss.

★★★★★ *How to Go on Living When Someone You Love Dies* (1991) by Therese Rando. New York: Bantam.

Originally published as *Grieving* in 1988, this book advises people about ways to grieve, effectively when someone they love dies. Rando believes that there is no wrong or right way to grieve because people are so different. She describes a variety of ways to grieve and encourages readers to select the coping strategy best for them. Part I, Learning about Grief, identifies what grief is, how it affects people, what factors influence grief, and how women and men experience grief differently. Part II, Grieving Different Forms of Death, explains how grief often varies depending on what caused the death. Part III, Grieving and Your Family, addresses the inevitable family reorganization following a family member's death and how to cope with the death of specific family members: spouse, adult loss of a parent, adult loss of a sibling, and loss of a child. Part IV, Resolving Your Grief, offers specific recommendations for getting through bereavement rituals and funerals, including information about funeral arrangements and talking about loss to others. Part V, Getting Additional Help, explains how to find effective professional and self-help groups. This five-star resource is an excellent self-help book for learning how to cope with the death of a loved one. There are no pat, overgeneralized suggestions on how to grieve. Rando covers a variety of grief circumstances and dispenses easy-to-understand, practical advice for each.

★★★★★ *When Bad Things Happen to Good People* (1981, reissued 1997) by Harold Kushner. New York: Schocken.

Rabbi Kushner provides a spiritual perspective on death, dying, and grief. He addresses the historic question: If God is just and all-powerful, why do good people suffer? Some conventional explanations of why bad things happen are that it's God's punishment for our sins, God is teaching us a lesson, or it's all part of a divine plan that is beyond our comprehension. Kushner writes that God provides us with the strength to endure. Although theologically guided, this is not a book about God and theology, but rather one about man's personal tragedy and his view of God, humans, and life, written in an informal and easy style. The mystery of tragedy is not answered, but readers are brought a little closer to accepting the mystery and, in turn, feel a little more comforted. A book for any adult, but especially for those experiencing the emotional and spiritual conflicts that accompany life's many tragedies. A highly regarded, best-selling source of solace.

★★★★★ *On Children and Death* (reprinted ed., 1997) by Elisabeth Kübler-Ross. New York: Collier.

This internationally known thanatologist writes about how children and their parents can cope with death. Death is the culmination of life, the graduation, the good-bye before another hello, the great transition. The material in this book represents a decade of working with dying children of all ages, their families, and friends. Kübler-Ross advises not to shield surviving children from the pains of death, but to let them share to the extent that they can. Among the topics addressed are death's influence on having other children, the spiritual aspects of working with dying children, and attending funerals. A valuable four-star book for the general public, particularly for people caring for a dying child.

★★★★ *The Grief Recovery Handbook: A Step-by-Step Program for Moving beyond Loss* (1988) by John W. James and Frank Cherry. New York: Harper & Row.

The coauthors stress that grief is a growth process. In this book, acceptance of grief is presented as a positive reaction to loss that helps prepare the griever for recovery. The five stages of grief are gaining awareness, accepting responsibility, identifying recovery communications, taking action, and moving beyond loss. This book is for adults who are dealing with the approaching reality of death or in the process of dealing with loss. Although it received a four-star rating in the national studies, its rating was high enough for five stars, but insufficient numbers of experts were familiar with it. A fine, practical resource.

★★★★ *Life Lessons* (2000) by Elisabeth Kübler-Ross and David Kessler. New York: Simon & Schuster.

The two authors write poignantly and passionately about life lessons, the ultimate truths that are the secrets to life itself. Kübler-Ross wanted this, her declared last book, to be about life and living, not death and dying. Each chapter includes richly described stories of people who experienced one of these life lessons. The perspective of the book might best be conveyed by citing some of the messages of life stories. On love: If you are loved by many, surely you would love yourself—but alas this is often not true. On relationships: We think we have relationship with relatively few people, but we have relationships with everybody we meet. On power: Power is not derived from position in life or money, but from authenticity, strength, integrity, and grace externalized. On the final lesson: Michelangelo said that beautiful sculptures were already there inside the stones. He simply removed the excess.

★★★★ *Learning to Say Good-By* (1976) by Eda LeShan. New York: Macmillan.

This book was written to help children cope with the death of a parent. LeShan believes that children are resilient and can live through anything as long as they are told the truth and allowed to share their suffering with loved ones. The book, a letter to children from LeShan, helps children understand what they are probably feeling, what their surviving parent is probably feeling, and why family members are behaving so strangely. Topics addressed include what happens immediately following a parent's death, feelings of grief, recovering, and how death teaches us about life. Although written for children, *Learning to Say Good-By* can help a surviving parent better understand children's feelings during this time of emotional upheaval. In our death-avoiding culture, LeShan's message is an important one: Children should be allowed to see our grief and have the privilege of expressing their own grief in their own time. LeShan is an excellent writer, and she sensitively communicates with children.

★★★★   *Talking about Death: A Dialogue between Parent and Child* (3rd ed., 1991) by Earl
         Grollman. Boston: Beacon.

This brief book (about 100 pages) is appropriate for children of all faiths. It consists of
dialogues between parents and children and is divided into two main parts: The
Children's Read-Along, which uses simple language so that even five- to nine-year-olds
can understand its messages about death and dying; and The Parent's Guide to Talking
about Death, which provides answers for children's anticipated questions about death.
Parents are urged to be straightforward with their children and are also helped to come
to terms with their own feelings of loss. Highly regarded by our mental health experts,
it received a four-star rating and is a solid self-help resource.

★★★★   *Recovering from the Loss of a Child* (1982) by Katherine Donnelly. New York:
         Macmillan.

This book tells parents and other family members how to cope with the death of a child.
It features excerpts from interviews with parents and siblings of children who died from
illness, accident, and suicide. Part I describes family members' and friends' experiences
with grief. Part II is devoted to organizations that help bereaved families. A basic theme
of the book is that the loss of a child of any age is tragic and a terrible loss for all members of the family. This four-star book presents a sensitive portrayal of a family's struggle to cope with the loss of a child; there is also an extensive list of support organizations.

★★★★   *Working It Through* (1982) by Elisabeth Kübler-Ross. New York: Macmillan.

Another, earlier Kübler-Ross book on death and grieving, *Working It Through* is based
on workshops for people dealing with death, people who are terminally ill, people who
have lost a loved one, and people who are involved with the dying. Sensitive photographs by Mal Warshaw complement the personal and emotional stories. The narratives cover a wide range of grieving experiences, such as emotions as our friends, the
significance of music, the loss of a child, suicide, and spiritual awareness. A book especially for those touched by death or wishing to understand the dying process more fully.

★★★★   *Helping Children Grieve* (1991) by Theresa Huntley. Minneapolis: Augsburg
         Fortress.

As the title suggests, this book is about helping children cope with death—their own
and the death of a loved one. Huntley presents a developmental approach: She begins
by discussing how children under 3 years of age understand death and then describes
how death is perceived by children ages 3–6 years, 6–10 years, 10–12 years, and in adolescence. Huntley says that children of different ages have different thoughts about the
nature of death. For example, toddlers come to understand death as an extension of
"all gone," whereas 10-year-olds often view a loved one's death as a punishment for some
misdeed. Advice is given on how to talk about death with children, and common behaviors and feelings children show when faced with death are discussed. Adults are advised
to encourage children to ask them questions about death and to answer these questions
as honestly as possible. This four-star resource gives adults sound, clear advice about
helping children cope with their own death or the death of a loved one.

Recommended

★★★ *A Time to Say Good-Bye: Moving Beyond Loss* (1996) by Mary McClure Goulding. Watsonville, CA: Papier-Mache.

In this book, a psychotherapist recounts her own journey of mourning the death of her husband. Goulding shares what she has learned in her years of experience, covering such topics as grief, loneliness, and retirement unshared with the mate she worked beside for so long. The book is her narrative of her 3½ years of mourning at her own speed. She speaks about the love of family, friends, and community, and the love of self that nurtured her and still supports her today. She no longer defines herself solely by whom she lost. For widows and widowers working out feelings of mourning and at the same time going on with living, this book can be an encouraging reminder to be patient and loving to themselves. Highly rated but not well-known by mental health professionals.

★★★ *How We Die* (1994) by Sherwin B. Nuland. New York: Knopf.

The author attempts to show that death with dignity is a myth and talks about the painful realities of death. His intention is to depict death in its biological and emotional reality, as seen by those who are witness to it and felt by those who experience it. His hope is that frank discussion will help us deal with the aspects of death that frighten us the most. Nuland also talks about responsibility and choices that we have as we exit our own lives. Ultimately, the dignity that we see in dying must grow out of the dignity with which we have lived our lives. For those interested in the physiological process of death and the accompanying emotions, this is an informative and insightful book.

★★★ *Living through Personal Crisis* (1984) by Ann Stearns. Chicago: Thomas More.

This self-help resource provides advice about coping with many different kinds of loss, especially the death of a loved one. Using case studies to document her ideas, Stearns stresses that it is common for the bereaved to blame themselves, and that the grieving person will undoubtedly experience physical symptoms such as aches and pains or eating and sleeping problems. Stearns advises readers not to hide their feelings but to get them out in the open, to be good to themselves, and to surround themselves with caring people. Stearns suggests when to seek professional help, how to find it, and how to evaluate progress. She closes the book with the image of a bird rising from the ashes as a metaphor for successfully overcoming the sense of loss, but she reminds readers that their scars will never completely disappear. An appendix answers commonly asked questions about grieving. This book provides a good overview of how grief works in variety of loss circumstances (loss of a limb, rape, loss of personal possessions in a fire, as well as the death of a loved one).

★★★ *Sudden Infant Death: Enduring the Loss* (1991) by John DeFrain, Linda Ernst, Deanne Jakub, and Jacque Taylor. Lexington, MA: Heath.

Sudden infant death (SIDS) occurs when an infant stops breathing, usually during the night, and dies suddenly without apparent cause. SIDS is the major cause of infant death from birth to one year of age. The tragic loss of a baby to SIDS affects families in many ways, and it is the authors' intention to help these families recapture the meaning and direction of their lives. The book's contents are based on interviews with 392 mothers, fathers, and siblings who have directly experienced the devastation of SIDS. The book recounts stories of the day the baby died and how parents mistakenly feel an overwhelming sense of guilt that their baby died of neglect. Grief symptoms, the effects of SIDS on marital relationships, and the suffering of grandparents are also covered. Suggestions are given for how friends and family members can be supportive. The fear of having another child and having it die is dealt with at length. This three-star book provides extensive knowledge and personal stories about SIDS. The book also will prove helpful to friends of a family that experiences SIDS, providing them with knowledge and support.

★★★   *On Death and Dying* (1969) by Elisabeth Kübler-Ross. New York: Macmillan.

This best-seller is about facing one's own death and negotiating the stages of dying. In the 1960s, Kübler-Ross and her students studied terminally ill patients to learn how they faced and coped with the crisis of their own impending death. Kübler-Ross and her staff interviewed 200 patients, focusing on them as human beings rather than bodies to be treated. Kübler-Ross concluded that people go through five stages as they face death:

1. Denial and isolation: The person denies that death is really going to take place.
2. Anger: The dying person's denial can no longer be maintained and gives way to anger, resentment, rage, and envy.
3. Bargaining: The person develops the hope that somehow death can be postponed or delayed.
4. Depression: The person accepts the certainty of death but is unhappy about it.
5. Acceptance: The person develops a sense of peace about accepting the inevitable and often wants to be left alone.

Kübler-Ross presents the five stages in considerable detail and discusses the effects of impending death on the dying person's family. Suggestions for therapy with the terminally ill are included. *On Death and Dying* received a three-star rating in our studies, just missing the four-star category. The book was one of the most frequently rated in our first study: 355 mental health professionals evaluated it. It is a classic in the field of death and dying, and Kübler-Ross's approach has helped millions of people cope effectively with impending death. Critics of the book say that no one has been able to confirm that people go through the stages of dying in the order Kübler-Ross proposes, but she feels that she has been misinterpreted, saying that she never intended the stages to be taken as an invariant sequence toward death. Her other two books reviewed in this chapter fared better in our national studies.

★★★   *The Widows Handbook* (1988) by Charlotte Foehner and Carol Cozart. Golden, CO: Fulcrum.

Following the deaths of their husbands, Foehner began studying financial investment and tax preparation, and Cozart started her first full-time job. The book provides emotional support for widows, offers suggestions for rearing children, tells widows how to care for themselves, and discusses changes in relationships, but its main emphasis is on the financial and procedural issues widows are likely to encounter. Making funeral arrangements, selecting an attorney and a financial advisory team, performing an executor's duties, filing claims for life insurance and survivor benefits, getting credit and checking accounts in order, and maintaining a house and auto are some of the practical topics covered. The authors include sample letters widows need to write and examine questions that crop up. This three-star book is very good at what it attempts—to provide widows with sound advice about financial and procedural matters—but it includes only minimal advice about the psychological and emotional dimensions of coping with the loss of a husband.

Diamonds in the Rough

♦ *Ambiguous Loss: Learning to Live with Unresolved Grief* (1999) by Pauline Boss. Cambridge, MA: Harvard University Press.

Ambiguous loss is defined as one of two conditions: (1) Individuals are physically absent but psychologically present, as in the case of MIAs, kidnapped victims, and immigrants who leave their families for better lives; or (2) individuals are physically present but psychologically absent, as in the case of those with Alzheimer's, addictions, chronic mental illness, and traumatic brain injury. The grief of loved ones is frozen and cannot be resolved. Family therapy is described as a means of working with the family in making decisions in the face of uncertain and incomplete information, of understanding that ups and downs become more accentuated and frequent, and of the value of family members hearing each other out. Boss discusses resolving loss and the difficulty in making sense of it. The hopeful message conveyed is that ambiguity can make people less dependent on stability and more tolerant of spontaneity and uncertainty. The author calls this concept the "benefits of doubt." This book accurately identifies and sensitively portrays the struggles of those living with ambiguous loss. As with the following two books in this chapter, *Ambiguous Loss* was very favorably but infrequently rated in our studies, thus achieving a Diamond in the Rough designation.

♦ *The Healing Journey Through Grief* (1999) by Phil Rich. New York: Wiley.

This workbook is a guided personal journal designed to assist readers in working through the loss of a loved one, either in a self-directed or bibliotherapeutic manner. The goal of the journal is to explore loss, identify feelings, and learn how to rebuild one's life. In an early section, an explanation of the stages of grief (e.g., adjustment, emotional immersion/deconstruction and reconciliation) sets the stage for subsequent topics, including acceptance, coping with feelings, finding meaning, recording shared history, and resolving unfinished relationships. Each chapter contains a short case vignette, defining terms, bullet point recommendations, and concepts about which to think. This workbook attends to the elements of grieving in a sequential and developmental way. Homework and outside activities are numerous, and the variety of experiential exercises ensure that any reader can find a means of dealing with grief. This book is a Diamond in the Rough because of its high but infrequent evaluations.

♦ *When Children Grieve* (2001) by John W. James and Russell Friedman with Leslie Landon Matthews. New York: HarperCollins.

How adults can help children deal with loss is the purpose of this book. Losses include death of grandparents, death of a pet, a major move, divorce of parents, injury to the child, or death of a friend or relative. Six myths keep adults and children stuck in grief: Don't feel bad, replace the loss, grieve alone, be strong, keep busy, and time heals all wounds. These concepts form the foundation for a stepwise instruction through grieving and recovery. The authors define completion of a grieving experience as communicating the undelivered emotions that attach to any relationship that changes or ends. Adults are urged to help children identify those relationships that are incomplete, and an emotional energy checklist is provided for guidance in talking through the energy-laden experiences. A 74-item questionnaire is offered to help adults understand how they are communicating with children about loss.

Strongly Not Recommended

† *Widowed* (1990) by Joyce Brothers. New York: Simon & Schuster.

† *Final Exit: The Practicalities of Self-Deliverance and Assisted Suicide for the Dying* (1991) by Derek Humphrey. Eugene, OR: Hemlock Society.

AUTOBIOGRAPHIES

Strongly Recommended

★★★★★ *Letting Go: Morrie's Reflections on Living While Dying* (1997) by Morrie Schwartz. New York: Dell.

Also published under the title *Morrie: In His Own Words,* this book describes the last years of sociologist Morrie Schwartz after he learned at age 75 that he had Lou Gehrig's disease, which is progressive and incurable. Schwartz became a participant–observer as his physical abilities declined, tape recording his observations, impressions, and memories. He became widely known after appearing three times on Ted Koppel's TV show *Nightline* to discuss his life, dying, and Lou Gehrig's disease. The book is a wise, compassionate account of the living of dying.

★★★★★ *A Grief Observed* (1961) by C. S. Lewis. New York: Seabury.

This is a poignant tale of loss and spiritual search following the death of a spouse. The movie *Shadowlands* is based on it. Both the book and the movie describe the humanizing of Oxford don and famed writer C. S. Lewis following the death of his wife, Joy Gresham, from cancer. Originally published under the pseudonym of N. W. Clerk just before Lewis's own death, *A Grief Observed* reveals the inner turmoil of his grief. The author says that he wrote these memoirs as a "defense against total collapse, a safety valve." This five-star autobiography presents profound human experience from the spiritual perspective of a gifted writer. It offers no advice for recovery but presents a moving description of human vulnerability. Lewis's personal loss will benefit many readers, especially those who feel themselves distant from ordinary human affairs.

★★★★★ *Death Be Not Proud: A Memoir* (1998) by John Gunther. New York: HarperCollins.

Classic, moving story of Johnny Gunther, a promising 16-year-old diagnosed with a serious brain tumor. Written by his father, it is a chronicle of hope as the tumor shrinks, pain as it resumes growing, the nobility of the struggle, Johnny's optimism and patience during a succession of invasive treatments, and courage as he says his final good-byes. An inspiring and affirming account, especially good for parents and for teens. The key message is to live life to the fullest as Johnny did.

★★★★ *The Wheel of Life: A Memoir of Living and Dying* (1998) by Elisabeth Kübler-Ross and Todd Gold. New York: Touchstone.

The noted authority on dying and promoter of the hospice movement, Elisabeth Kübler-Ross recounts her life growing up in Switzerland, becoming a physician and psychiatrist, moving to the United States, and her pioneering studies of death and dying. Her research initially encountered considerable opposition because, she maintains, people refuse to accept their own mortality. Having had several strokes, she is prepared to face her end and considers this to be her final book. There are also sections more controversial than the description of her career and strokes, and these deal with near death and out-of-the-body experiences, communicating and channeling spirits, and other aspects of the paranormal.

★★★★ *Motherless Daughter* (1995) by Hope Edelman. New York: Delta.

The author was 17 when she lost her mother. After finishing college and working as a journalist, Edelman realized that she was still grieving. She turned this experience first into a magazine article and then into this book, which attracted a large amount of media attention. Often described as the first book specifically on loss of a mother, *Motherless Daughter* discusses the experience of women who lost their mothers either as children or as adults.

Recommended

★★★ *After the Death of a Child: Living with Loss through the Years* (1998) by Ann Finkbeiner. Baltimore: Johns Hopkins University Press.

The author's only child died in 1987. She describes her grief and the methods she used to cope with the loss. She interviewed other parents who had lost children to collect additional material for this book. Highly rated, but infrequently so, in our national studies.

Diamonds in the Rough

◆ *Eric* (2000) by Doris Lund. New York: HarperCollins Perennial.

The death of a child isn't easy to understand or write about. *Eric* is the reissue of a classic book made into a movie in the 1970s about a vibrant and athletic 17-year-old diagnosed with leukemia. Written by his mother, it chronicles Eric's struggle to avoid despair and make the most of the remaining time, to live while dying, and sensitively portrays the pain of family members as they pass through stages of shock, disbelief, rage, depression, and acceptance. A moving and cathartic book for anyone who has a family member with leukemia or is faced with a child's death.

♦ *Hannah's Gift: Lessons from a Life Fully Lived* (2002) by Maria Housden. New York: Doubleday Dell.

Beautifully written story of a three-year-old girl diagnosed with terminal cancer, the succession of unsuccessful treatments, her death, and the family's coming to terms. Hannah was an outgoing, excited child whose infectious curiosity and joy changed the lives of those who met her. Hannah demanded to be treated in the hospital as an individual, to wear her Mary Janes in the operating room, and to know the names of her physicians. The book is about child as teacher and about a parent's pain, joy, and dignity when faced with the incomprehensible. A touching, uplifting book.

FILMS

Strongly Recommended

★★★★★ *Ordinary People* (1980) directed by Robert Redford. R rating. 124 minutes.

This is a movie about grieving and the denial of grief. A privileged family loses its prize son and the parents' withdrawal becomes too extreme for their other son. In his isolation, he cuts his wrists and is hospitalized for months. When he returns, nothing has changed. His father's cheerfulness is all pretense; his mother's self-preoccupation is a stone wall. This stirring but ultimately hopeful film, winner of a bushel of Academy Awards, tragically illustrates how some families respond psychologically and interpersonally to loss, and how the stress of loss makes them more of what they were before.

★★★★★ *Corrina, Corrina* (1994) directed by Jessie Nelson. PG rating. 115 minutes.

A light-hearted and warm-hearted film focusing on a withdrawn eight-year-old child whose mother has died. Her father hires Corrina, a sassy housekeeper played by Whoopi Goldberg, who coaxes the daughter back to life and shows the survivors a whole new way of living. It is a valuable resource for demonstrating children's reactions toward death and for reminding us all that life can again blossom following death of a family member.

★★★★ *Steel Magnolias* (1990) directed by Herbert Ross. PG rating. 118 minutes.

This is both a woman's picture and a picture of women. Six friends joke, gossip, and support each other for several years in a small Louisiana town in the early 1980s. They cry, fight, make up, and get their hair done at the beauty parlor that is the center of their lives. When a tragic death strikes, their grieving is wonderful to watch: Character tells, and strength is required. This may be an excellent movie to show survival in the face of tragedy, although comedy is the main focus of the movie.

★★★★ *In the Bedroom* (2001) directed by Todd Field. R rating. 130 minutes.

The Fowlers (Sissy Spacek, Tom Wilkinson) are a respectable, upper-middle-class Maine couple whose 21-year-old son falls in love with a young woman separated but not yet divorced from her husband. The separated husband is pathologically jealous and violent, resulting in the murder of the Fowlers' son. The unthinkable tragedy tears the Fowlers apart, and the film traces their loss, rage, and quest for revenge. The grief is palpable; Wilkinson's character expresses more loss and helplessness than any words could ever convey. *In the Bedroom* is wrenching emotional drama, as sensitive and accurate a portrayal of grief for a child as ever filmed. The movie was nominated for an Oscar for best picture, and its two main characters were also nominated for best actress and best actor.

★★★★ *A River Runs through It* (1988) directed by Robert Redford. PG rating. 123 minutes.

This movie is about how one can chose to live one's life. In the words of movie critic Roger Ebert, "Fly-fishing stands for life in this movie. If you can learn to do it correctly, to read the river and the fish and yourself, and to do what needs to be done without one wasted motion, you will have attained some of the grace and economy needed to live a good life. If you can do it and understand that the river, the fish and the whole world are God's gifts to use wisely, you will have gone the rest of the way."

★★★★ *Truly, Madly, Deeply* (1991) directed by Anthony Minghella. PG rating. 105 minutes.

A London couple is truly, madly, and deeply in love but then one of them dies. The spouse is heartbroken, left alone in a house filled with rats and repair men, until her love reappears as a ghost. This romantic comedy centers on the memory of a loved one and ignoring life for the dead. An intelligent and realistic film for people who have suffered the loss of a true love, and for those who need to let the past go in order to move forward.

Recommended

★★★ *Unstrung Heroes* (1995) directed by Diane Keaton. PG rating. 93 minutes.

A dramatic comedy in which a boy coming of age grapples with a dying mother and rebels against his father. He goes to live with his two pleasantly crazy uncles, who support him through his ordeal and help him thrive. The mother is very loving, but sadly abandons him by dying. A quirky yet moving film, probably best as a self-help resource for those who have relocated following a parent's death.

★★★ *My Life* (1993) directed by Bruce Joel Rubin. PG-13 rating. 112 minutes.

A successful advertising executive whose wife is pregnant learns that he is dying and doesn't know how to deal with the unfinished business in his life (particularly his feelings of anger toward his family) or the fact that he may never see his child. He is able to reach out to his unborn child by making videotapes. His wife is shown as a pillar of strength, his doctors as automatons. There are many truthful and poignant moments in this unabashed tearjerker, but contrivances ultimately take over, especially toward the end. The film could be used to illustrate loss, grief, and unfinished business, if the responses to them are not taken too realistically.

★★★ *The Accidental Tourist* (1989) directed by Lawrence Kasdan. PG rating. 121 minutes.

On the surface, this acclaimed film is about a man who is shattered by the death of his son and withdraws from any emotional contact. His wife leaves him, and he lives a safe but routine life until he meets a kooky, assertive woman who draws him out of his shell. Sounds like a typical Hollywood romance. This film could illustrate a style of coping with death and its negative consequences. It also shows how the man brings himself finally to choose between isolation and routine in his shell or love and risk in a new relationship. The film can be used with couples because it illustrates how the nature of the man's marriage, calm but distant, is too weak to support the couple's needs after their tragedy. The wife needs to talk, but the husband needs to be alone and deny his feelings.

★★★ *The Summer of '42* (1971) directed by Robert Mulligan. PG rating. 103 minutes.

A nostalgic look back at an adolescent boy's infatuation with an older woman who shares a sexual experience with him after her husband is killed in World War II, and then disappears. The film illustrates how she, desperate for companionship in her despair over her husband's absence and then his sudden and tragic death, reaches out to the boy.

★★★ *The Lion King* (1995) directed by Roger Allers and Robert Minkoff. G rating. 87 minutes.

Sure, it is a cartoon, and one without people in it, too. But the story is a wonderful one of how courage, assumption of adult responsibilities, and friends can triumph over loss, evil, and treachery. The evil Scar has the king killed and drives the young prince out so that he can become king. The prince lives a carefree life until his father's ghost commands him to return and seek revenge. The film can illustrate how an individual need not be defeated by deaths and losses, and can prevail by "growing up" and taking on social responsibilities.

★★★ *My Girl* (1992) directed by Howard Zieff. PG rating. 102 minutes.

An 11-year-old girl has become hypochondrical and as eccentric as her father. He copes with her mother's death in childbirth by isolation and has contact only with the dead; she copes by a preoccupation with death, the meaning of life, and her imaginary diseases. She becomes close to a boy and shares puppy love, philosophical questions, and much of her time. When he dies, she is submerged in guilt—she feels like she killed him and her mother—and she is alone. Through her grieving and sharing with others, she develops new friends and accepts her father's new girlfriend. She struggles and achieves a normal (early) adolescent's life. While imperfect, this film can be valuable in suggesting the complexities of grief in families.

Not Recommended

★★ *Message in a Bottle* (1999) directed by Luis Mandoki. PG-13 rating. 126 minutes.

★★ *Ghost* (1991) directed by Jerry Zucker. PG-13 rating. 122 minutes.

INTERNET RESOURCES

Metasites

★★★★★ *Growth House* http://www.growthhouse.org

This rich site has thousands of links covering end-of-life care. Although there are few publications available here and the resources require clicking through several levels, the organization is functional and clear, and the resources are well described. This site should be the starting point for searches.

★★★★ *Last Acts* http://www.lastacts.org

Perhaps a little too comprehensive, this site is nevertheless ideal for those who are searching for information and support.

★★★★ *GriefNet* http://rivendell.org

In the *Library*, under Articles and Manuscripts, are many useful papers on gender differences, helping others cope with loss, and so on.

★★★★ *The Compassionate Friends* http://www.compassionatefriends.org

This is the major organization for those who have lost a child. The 15 brochures are excellent and comprehensive, with many published books and booklets (see Resources) for all who are bereaved.

Psychoeducational Materials for Clients and Families

These resources are grouped separately under Grieving and Dying.

Grieving

★★★★ *Counseling for Loss and Life Changes* http://www.counselingforloss.com

Under Articles, Jane Bissler's site offers reprints of about 30 short writings and links to perhaps 50 more.

★★★★ *Life after Loss: Dealing with Grief*
        http://www.utexas.edu/student/cmhc/booklets/Grief/grief.html

A six-page overview written for college students.

★★★★ *Grief and Loss* http://www.couns.uiuc.edu/brochures/grief.htm

A three-page set of guidelines suitable as a handout for explaining the nature and process of grief and loss.

★★★★ *Safe Crossings* http://www.providence.org/resources/safecrossings

This site is operated by a hospice and is for children facing the loss of a loved one. Not cute, it interactively explores many feelings, and offers activities and ways to memorialize the loss. See also *Julie's Place* at http://www.juliesplace.com, a site for children who have lost a brother or sister that is perhaps too cute but does offer support and chat.

★★★★ *Grief and Loss* http://www.aarp.org/griefandloss/home.html

This rather comprehensive site from the American Association of Retired Persons contains many leads. Probably best for a trusted introduction to the issues.

★★★★ *Pet Loss* http://www.avma.org/care4pets/losspetl.htm

The pain associated with the death of a beloved pet is often underappreciated. The brochure, Making the Decision, is complete. Also useful is the brochure "Grief and Pet Loss"by Margaret Muns, DVM, at http://www.petloss. com/muns.htm.

★★★ *Grief and Bereavement* http://www.psycom.net/depression.central.grief.html

Many links of value, including material on teens, pet loss, and widowhood.

★★★ *Bereavement* http://www.rcpsych.ac.uk/info/help/bereav/index.htm

A good, six-page overview aimed at general readers.

★★★ *Mothers in Sympathy and Support (MISS) Foundation*
    http://www.misschildren.org

Oriented around the loss of a child, this site includes several useful articles and advice for friends and professionals.

★★★ *WidowNet* http://www.fortnet.org/WidowNet

The first three articles are helpful: Dumb Remarks and Stupid Questions, Getting through the Holidays, and You Know You're Getting Better When . . . Readers can also find a nearby support group here.

★★★ *Grief Journey* http://www.griefjourney.com/help1.htm

The six articles by Bill Webster are useful, short readings for clients.

Dying

★★★★ *Partnership for Caring* http://www.partnershipforcaring.org/HomePage/

The site offers readings about end-of-life issues, legal aspects, and state-specific advance directives.

★★★★ *National Hospice Foundation* http://www.hospiceinfo.org/index.cfm?weburl=/
    public/articles/index.cfm?cat=2

The brochures here explain what a hospice is and is not, its benefits and logic, Medicare coverage, and clarifying one's end-of-life wishes. Essential structuring and calming information.

★★★★ *A Dying Person's Guide to Dying*
http://www.acponline.org/public/h_care/dying-gd.htm

This page provides superb advice. The entire book is available for download with much specific and tender advice for dying as well as possible.

★★★★ *FAMSA: Funeral Consumers Alliance* http://www.funerals.org/

A consumer-oriented site with lots of information to help make responsible and efficient choices about funerals, cemeteries, and caskets.

Other Resources

★★★★ *Hospice Net* http://www.hospicenet.org

This site provides more than 50 articles on end-of-life issues.

★★★ *A Heartbreaking Choice* http://www.aheartbreakingchoice.com/

"For parents who have terminated a pregnancy after learning their baby has severe birth defects."

NATIONAL SUPPORT GROUPS

Compassionate Friends
PO Box 3696
Oak Brook, IL 60522-3696
Phone: 630-990-0010
E-mail: elaine@compassionatefriends.org
http://www.compassionatefriends.org

This is the major organization for parents who have lost a child.

Compassion in Dying
6312 SW Capital Highway, Suite 415
Portland, OR 97239
Phone: 503-221-9556
E-mail: info@compassionindying.org
http://www.CompassionInDying.org

Offers information, emotional support, and referrals for all end-of-life options.

Concerns of Police Survivors (COPS)
COPS National Office
PO Box 3199
Camdenton, MO 65020
Phone: 573-346-4911
E-mail: cops@nationalcops.org
http://www.nationalcops.org

This group was created to reach out to surviving families of America's law enforcement officers killed in the line of duty.

Mothers against Drunk Driving (MADD)
511 Carpenter Freeway, Suite 700
Irving, TX 75062
Phone: 800-GET-MADD
http://madd.org/home

For victims of drunk drivers.

Parents of Murdered Children
100 East Eighth Street, Suite B-41
Cincinnati, OH 45202
Phone: 513-721-5683
E-mail: natlpomc@aol.com
http://www.pomc.org

Partnership for Caring: America's Voices for the Dying
1620 Eye Street NW, Suite 202
Washington, DC 20006
Phone: 202-296-8071
E-mail: pfc@partnershipforcaring.org
http://www.partnershipforcaring.org

"The inventor of living wills in 1967, it is dedicated to fostering communication about complex end-of-life decisions. The nonprofit organization provides advance directives, counsels patients and families, trains professionals, advocates for improved laws, and offers a range of publications and services."

Pet Loss Hotline
College of Veterinary Medicine
Washington State University
Pullman, WA 99164-7010
Phone: 509-335-5704
E-mail: plhl@vetmed.wsu.edu
http://www.vetmed.wsu.edu/plhl/
  index.htm

"It's okay to love and miss your pet." Provides a support mechanism for grieving people who have experienced pet loss.

Sudden Infant Death Syndrome Alliance (SIDS Alliance)
1314 Bedford Avenue, Suite 210
Baltimore, MD 21208
Phone: 800-221-SIDS
E-mail: info@sidsalliance.org
http://www.sidsalliance.org

SHARE Office (Pregnancy and Infant Loss Support)
St. Joseph Health Center
300 First Capitol Drive
St. Charles, MO 63301-2893
Phone: 800-821-6819
E-mail: share@nationalshareoffice.com
http://www.nationalshareoffice.com

Society of Military Widows
5535 Hempstead Way
Springfield, VA 22151
Phone: 800-842-3451
E-mail: shirleydalton@attbi.com
http://www.militarywidows.org

TAPS (Tragedy Assistance Program for Survivors)
2001 S Street NW, Suite 300
Washington, DC 20009
Phone: 800-959-TAPS
E-mail: info@taps.org
http://taps.org/

"TAPS serves all those affected by a death in the line of military duty and works with parents, children, spouses, and friends."

CHAPTER 16

Dementia/Alzheimer's

The majority of older adults are living longer, more active, and fulfilling lives, but some older adults are declining mentally and physically to the point of needing continuous help. Many of these older adults are suffering from dementia, which commonly refers to global decline involving impairment in cognitive functioning, always including memory dysfunction and personality alterations (Lezak, 1995).

By far, the most prevalent and best known of the dementias is Alzheimer's disease, a progressive and irreversible brain disorder characterized by a gradual deterioration in memory, reasoning, language, and physical functioning. About 19% of people ages 75 to 84 suffer from Alzheimer's, and the disease afflicts nearly half of those 85 and older. Some research suggests that, as people live longer, the incidence of Alzheimer's could triple within the next 50 years.

A family caring for a dementia patient assumes a great deal of responsibility. The condition typically begins so gradually that the family is often unaware that anything is wrong until work problems pile up or a sudden disruption in routine leaves the patient disoriented, confused, and unable to deal with the unfamiliar situation. Families caring for loved ones diagnosed with dementia need to be educated and prepared to cope with a number of predictable and unpredictable behaviors. Family distress tends to be chronic and high. There will come a time when the family has to decide what level of care its family member needs and the most appropriate setting in which to provide that care.

In this chapter, we present the experts' consensual ratings and our brief descriptions of self-help books, autobiographies, and films on this crippling disease. Listings of Internet resources and national support groups round out the resources.

RECOMMENDATION HIGHLIGHTS

Self-Help Books

- For families caring for a person with Alzheimer's:

    ★★★★★ *The 36-Hour Day* by Nancy Mace and Peter Rabins

    ★★★ *The Hidden Victims of Alzheimer's Disease* by Steven Zarit et al.

    ◆ *When Your Loved One Has Alzheimer's* by David L. Carroll

Autobiographies

- For moving accounts of caring for a spouse with Alzheimer's:

    ★★★★ *Elegy for Iris* by John Bayley

    ★★★ *The Diminished Mind* by Jean Tyler and Harry Anifantakis

    ◆ *Alzheimer's, A Love Story* by Ann Davidson

- Ongoing diary record of the early stages:

    ◆ *Losing My Mind* by Thomas DeBaggio

Films

- For superb portrayals of Alzheimer's and its impact on the spouse:

    ★★★★★ *Iris*

    ★★★ *Do You Remember Love?*

- For repairing relationships while a parent descends into dementia:

    ★★★ *Memories of Me*

Internet Resources

- For extensive materials for patients and caregivers:

    ★★★★★ *The Alzheimer's Association* http://www.alz.org

    ★★★★★ *Alzheimer's Outreach*
    http://www.zarcrom.com/users/alzheimers/dirs.html

    ★★★★★ *Alzheimer's Australia*
    http://www.alzheimers.org.au/content.cfm?topicid=26

- For great ideas for caregivers of Alzheimer's patients:

    ★★★★ *The Caregiver's Handbook*
    http://www.acsu.buffalo.edu/~drstall/hndbk0.html

- For managing memory limitations:

    ★★★★ *Memory and Dementia*
    http://www.rcpsych.ac.uk/info/help/memory/

SELF-HELP BOOKS

Strongly Recommended

★★★★★ *The 36-Hour Day: A Family Guide to Caring for Persons with Alzheimer's Disease, Related Dementing Illness and Memory Loss in Later Life* (3rd ed., 1999) by Nancy Mace and Peter Rabins. Baltimore: Johns Hopkins University Press.

This book, now in its third edition, is a family guide to caring for persons with Alzheimer's and related diseases. The authors say that for those who care for a person with Alzheimer's or related diseases, every day seems as if it is 36 hours long. This is a guide for the home care of older adults in the early and middle stages of these diseases. The family is assisted in recognizing the point beyond which home care is no longer enough and is guided in choosing a nursing home or other care facility. Various support groups formed to help families with an Alzheimer's member are also described. This five-star book is an excellent guide for families who have a relative with Alzheimer's. It provides practical advice with specific examples that help readers learn how to care for an impaired relative on a day-to-day basis. *The 36-Hour Day* is one of the highest rated self-help books in our national studies.

Recommended

★★★ *The Hidden Victims of Alzheimer's Disease: Families under Stress* (1985) by Steven Zarit, Nancy K. Orr, and Judy M. Zarit. New York: New York University Press.

The authors offer families support and advice in caring for a person with Alzheimer's disease. Specific situations and interventions are addressed, including stealing, incontinence, asking repetitive questions, lowered sexual inhibitions, and inappropriate public behavior. Also covered are positive psychosocial approaches to dementia, causes of memory loss, and how to assess for dementia. The section on caring for the caregivers is especially good. This book was written primarily for practitioners working with patients and their families in community settings. It may also serve the needs of family members working with organizations devoted to Alzheimer's. Besides recognizing and dealing with Alzheimer's, the book addresses individual counseling, family meetings, support groups, and special treatment concerns (e.g., drugs, placement, and patients without families). This valuable three-star resource would have received four stars if it had been more frequently rated.

★★★ *The Alzheimer's Caregiver: Dealing with the Realities of Dementia* (1998) by Harriet Hodgson. Minneapolis: Chronimed.

The chronic and debilitating nature of Alzheimer's is sensitively captured in Hodgson's book. As a patient's mental abilities deteriorate, the caregiver's responsibilities and emotional challenges escalate. The caregiver needs to learn how to cope with this consuming process and to care for him- or herself without guilt. Various problems covered in the book are home care, assisted living, anticipatory grief, legal complications, personal struggles, Alzheimer's depression, health care costs, and the family system. Appendixes provide self-assessment. This three-star book is clearly and effectively aimed at caregivers.

Diamond in the Rough

♦ *When Your Loved One Has Alzheimer's: A Caregiver's Guide* (1989) by David L. Carroll. New York: Harper & Row.

The author covers a variety of Alzheimer's topics, notably, understanding the disease, reviewing medical care and coverage, preparing the family home, maintaining the caregiver's emotional health, and getting help. The information and techniques in these pages are designed to be used on several levels—practical, psychological, and spiritual. Some of the day-to-day problems discussed in the book include the person's temper tantrums, incontinence pads, embarrassing scenes in public settings, motor difficulties, and impaired memory. This book is written expressly for caregivers as a how-to manual. Favorably rated but not widely known by the mental health experts in our studies, thus meriting the Diamond in the Rough designation.

AUTOBIOGRAPHIES

Highly Recommended

★★★★ *Elegy for Iris* (1999) by John Bayley. New York: St. Martin's Press.

This is a moving account of the literary courtship and unconventional union between Oxford don and literary critic John Bayley and renowned philosopher and novelist Dame Iris Murdoch. Using his talents for elegant prose, Bayley recounts his wife's descent into unknowing darkness and the caretaking role he was forced to take and performed nobly. Impressive not only for the perceptive account of Alzheimer's but also because the author and the subject are important literary figures. This beautiful book shows how Bayley played the hand he was dealt with grace and dignity, never losing respect or love for his partner.

Recommended

★★★ *The Diminished Mind: One Family's Extraordinary Battle with Alzheimer's* (1991) by Jean Tyler and Harry Anifantakis. Blue Ridge Summit, PA: TAB.

Jean Tyler tells the true story of her husband Manley's devastating battle with Alzheimer's disease. Manley Tyler was a loving husband and a respected elementary school principal before the onset of Alzheimer's. Jean Tyler sensitively describes the pain and grief of her husband's slow, 15-year decline and eventual death. Alzheimer's hits most older adults much later than it did Manley Tyler. He was only 42 years old when he first showed symptoms. Jean Tyler relates the progressive deterioration of memory and judgment that made it impossible for him to complete even the simplest of tasks, and made him increasingly prone to hostile behavior and paranoia. This three-star autobiography not only speaks volumes about the emotionally draining losses involved in Alzheimer's but it also carries some important messages for the survivors of an Alzheimer's victim, who can emerge from the experience with fond memories of their loved one and a stronger understanding of what it means to be human.

Diamonds in the Rough

◆ *Alzheimer's, A Love Story: One Year in My Husband's Journey* (1997) by Ann Davidson. Secaucus, NJ: Birch Lane.

At the age of 50, Julian Davidson, a well-known Stanford professor of physiology and medical researcher, was diagnosed with Alzheimer's. This book is his wife's account of the year in which she and her husband came to terms with his increasing deficits. Together, sharing what was happening, they went through stages of confusion, anger, grief, mourning for what was lost, to acceptance. Told in 56 vignettes, some bittersweet, even humorous, and rich with honest dialogue, this splendid book captures the progressively debilitating effects of this disorder on the daily lives of clients and their families. It was very favorably rated by mental health professionals but unfortunately not well-known by them.

◆ *Losing My Mind: An Intimate Look at Life with Alzheimer's* (2002) by Thomas DeBaggio. New York: Free Press.

Most books on progressive memory loss have been written by family members. DeBaggio had several things going for him in this remarkable autobiography. A journalist, freelance writer, and author of several garden books, he was diagnosed with Alzheimer's at a relatively early age (57) and started writing the book on the day he received the diagnosis. He describes the cognitive deficits as they appear on a daily basis, especially the losses in communication skills and how they affected his life and his family. Long-term memories of his childhood seem more vivid than what is happening around him. He tells of the hopelessness he feels, knowing that things will only get worse. Keeping a journal helped DeBaggio cope. Sometimes he writes out of desperation, to attempt to record even if he cannot comprehend what is occurring. This is a wonderful book for caregivers and those fearful of developing Alzheimer's. It does not sugar coat the condition, but shows that sentience (reflection) and family life can continue. Brand new book, not well known by our mental health experts.

FILMS

Strongly Recommended

★★★★★ *Iris* (2001) directed by Richard Eyre. R rating. 97 minutes.

A tender depiction of novelist Iris Murdoch's descent into Alzheimer's. The film is a series of flashbacks from the perspective of Iris's husband, John Bayley, and is based on his acclaimed book *Elegy for Iris* (reviewed above). The earlier scenes depict Iris as a vibrant young woman, a revered British writer and philosopher; the later scenes, in stark and sad contrast, depict a helpless and confused victim of Alzheimer's ravages. Sensitively rendered, it is simultaneously a love story and a dementia tale. *Iris* was deservedly one of highest rated movies in our national studies.

Recommended

★★★ *Do You Remember Love?* (1985, made for TV) directed by Jeff Bleckner. Not rated.

Joanne Woodward won an Emmy for her portrayal of a middle-aged college professor who begins to suffer from Alzheimer's disease. The effect on her husband and family are superbly shown in an Emmy-winning script. Realistic and touching at the same time.

★★★ *Memories of Me* (1989) directed by Henry Winkler. PG-13 rating. 105 minutes.

After his own heart attack, a heart surgeon seeks to reconcile with his father in order to put his own life back in order. That fathers and sons have superficial and (especially in this movie) joking relationships is not news, but the way these men struggle and partly succeed in deepening their relationship is funny and memorable. The son's response to his father's early Alzheimer's is also illuminating at times.

INTERNET RESOURCES

Metasites

★★★★★ *The Alzheimer's Association*   http://www.alz.org

The informational materials are extensive and address all the right issues for patients and caregivers. This is the best place to start learning about the disease. Take the time to understand the excellent organization of the resources.

★★★★★ *Alzheimer's Outreach*   http://www.zarcrom.com/users/alzheimers/dirs.html

Go to the four Alzheimer's directories: Caregiving, Alzheimer's, Nursing/Nursing Home Information, and Health Care Issues to find massive, detailed, and, best of all, practical information.

★★★★★ *Alzheimer's Australia*
      http://www.alzheimers.org.au/content.cfm?topicid=26

There are about 100 "Help Sheets" under nine headings. Solid information is briefly presented. Those under "Information for people with dementia" are particularly valuable.

★★★★ *The Alzheimer's Disease Education and Referral (ADEAR)*
      http://www.alzheimers.org

This is the Alzheimer's section of the National Institute on Aging of the National Institutes of Health. The nine Fact Sheets (under Publications) offer solid information and are a good starting place. A list of the 29 federally funded Alzheimer's disease centers for referral, evaluation, and treatment appears at http://www.alzheimers.org/adcdir.htm.

Psychoeducational Materials for Clients and Families

★★★★ *Alzheimer's Center*
http://www.mayoclinic.com/findinformation/conditioncenters/
centers.cfm?objectid=0007c524-3895-1b32-82d780c8d77a0000

From the Mayo Clinic, this site offers about a dozen short articles about different aspects of the disease. The sections on risk assessment and genetics seem unique. The papers on Caregiving are well done but brief.

★★★★ *Memory and Dementia* http://www.rcpsych.ac.uk/info/help/memory/

Fact sheets and brochures discussing appropriate memory expectations, the role of anxiety and depression in lessening recall, aspects of dementia, self-help tips, and readings.

★★★★ *AARP Andrus Foundation* http://www.andrus.org/index.shtml

This site features a different approach: focusing on living well and independently despite the burdens of age, loss, and disease. It requires looking through the whole site but is greatly rewarding. Ideal for the worried and confused, but not for those in crisis.

★★★★ *ALZwell Alzheimer's Caregivers' Page* http://www.alzwell.com

A comprehensive site with many resources especially designed for supporting caregivers.

★★★★ *Ageless Design* http://www.agelessdesign.com

Alzheimer's-proofing your house, special products, a newsletter, and the like.

★★★★ *The Caregiver's Handbook: Assisting Both the Caregiver and the Elderly Carereceiver*
by Robert S. Stall, MD
http://www.acsu.buffalo.edu/~drstall/hndbk0.html

This is a book of about 100 pages, with detailed and practical ideas for caregivers about nutrition, emotions, personal care, and legal and financial issues.

★★★★ *Awakenings* http://www.parkinsonsdisease.com

A comprehensive Parkinson's disease site. There are materials for primary care physicians, as well as the public, support, and advice under Living with PD.

★★★ *The Elderly Place* http://www.geocities.com/~elderly-place

A Caregiver's Guide to Alzheimer's and the nursing homes section are practical and specific.

★★★ *Caring for People with Huntington's Disease*
http://www.kumc.edu/hospital/huntingtons/

This site contains information, such as inheritance patterns, specific to Huntington's.

★★★ *Alzheimer's Disease Fact Page* by David S. Geldmacher, MD
http://www.ohioalzcenter.org/facts.html

A good, four-page overview, providing unique autopsy information.

Other Resources

★★★★★ *The Alzheimer's Disease Bookstore*
http://www.alzheimersbooks.com/102.Alzheimerbookstore.html

This site has every book for caregivers and children on designing a safe environment, legal issues, activities, and other practical advice. A real find. Videotapes are available at http://www.alzheimersbooks.com/AlzVideos.html.

★★★ *Practice Guidelines for the Treatment of Patients with Alzheimer's Disease and Other Dementias of Late Life* http://www.psych.org/clin_res/pg_dementia.cfm

This Practice Guideline from the American Psychiatric Association is a minitextbook, and the sections on features, natural history, treatments, and treatment planning may be useful.

NATIONAL SUPPORT GROUPS

Alzheimer's Association National Office
919 North Michigan Avenue, Suite 1100
Chicago, IL 60611-1676
Phone: 800-272-3900, 312-335-8700
E-mail: info@alz.org
http://www.alz.org

Provides information, publications, and support to patients and their caregivers.

Alzheimer's Disease and Related Disorders Association
919 North Michigan Avenue, Suite 1100
Chicago, IL 60611-8700
Phone: 312-335-8700
E-mail: info@alz.org
http://www.alz.org

For caregivers of Alzheimer's patients.

Alzheimer's Disease Education and Referral Center (ADEAR)
National Institute on Aging
PO Box 8250
Silver Spring, MD 20907-8250
Hotline: 800-438-4380
E-mail: adear@alzheimers.org
http://www.alzheimers.org

Information, referrals, publications, and information about clinical trials.

National Family Caregivers Association
10400 Connecticut Avenue, Suite 500
Kensington, MD 20895-3944
Phone: 800-896-3650
E-mail: info@nfcacares.org
http://www.nfcacares.org

National Niemann–Pick Disease Foundation
PO Box 49
415 Madison Avenue
Ft. Atkinson, WI 53538
Phone: 877-287-3672
E-mail: nnpdf@idcnet.com
http://www.nnpdf.org

See also Aging (Chapter 5) and Death and Grieving (Chapter 15).

CHAPTER 17

Depression

Depression is a frequently used and abused term. When someone asks you what is wrong as they look at your gloomy face, you might respond, "I feel depressed about myself, about my life." Everyone is down in the dumps some of the time, but most people, after a few hours, days, or weeks, snap out of their despondent moods.

However, some people are not as fortunate. They suffer from major depression, a mood disorder that involves feeling deeply unhappy, demoralized, self-derogatory, and apathetic. A person who has major depression often does not feel physically well, loses stamina, has a poor appetite, is listless, and experiences a sleep disorder. Major depression is so common in the United States that it has been called the flu of mental disorders. (The extreme mood swings of bipolar disorder, or manic–depression, are covered in Chapter 10).

Just as with anxiety, there is a swirl of controversy about the etiology and treatment of depression. Some experts believe that most depressions are psychologically and experientially determined and therefore best treated through psychotherapy. Others believe that depression is largely biologically determined and should be treated mainly with medication. But all experts acknowledge the reciprocal interaction of both psychology and physiology, and most believe in the superiority of a combination of medication and psychotherapy.

In this chapter, we critically review the voluminous body of self-help books, autobiographies, films, and Internet resources related to depression. Our primary concern is with major depression, but we also cover seasonal affective disorder (SAD), dysthymia, and postpartum depression.

SELF-HELP BOOKS

Strongly Recommended

★★★★★ *Feeling Good: The New Mood Therapy* (revised ed., 1999) by David Burns. New York: Avon.

The cognitive therapy that psychiatrist Burns describes in this updated self-help classic is the most popular form of psychological treatment for depression. Cognitive thera-

RECOMMENDATION HIGHLIGHTS

Self-Help Books

- For alleviating depression through cognitive-behavioral methods:

  ★★★★★ *Feeling Good* by David Burns

  ★★★★★ *The Feeling Good Handbook* by David Burns

  ★★★★★ *Mind Over Mood* by Dennis Greenberger and Christine A. Padesky

  ★★★★★ *Control Your Depression* by Peter Lewinsohn et al.

  ★★★★★ *Cognitive Therapy and the Emotional Disorders* by Aaron Beck

- For reducing depression by brief and practical directives:

  ★★★★ *When Living Hurts* by Michael D. Yapko

- For converting depression into new sources of growth:

  ★★★★ *When Feeling Bad Is Good* by Ellen McGrath

- For treating seasonal affective disorders:

  ★★★ *Winter Blues: Seasonal Affective Disorder* by Norman E. Rosenthal

- For identifying and remediating men's depression:

  ★★★ *I Don't Want to Talk about It* by Terrence Real

- For helping parents cope with teenager's depression:

  ◆ *Overcoming Teen Depression* by Miriam Kaufman

Autobiographies

- For sensitive descriptions of severe depression and near suicide:

  ★★★★★ *Darkness Visible* by William Styron

  ★★★★ *Undercurrents* by Martha Manning

  ★★★ *The Beast* by Tracy Thompson

- For a personal yet comprehensive look at depression:

  ★★★ *The Noonday Demon* by Andrew Solomon

Films

- For a harrowing and systemic portrait of depression:

  ★★★★ *A Woman under the Influence*

Internet Resources

- For accurate and comprehensive information on depression:

  ★★★★★ *Dr. Ivan's Depression Central*
  http://www.psycom.net/depression.central.html

  ★★★★★ *Wing of Madness* http://www.wingofmadness.com

  ★★★★ *Psychology Information Online: Depression*
  http://www.psychologyinfo.com/depression

- For medication and/or psychotherapy for mood disorders:

  ★★★★★ *Are You Considering Medication for Depression?*
    http://www.utexas.edu/student/cmhc/booklets/meds/meds.html

  ★★★★★ *Psychotherapy versus Medication for Depression*
    http://www.apa.org/journals/anton.html

- For information on cognitive-behavioral therapy:

  ★★★★★ *The Cognitive Therapy Pages*
    http://www.habitsmart.com/cogtitle.html

  ★★★★ *Cognitive Behavior Therapy*
    http://www.cognitive-behavior-therapy.org

- For understanding depression in children:

  ★★★★★ *Depression in Children and Adolescents* http://www.klis.com/
    chandler/pamphlet/dep/depressionpamphlet.htm

pists believe that people become depressed because of faulty thinking that triggers self-destructive moods. Examples of faulty thinking are all-or-nothing thinking (if a situation is anything less than perfect, it is a total failure), discounting the positive (positive experiences don't count), magnification (exaggerating the importance of problems and shortcomings), and personalization (taking personal responsibility for events that aren't entirely under one's control). In *Feeling Good*, Burns outlines techniques people can use to identify and combat their faulty thinking. These techniques have been extensively tested in published research studies; indeed, this is one of the few books in the entire self-help literature that can boast about its demonstrated effectiveness (Ackerson, Scogin, McKendree-Smith, & Lyman, 1998; Cuijpers, 1997). It is peppered with self-assessment tests, self-help forms, and charts. The self-assessment techniques include the widely used Beck Depression Inventory, an anger scale, and a dysfunctional attitudes scale. The self-help forms and charts include a daily record of dysfunctional thoughts, an antiprocrastination sheet, a pleasure-predicting sheet, an anger cost–benefit analysis, and an antiperfection sheet. Updated in 1999 with a new section on antidepressant medications, this was the highest-rated book in the depression category of our national studies. An outstanding self-help book that has sold more than 2 million copies since its original publication in 1980, Burns's easy-to-read writing style, extensive use of examples, and enthusiasm give readers a clear understanding of cognitive therapy and the confidence to try its techniques.

★★★★★ *The Feeling Good Handbook* (revised ed., 1999) by David Burns. New York: Plume.

In this sequel to *Feeling Good*, Burns says that one of the most exciting recent developments is the discovery that cognitive therapy, which he calls the new mood therapy, can help people with the entire range of mood problems they encounter in their everyday lives. These include feelings of insecurity and inferiority, procrastination, guilt, stress, frustration, and irritability. In this handbook, Burns explains why we are plagued by irrational worries and how to conquer our worst fears without having to rely on addictive tranquilizers or alcohol. Burns also describes the important application of cognitive therapy in recent years to problems in personal relationships, especially marital and couple relationships. *The Feeling Good Handbook* asks readers to complete a number of self-assessment tests once a week, just as patients do, to monitor progress. The tests ask about thoughts, feelings, and actions in a variety of circumstances that typically make people feel angry, sad, frustrated, or anxious. There are two main differences in *The Feeling Good Handbook* and the original book: It covers a wider array of problems (anxiety and relationships, as well as depression), and includes daily logs to fill out. This five-star resource can be used as an adjunct to *Feeling Good* or independent of it. In either case, it is a very valuable and prized self-help book.

★★★★★　*Mind Over Mood: Change How You Feel by Changing the Way You Think* (1995) by Dennis Greenberger and Christine A. Padesky. New York: Guilford Press.

The authors have taken the nuts and bolts of cognitive therapy and spelled out in a step-by-step fashion how a layperson can utilize these methods in dealing with depression, anxiety, guilt, and shame. Strategies described in this book can also help people solve relationship problems, handle stress better, improve self-esteem, and become less fearful and more confident. The book helps people identify and make necessary changes in the relationship among thoughts, emotions, behavior, body changes, and events in their lives. Each chapter contains practice exercises. This five-star cognitive therapy manual can be truly helpful for adults suffering from depressive complaints—truly a matter of "mind over mood."

★★★★★　*Control Your Depression* (1996) by Peter Lewinsohn, Ricardo Munoz, Mary Ann Youngren, and Antonette Zeiss. Englewood Cliffs, NJ: Prentice-Hall.

This self-help resource, also in the cognitive-behavioral tradition, is intended to teach a way of thinking about depression as well as controlling it. The book is divided into three parts: Part I explains how depressed people think; Part II provides step-by-step procedures to control depression; and Part III is about ensuring success. Techniques include self-control, relaxation, planning pleasant activities, and modifying self-defeating thinking patterns. There are illustrations of how to gauge progress, maintain gains, and determine the need for further help. *Control Your Depression* has been shown in controlled research to work effectively in many cases (Cuijpers, 1998). This five-star resource is a solid, research-based self-help book for treating depression.

★★★★★　*Cognitive Therapy and the Emotional Disorders* (1976) by Aaron Beck. New York: International Universities Press.

This text, as the title implies, presents a cognitive therapy approach to depression and other emotional disorders. Aaron Beck pioneered the cognitive therapy approach to depression. He describes the cognitive triad, which consists of negative thoughts about the self, ongoing experience, and the future. Beck believes that systematic errors in thinking, each of which darkens the person's experiences, produce depression. These errors include drawing a conclusion when there is little or no evidence to support it; focusing on an insignificant detail while ignoring the more important features of a situation; drawing global conclusions about worth or performance on the basis of a single fact; magnifying small bad events and minimizing large good events; and incorrectly engaging in self-blame for bad events. Cognitive therapy attempts to counter these distorted thoughts. People are taught to identify and correct the flawed thinking, and are trained to conquer problems and master situations they previously thought were insurmountable. This valuable five-star book was written primarily for professionals rather than a self-help audience. Many of the ideas in Beck's book are presented in a much easier to read fashion in Burns's *Feeling Good* and Greenberger and Padesky's *Mind Over Mood*. Beck's book will thus appeal primarily to the clinical community and to the knowledgeable layperson.

★★★★ *When Living Hurts: Directives for Treating Depression* (1994) by Michael D. Yapko. New York: Brunner/Mazel.

This book addresses brief and practical methods for treating depression. Yapko believes that depression can be managed, and that when it is well-managed, it doesn't hurt as much or as long. He gives directives and strategies intended to help the clinician intervene actively and provide catalysts for learning to interrupt the cycle of depression. The first part of the book provides a theoretical overview; the second part describes 91 directives; and the third part presents case narratives that illustrate applications of the directives. This excellent, four-star book is largely a reference volume for clinicians; if a client were to use it as a self-help resource, it should probably be used in conjunction with a professional. Yapko's *Breaking the Patterns of Depression* (reviewed below) is a more conventional self-help book.

★★★★ *When Feeling Bad Is Good* (1994) by Ellen McGrath. New York: Bantam.

This book provides a program for women to convert "healthy depression" into new sources of growth. McGrath challenges the cultural myth that feeling bad must necessarily be negative and introduces a new perspective on women's depression. A woman's healthy depression may be a realistic and appropriate emotional response to the unhealthy culture in which she lives. McGrath identifies six types of healthy depression: victimization depression, relationship depression, age-range depression, depletion depression, body image depression, and mind–body depression. This valuable four-star book is appropriate for women of all ages, ethnicities, and socioeconomic strata.

Recommended

★★★ *You Can Beat Depression: A Guide to Prevention and Recovery* (3rd ed., 2001) by John Preston. San Luis Obispo, CA: Impact.

In the third edition of this valuable book, the author helps readers appreciate that all depression is not alike (for example, chronic vs. acute depression). After providing a clearer understanding of depression, Preston guides readers through various treatment choices, such as brief therapy, self-help approaches, family therapy, medication, and cognitive changes. Relapse prevention programs are also addressed for the person working to maintain or improve gains. This three-star book would actually be a four-star selection if not for the fact that relatively few mental health professionals rated it. A very useful resource for people trying to understand and make choices about treating their depression.

★★★ *Winter Blues—Seasonal Affective Disorder: What It Is and How to Overcome It* (1998) by Norman E. Rosenthal. New York: Guilford Press.

A book for patients, spouses, and family members who wish to better understand and cope with seasonal affective disorders (SADs). Psychiatrist Rosenthal begins with a self-test to evaluate the level of SAD and then reviews the effectiveness of antidepressant medication, light therapy, St. John's wort, and a nutritional regimen. Light therapy, the author's research area, is particularly favored. There is also a step-by-step guide on coping with SADs all year round. This is probably the best self-help book on SADs.

★★★ *Getting Un-Depressed: How a Woman Can Change Her Life through Cognitive Therapy* (revised ed., 1988) by Gary Emery. New York: Touchstone.

The cognitive therapy approach of this book is designed to help women cope effectively with depression. Women's risk of developing depression is about double that of men. Emery explains what depression is and how cognitive therapy can help. He describes how women can get immediate relief from their symptoms and improve their state of mind. Next, the author focuses on ways to overcome common complications of depression (weight gain, alcohol and drug dependence, and relationship problems). After this, women learn that they can avoid future depression by working on the psychological causes of depression, which, according to Emery, are underlying negative beliefs and ineffective ways of handling stress. Finally, Emery outlines how women can lead more self-reliant and self-directed lives. This three-star book, just missing the four-star rating, is a popular and practical application of cognitive therapy to depression for women.

★★★ *I Don't Want to Talk about It: Overcoming the Secret Legacy of Male Depression* (1997) by Terrence Real. New York: Scribner.

Feeling the stigma of depression's "unmanliness," many men hide their condition not only from family and friends but also from themselves. Real believes that by directing their pain outward, depressed men hurt the people they love and frequently pass their condition on to their children. Real mixes in his own experiences with depression, as a son of a depressed, violent father and the father of two young sons. By integrating personal and professional experiences, Real teaches men how they can unearth their pain, heal themselves, restore relationships, and break the legacy of abuse. A useful self-help book specifically for men.

★★★ *How to Stubbornly Refuse to Make Yourself Miserable about Anything, Yes Anything!* (1988) by Albert Ellis. New York: Lyle Stuart.

This internationally respected psychologist, originator of Rational–Emotive Behavioral Therapy (REBT), contends that we create our own feelings and choose to think and feel in self-harming ways. Ellis's goals here are to show people how to express and control their emotional destinies, how to stubbornly refuse to make themselves miserable, how to use scientific reasoning, and how to effectively change their emotional and behavioral problems. The book certainly covers depression and misery, but it is broader in its coverage. This three-star book can be helpful for laypersons who are self-motivated or already involved in cognitive-behavior therapy.

★★★ *Hand-Me-Down Blues: How to Stop Depression from Spreading in Families* (1999) by Michael D. Yapko. New York: Golden.

The family is a powerful system, both for unwittingly teaching depression and for helping to overcome it. Psychologist Yapko advocates a shift away from medications as the sole solution for depression toward the curative role of family therapy. He emphasizes that "depression can be relieved with a family approach as family members are brought together to relieve their distress by learning to help each other and to avoid blame as the whole family reacts to depression." A realistic and family approach to the management of depression.

★★★ *Overcoming Depression: A Cognitive Therapy Approach for Taming the Depression BEAST* (1999) by Mark Gilson and Arthur Freeman. Albany, NY: Graywind. (Also distributed by the Psychological Corporation.)

The depression BEAST is a treatment acronym: one chapter addresses "B" for body and biology; "E" for emotions; "A" for action; "S" for situations and vulnerability; and "T" for thoughts. A final chapter focuses on the role of hope. The book adopts an integrative but largely cognitive perspective in the treatment of depression. It is educational, easy to read, and quite practical. A useful self-help resource for depressed persons and their families.

★★★ *How to Cope with Depression* (1989, reprinted 1996) by Raymond DePaulo and Keith Ablow. New York: Ballantine.

Subtitled *A Complete Guide for You and Your Family*, this book is primarily about the biological causes of depression and the treatment of depression through drug therapy. Part I, Depression: What We Know, defines depression and bipolar disorder (the authors call it manic–depressive illness) and describes the causes of depression as biological. Part II, The Experience of Depression, portrays the nature of depression from the perspective of the patient, the family, and the physician. Part III, The Four Perspectives of Depression, evaluates the disease perspective, the personality perspective, the behavior perspective, and the life-story perspective, and Part IV, Current Treatments, presents the authors' view of how depression should be treated. This three-star book was not widely known in our studies, and its title notwithstanding, it is less a guide to coping with depression than a primer on possible causes, treatments, and professional perspectives. The authors make clear their own view: Depression is a physical disease with genetic and biological causes that can be successfully treated only through drug therapy. Other therapies are given token discussion.

★★★ *When the Blues Won't Go Away* (1991) by Robert Hirschfeld. New York: Macmillan.

This book concerns one form of depression—dysthymic disorder—that is long-lasting and relatively mild. In the early chapters, Hirschfeld describes the rut that people with dysthymic disorder (DD) get themselves into and what they do to stay in that rut. Many characteristics of DD resemble those of major depression, but DD's symptoms are less severe and usually last longer. People with DD continue to function at home and work, but not at the level they once did. Most of the book is devoted to getting rid of DD, and Hirschfeld does an excellent job of presenting a variety of treatment strategies. The author outlines self-help strategies and tailor-made therapies for such problems. He also discusses antidepressant medications and shows how a combination of drug therapy and psychotherapy can be effective. This three-star resource came out just before one of our studies was conducted, so only a small number of mental health professionals rated it. We believe that *When the Blues Won't Go Away* provides a well-balanced analysis of a specific type of depression—long-lasting, relatively mild depression.

★★★ *Breaking the Patterns of Depression* (1997) by Michael D. Yapko. New York: Doubleday.

The author's dual foci are the initial treatment and the prevention of depressive disorders. Yapko provides over 100 activities to help learn the skills necessary for becoming and remaining depression-free. Readers are asked to participate in the activities listed in each chapter. Action steps are emphasized throughout.

★★★ *Understanding and Overcoming Depression: A Common Sense Approach* (1999) by Tony Bates. Freedom, CA: Crossing.

The author offers a heartwarming message that builds self-esteem and gives us trust in ourselves. In 128 pages, Bates overviews the signs and causes of depression, and argues that hopelessness is the major obstacle to overcoming depression. The recovery plan includes cognitive work on self-image and a relapse prevention/maintenance plan. Pharmacological and psychotherapy are briefly addressed. A useful and—as the title declares—common sense self-help book.

★★★ *Listening to Prozac* (1997) by Peter D. Kramer. New York: Penguin.

This best-selling author guides us into the scientific study of biology and personality. Kramer explains the historical debate over what drives us as human beings—nature versus nurture. He then shares his psychiatric and philosophical observations about the influence of a medication such as Prozac on a patient's outlook and self-image. His focus is limited mainly to explaining the impact of mood-altering drugs on the modern sense of self: What is Prozac's influence on personality, work performance, memory, dexterity? Does it affect character rather than illness? For the professional and the layperson interested in the ongoing debates about mind versus body and nature versus nurture, this is a stimulating read. However, it is not intended as a self-help guide.

Diamond in the Rough

◆ *Overcoming Teen Depression: A Guide for Parents* (2001) by Miriam Kaufman. Buffalo, NY: Firefly.

This self-help book was explicitly written for the parents of depressed teenagers. The author reviews the signs of teen depression, its various types, comorbid conditions, and suicide risks. She usefully discusses indications for psychotherapy, selection of a therapist, the purposes of psychopharmacology, and the possibilities of alternative treatments, such as herbal medicines. It is a practical and reassuring book for parents and family members. If *Overcoming Teen Depression* had been read by more experts in our national studies, it would have certainly received a rating of three or more stars.

Not Recommended

★★ *You Mean I Don't Have to Feel This Way?* (1991) by Colette Dowling. New York: Scribner.

★ *The Good News about Depression: Cures and Treatments in the New Age of Psychiatry* (revised ed., 1995) by Mark S. Gold. New York: Villard.

AUTOBIOGRAPHIES

Strongly Recommended

★★★★★ *Darkness Visible: A Memoir of Madness* (1992) by William Styron. New York: Vintage.

In beautifully written prose, novelist William Styron describes his gradual recognition of debilitating depression, his descent into despair, his suicidal impulses, hospitalization, and recovery. In one of the best portrayals of the loneliness and despair of major depression ever written, the book illustrates the benefits of brief hospitalization; "For me," Styron writes, "the real helpers were seclusion and time" afforded by brief hospital stays. This book is widely known and very positively evaluated in our national studies—and short enough to be read by someone suffering from depression.

★★★★ *Undercurrents: A Therapist's Reckoning with Her Own Depression* (1994) by Martha Manning. San Francisco: Harper.

In her late 30s, psychotherapist Manning experienced a severe unipolar depression. Symptoms included sleep disturbance, lack of energy, and suicidal impulses. Neither psychotherapy nor drugs seemed to help. Reluctantly, she underwent electric shock therapy (EST), described in detail, which lifted the depression. Afterwards, she learned that it was difficult to convince her colleagues and her friends that EST was a beneficial treatment. The book takes some of the fear out of EST and demonstrates how the experience of depression can deepen understanding of the human condition. Manning writes, "In these flashes of insight, I understand for a moment that one of the great dividends of darkness is an increased sensitivity to light." A very sensitive account by a therapist who was compelled to switch roles and become a patient.

★★★★ *Leaves from Many Seasons: Selected Papers* (1983) by O. Hobart Mowrer. New York: Praeger.

As a psychologist, the author is best known for his research on learning. This book is a collection of his essays, one of which describes his history of depressive episodes. The first occurred when he was a freshman in high school, the second when he graduated from college and entered graduate school (where he tried psychoanalysis), the third as a postgraduate fellow when he began teaching at Yale, and again, in Washington, DC (where he again tried psychoanalysis). The last depression episode occurred when he was at the pinnacle of his career, as president-elect of the American Psychological Association. He became a voluntary patient at a small Chicago psychiatric hospital. This last episode was the beginning of Mowrer's interest in the relation between religion and psychopathology. Although the book received a four-star rating from professionals, the fact that only a single chapter concerns his depression limits the usefulness of the book as a self-help resource for depression.

Recommended

★★★   *The Beast: A Journey through Depression* (1996) by Tracy Thompson. New York: Plume.

Drawing on notes in a journal she kept from adolescence onward and her considerable research skills as a reporter for the *Washington Post*, Thompson writes of her struggles with the depression, suicidal thoughts, and inner demons that have been with her since adolescence. She was treated with psychotherapy and various drugs, including Prozac and imipramine. A compassionate and well-written account, told with candor that captures the emotional depths of depression, the book is particularly useful in showing that one can have a serious, chronic depression and still maintain a successful career. Very high but infrequent rating by the mental health experts in our studies resulted in the three stars.

★★★   *The Noonday Demon: An Atlas of Depression* (2002) by Andrew Solomon. New York: Simon & Schuster.

Superbly written and well researched, this combined memoir and compendium by National Book Award winner Andrew Solomon has become an instant classic on depression. His own serious bouts of depression, his desire to end his life, and the many treatments he had undergone led him to explore the condition in medical, historical, and cross-cultural contexts. He interviewed psychotherapists and researchers, other people with depression, drug makers, and philosophers, and read accounts of famous literary figures who had serious depression. To understand the many expressions of depression, he visited mental hospitals and traveled to Senegal, Cambodia, and Greenland. The book covers both unipolar and bipolar disorders, and describes treatment modalities across the spectrum, including drugs, talk therapies, alternative herbal and homeopathic remedies, diet and exercise, and electroconvulsive therapy. Concluding with a chapter titled "Hope," this moving, empathic, and comprehensive work is a milestone among books on depression. Although its average rating would have merited five stars, this autobiography is not yet widely known and did not collect sufficient ratings for a five-star designation.

★★★   *On the Edge of Darkness* (1995) by Kathy Cronkite. New York: Dell.

Following her own bout with depression, Kathy Cronkite undertook research into the disorder and produced this combination autobiography and self-help book. Most of the book involves interviews with celebrities who have suffered from depression, including Mike Wallace, Kitty Dukakis, Rod Steiger, and William Styron. Cronkite also talked to researchers and describes therapeutic options for adults and children with depression. The interviewees recommend seeking treatment sooner rather than later, because untreated depression is likely to worsen, bringing with it risks of suicide. Learning that successful people have suffered from the disorder and come through the experience will benefit many readers, especially in overcoming the "No one has ever felt like this before" feelings so typical of serious depression.

★★★   *The Bell Jar* (1995) by Sylvia Plath. Cutchogue, NY: Buccaneer.

Plath was a prize-winning poet who received much acclaim during her lifetime and afterward. This autobiographical novel, published only a month before her suicide in 1963, recounts the young woman's hospitalization for severe depression while she was a summer intern at a New York City magazine. She was given shock treatments and spent time in private psychiatric hospitals. Her multiple hospitalizations left her fearful of treatment, especially shock treatment. The book is regarded as a literary classic in its sensitive description of inner pain so great that it leads to suicide. This is not a hopeful book—Plath's tragic end is already known—but it can awaken readers to danger signs in themselves and others.

Diamond in the Rough

♦   *Composing Myself: A Journey through Postpartum Depression* (1998) by Fiona Shaw. South Royalton, VT: Steerforth.

Composing Myself is a autobiographical journey into a depression after the birth of the author's second child. The chronic nature of the depression led the author to hospitalization and extended psychiatric care. During this process, her childhood alienation, loneliness, and estranged parental relationship came to the surface; the story of her life was intertwined with her adult experience of postpartum depression. The literary ability of the author is evident in the expressive narrative her story takes. This book is written to provide a familiar voice and story to those who suffer postpartum depression and feel isolated, unique, and misunderstood. The author's perspective, coupled with the recent publication date, qualify this book as a Diamond in the Rough.

Not Recommended

★★   *Prozac Nation: Young and Depressed in America* (1997) by Elizabeth Wurtzel. New York: Riverhead.

FILMS

Strongly Recommended

★★★★   *A Woman under the Influence* (1974) directed by John Cassavetes. R rating. 155 minutes.

A harrowing film that charts the emotional breakdown of a housewife and the effects of her depression on her blue-collar family. Peter Falk plays a distant, inexpressive construction worker flummoxed by the fragile mental condition of his wife, Gena Rowlands. When her condition threatens the well-being of their children, he has her committed to a psychiatric hospital for several months. The film poignantly demonstrates one person's sense of depressive desperation, a partner's inability to provide emotional support, and the devastating consequences. The heart wrenching performances leave a lasting impression.

INTERNET RESOURCES

Metasites

★★★★★ *Wing of Madness: A Depression Guide* http://www.wingofmadness.com

An enormous collection of sensible and accurate information, with many clearly organized sections and links, designed for laypersons. A pleasure to explore. Support, personal experiences, advice, links, and so on.

★★★★★ *Dr. Ivan's Depression Central*
              http://www.psycom.net/depression.central.html

Offers about a million links, papers, and other materials under about 70 headings. Many are by Ivan K. Goldberg, MD, an expert on psychopharmacology. Although the site is medication-oriented, some subjects are free of this emphasis (e.g., Grief and Bereavement, Psychotherapy for People with Depression). Most materials are aimed at professionals and the sophisticated, but some can be used as introductory materials.

★★★★ *Psychology Information Online: Depression*
            http://www.psychologyinfo.com/depression

A very large site, organized by psychologists, full of accurate information about diagnosis, cognitive therapy, SAD, medication, and many other topics. Many articles are quite short but may be useful for people needing an overview. This is a product of Donald J. Franklin, PhD, and offers his *National Directory of Psychologists.*

★★★★ *Internet Mental Health: Major Depressive Disorder*
            http://www.mentalhealth.com/fr20.html

Click on Depression in the column on the left. The site has about a hundred clinically useful and educational papers, ranging from consensus guidelines to personal stories of recovery.

Psychoeducational Materials for Clients and Families

General Sites on Depression

★★★★★ *Depression* http://www.nimh.nih.gov/publicat/depressionmenu.cfm

From the National Institute of Mental Health, this page offers a dozen brochures organized by audience (adolescents, employers, senior citizens, and women) and by topic (bipolar disorder, suicide, comorbidity, etc.).

★★★★★ *Depression in Children and Adolescents: What It Is and What to Do about It* by Jim Chandler, MD
      http://www.klis.com/chandler/pamphlet/dep/depressionpamphlet.htm

About 20 pages of solid information and some vignettes written for the public and teens. The section What Can be Done? is about behavioral interventions.

★★★★ *Depression and Bipolar Support Alliance*
      http://www.dbsalliance.org/bookstore/brochures.html

This site offers about a dozen brochures on depression and bipolar disorder. A five-page brochure for teens about depressive illnesses is useful.

★★★★ *So You Don't Want to Go to a Psychiatrist!*
      http://www.mentalhealth.com/fr20.html

Click on Depression in the column on the left, then Stories of Recovery, then to this title. Although it never mentions nonpsychiatrists, this three-pager addresses the anxieties of our clients. It is perhaps best used for the ambivalent patient.

★★★★ *People with Depression Tend to Seek Negative Feedback*
      http://www.shpm.com/articles/depress/negfeed.html

A brief but useful handout because it addresses and teaches this important point about negativity.

★★★★ *Understanding and Treating Depression*
      http://www.couns.uiuc.edu/brochures/depression.htm

A brief, balanced, and complete overview.

★★★★ *Have a Heart's Depression Home* http://www.have-a-heart.com

Stephen L. Bernhardt, PhD, offers several fine essays: Depression: Understanding Suicidal Thoughts (he covers seven triggers for suicide); Helping a Depressed Friend; Emotional Thought Stopping (an exercise); and others. Very clear and useful for therapy.

★★★★ *Steven Thos's Mental Health Resources—Depression and Bipolar Disorder*
      http://www.thewritebrain.org/thow9903.html

About 40 questions very likely to be asked by patients or families, and annotated links to multiple answers.

★★★ *Best and Worst Things to Say to Someone Who Is Depressed*
      http://www.thewellspring.com/Journal/JWT/worstbestdepressed.html

There are 23 best and 99 worst. These might be useful for frustrated family members to consider.

Medication Treatment

★★★★★ *Are You Considering Medication for Depression?*
        http://www.utexas.edu/student/cmhc/booklets/meds/meds.html

About eight pages in a question-and-answer format on medications. Very relevant questions and good writing make this a useful handout before medication evaluation.

★★★★ *Pharmacological Treatment of Mood Disorders* by David M. Goldstein, MD
       http://www.healthyplace.com/communities/bipolar/nimh/bipolar_
       medications.htm

A rather sophisticated, six-page review of medications.

Against Solely Medication

★★★★★ *Psychotherapy versus Medication for Depression: Challenging the Conventional
        Wisdom with Data* by David O. Antonuccio, PhD, William G. Danton, PhD,
        and Garland Y. DeNelsky, PhD http://www.apa.org/journals/anton.html

"This article reviews a wide range of well-controlled studies comparing psychological and pharmacological treatments for depression. The evidence suggests that the psychological interventions, particularly cognitive-behavioral therapy, are at least as effective as medication in the treatment of depression, even if severe." Written for the reading level and sophistication of professionals.

★★★ *Placebo Effect Accounts for Fifty Percent of Improvement in Depressed Patients Taking
      Antidepressants* http://www.apa.org/releases/placebo.html

Summary written for the public.

Cognitive Therapy

★★★★★ *The Cognitive Therapy Pages* by Robert Westermeyer, PhD
        http://www.habitsmart.com/cogtitle.html

In six sections of two to six pages each, Westermeyer offers complete and accessible explanations. Suitable for introducing almost all patients to cognitive-behavioral therapy.

★★★★ *Cognitive Behavior Therapy*
       http://www.cognitive-behavior-therapy.org

There are excellent explanations of cognitive-behavioral therapy (CBT) in a format for the average reader, totaling about 25 pages, under What is CBT? Thank you, Dr. Bush.

★★★ *Cognitive Therapy: A Multimedia Learning Program* http://mindstreet.com/

In a series of 11 brief excerpts (downloadable as QuickTime movies), the basics of cognitive therapy for depression are presented. They are from a commercial CD-ROM, a sophisticated training program in CBT, that could serve as an introduction to treatment for the less-skilled reader or those who like computerized presentations.

Seasonal Affective Disorder (SAD)

★★★★ *Seasonal Light/SAD*
http://www.geocities.com/hotsprings/7061/sadhome.html

This site is about SAD only. It offers many links, bibliographies, organizations, and products. A similar site is *Outside In* at http://www.outsidein.co.uk/sadinfo.htm.

NATIONAL SUPPORT GROUPS

Depression and Related Affective Disorders Association
Johns Hopkins Hospital
600 North Wolfe Street
Baltimore, MD 21287-4647
Phone: 410-955-4647
E-mail: drada@jhmi.edu
http://www.drada.org

Emotional Health Anonymous
PO Box 2081
San Gabriel, CA 91778
Phone: 626-287-6260
E-mail: sgveha@hotmail.com
http://www.flash.net/~sgveha

Fellowship of people who meet to share experiences, strengths, and hopes to solve common mental health problems.

Emotions Anonymous
PO Box 4245
St. Paul, MN 55104
Phone: 651-647-9712
http://www.emotionsanonymous.org

Fellowship for people experiencing emotional difficulties.

National Alliance for the Mentally Ill
Colonial Place Three
2107 Wilson Boulevard, Suite 300
Arlington, VA 2201
Phone: 703-524-7600 or 800-950-NAMI
    (Hotline)
http://www.nami.org

National Depressive and Manic Depressive Association
730 North Franklin, Suite 501
Chicago, IL 60610
Phone: 800-826-3632
http://www.ndmda.org.

Prozac Survivors Support Group
PO Box 1727
Pacific Palisades, CA 90272
Phone: 800-392-0640
E-mail: skisun@earthlink.net
http://www.pssg.org

Postpartum Support International
927 North Kellogg Avenue
Santa Barbara, CA 93111
Phone: 805-967-7636

To increase awareness of the emotional changes women often experience during pregnancy and after the birth of a baby.

Recovery
802 North Dearborn Street
Chicago, IL 60610
Phone: 312-337-5661
http://www.recovery-inc.org

A community mental health organization that offers a self-help method of will training.

See also Bipolar Disorder (Chapter 10) and Suicide (Chapter 33).

CHAPTER 18

Divorce

Divorce has become epidemic in our society. Until recently, it was increasing annually by 10%, although its rate of increase has now leveled off.

For those involved, separation and divorce are complex and emotionally charged, and the stresses place men, women, and children at risk for psychological and physical difficulties. Separated and divorced adults have higher rates of behavioral disorders, admission to psychiatric hospitals, substance abuse, suicide, and depression than their married counterparts. Many separations and divorces immerse children in conflict and, as a consequence, the children are more likely to have school-related problems, especially at the beginning of the separation and divorce.

Self-help resources on divorce fall into four main categories: divorced or divorcing parents; the children of divorced or divorcing parents; divorced or divorcing adults in general; and child custody. This chapter presents self-help books, films, Internet resources, and national support groups for all those involved in divorce.

SELF-HELP BOOKS

Strongly Recommended

★★★★★ *The Boys and Girls Book about Divorce* (1985) by Richard Gardner. New York: Bantam.

This treasured book is written to help children cope with their parents' separation and divorce. It is appropriate for children of average or better intelligence who are 10 years of age and older. Most of what psychiatrist Gardner tells children in the book comes from his therapy experiences with children of divorce. Gardner talks directly to children about their feelings after the divorce, who is and is not to blame for the divorce, parents' love for their children, and how to handle angry feelings and the fear of being left alone. Then he tells children about how to get along better with their divorced

RECOMMENDATION HIGHLIGHTS

Self-Help Books

- For young children in divorced families:
  - ★★★★★ *Dinosaurs Divorce* by Laurene Brown and Marc Brown

- For older children and adolescents in divorced families:
  - ★★★★★ *The Boys and Girls Book about Divorce* by Richard Gardner
  - ★★★★ *How It Feels When Parents Divorce* by Jill Krementz

- For divorced parents to help children:
  - ★★★★ *Growing Up with Divorce* by Neil Kalter
  - ★★★ *Helping Your Kids Cope with Divorce* by M. Gary Neuman
  - ★★★ *For Better or for Worse* by E. Mavis Hetherington and John Kelly
  - ★★★ *Helping Children Cope with Divorce* by Edward Teyber
  - ★★★ *The Parents' Book about Divorce* by Richard Gardner

- For those undergoing divorce:
  - ★★★ *Crazy Time* by Abigail Trafford

- For those wanting to examine the research controversy on the effects of divorce:
  - ★★★★ *The Unexpected Legacy of Divorce* by Judith Wallerstein et al.
  - ★★★★ *Coping with Divorce, Single Parenting, and Remarriage* by E. Mavis Hetherington

Films

- On the pain of custody battles and the need to attend to children:
  - ★★★★ *Kramer vs. Kramer*

- On women making the postdivorce transition and redefining themselves:
  - ★★★★ *An Unmarried Woman*

- On inevitable changes in marriages and friendships:
  - ★★★ *The Four Seasons*

Internet Resources

- For complete and supportive sites for people going through divorce:
  - ★★★★★ *Divorce Central* http://www.divorcecentral.com
  - ★★★★ *Divorce Support* http://www.divorcesupport.com
  - ★★★★ *FAQ on Surviving the Emotional Trauma of Divorce* http://www.divorcecentral.com/lifeline/life_ans.html#notsaved

- For a short course about avoiding the courtroom:
  - ★★★★★ *Divorce Helpline* http://www.divorcehelp.com/index.html

- For guides on children who go through divorce:
  - ★★★★ *Coping with Separation and Divorce*
    http://www.nnfr.org/curriculum/topics/sep_div.html
  - ★★★ *Breaking the News*
    http://www.fsbassociates.com/fsg/whydivorce.html#excerpt

mothers and fathers. Gardner also covers the important topic of getting along with parents who live apart, sensitively handling difficult issues such as playing one parent against the other and what to do when parents try to use the child as a weapon. The final chapter explains to children what to expect if they see a psychotherapist. Written at an appropriate reading level for its intended audience, the book also features a number of cartoon-like drawings, which adds to its appeal for children. It has survived the test of time and remains a superb resource for divorced or divorcing parents to give to their 10-year-old and older children.

★★★★★ *Dinosaurs Divorce: A Guide for Changing Families* (1986) by Laurene Brown and Marc Brown. Boston: Little, Brown.

This book, designed for children living in divorced families, grew out of the Browns' experiences with divorce as parent and stepparent, and for Laurene, as a child herself. *Dinosaurs Divorce* is a 30-page, full-color picture book that takes children through the experience of divorce in a dinosaur family. The topics include why parents divorce, how children feel when their parents divorce, what happens after the divorce, what it's like to live with one parent, what it's like to visit the other parent, having two homes, celebrating holidays and special occasions, telling friends, meeting parents' new friends, and having stepsisters and stepbrothers. The book is simple and easy for children to understand. Much of it can be read and understood by children in elementary school. Parents can read and discuss the pictures and words with younger children.

★★★★ *How It Feels When Parents Divorce* (1984) by Jill Krementz. New York: Knopf.

Jill Krementz, a writer and photographer, presents 19 children's experiences with the divorces of their parents. Krementz interviewed and photographed 19 children ages 7 to 16. The title of each of the chapters is a child's name. Each chapter opens with a full-page photograph of the child, followed by the child's experience in a divorced family. The children talk about the changes in their lives, their hurt, their confusion, and the knowledge they gained. The book is mainly geared toward children and adolescents; it is at about the same reading level as Gardner's *The Boys and Girls Book about Divorce*, although divorced parents can also benefit from the children's descriptions of their experiences. The children's stories reflect their vulnerability and resilience. Eight-year-old Lulu reflects, "I suppose they needed the divorce to be happy, but there were times when I thought it was stupid and unfair and mean to me." Many mental health professionals find it an excellent self-help book for older children and adolescents.

★★★★ *The Unexpected Legacy of Divorce* (2001) by Judith Wallerstein, Sandra Blakeslee, and Julia Lewis. New York: Hyperion.

This book provides descriptions of people's experiences with divorce at different points in their lives. The authors describe how people still define themselves as children of divorce up to 30 years after their parents' divorce. The unexpectedly negative results of divorce reported here have made this book a somewhat controversial and certainly sobering reevaluation of the decision to divorce. The authors assert that many children of divorce make bad choices in relationships or avoid relationships altogether. The book is based on tracking approximately 100 children of divorce into their adult lives.

★★★★ *Coping with Divorce, Single Parenting, and Remarriage* (1999) edited by E. Mavis Hetherington. Mahwah, NJ: Erlbaum.

Leading divorce researcher Mavis Hetherington edited this book, and a number of leading researchers contributed chapters. It is more a research volume than a self-help book. However, if you want to read more about what leading researchers in this area are studying, this book is a good choice.

★★★★ *Surviving the Breakup* (1996) by Judith Wallerstein and Joan Kelly. New York: Basic Books.

Based on their Children of Divorce Project, Wallerstein and Kelly describe how children, adolescents, and their parents cope with divorce. Especially helpful are the authors' portrayals of how children of different ages cope with divorce and the ways that parents can help them. A fine, four-star self-help guide by the lead author of *The Unexpected Legacy of Divorce* (reviewed above).

★★★★ *Growing Up with Divorce* (1990) by Neil Kalter. New York: Free Press.

This book, written for divorced parents, provides information to help their children avoid emotional problems. It is especially designed to counteract the long-term effects of divorce on children, many of whom struggle with emotional difficulties for years after the actual divorce itself. Kalter's book offers parents practical strategies for helping children cope with the anxiety, anger, and confusion that can occur immediately or develop over a number of years. Kalter nicely shows how a child's level of psychological development influences the specific ways he or she experiences, understands, and reacts to the stress of divorce. The book includes in-depth accounts of the experiences of children from infancy through adolescence. Kalter gives step-by-step instructions to parents about how to speak to their children in indirect and nonthreatening ways and tells them what to say in specific situations. A splendid self-help book for divorced parents.

Recommended

★★★ *Crazy Time: Surviving Divorce* (1982) by Abigail Trafford. New York: Harper & Row.

As a result of her own painful experience with divorce, journalist Trafford began recording the many stories she heard from others who were going through divorce. Each story was different, yet each fit a pattern. Trafford identifies and describes the developmental stages of divorce, crazy time, and the recovery. *Crazy Time* is the author's term for the two years immediately following a divorce, in which unpredictable and inexplicable emotions take over and the roller-coaster ride begins. Each topic is approached through the true-life experiences of many interviewees. The personalized style of the book gives an intimate feeling to the stories and the people who lived them. *Crazy Time* received a sterling evaluation from those experts familiar with it, but the low number of ratings reduced its overall rating.

★★★ *Helping Children Cope with Divorce* (revised ed., 2001) by Edward Teyber. New York: Wiley.

Teyber provides good strategies for parents to help their children through a divorce as unscathed and emotionally strong as possible in the face of stressful circumstances. Parents learn about ways to minimize stress, explain the divorce, establish custody and visitation plans, and shield the children from parental conflicts. A wise and sensible book in the divorce field characterized by ideology and polarization. If this self-help book had been more widely known among metal health professionals, it might have reached five-star status.

★★★ *The Good Divorce* (1995) by Constance Ahrons. New York: HarperCollins.

Based on her longitudinal study of postdivorce families, Ahrons provides hope that divorced spouses can handle their breakup in a way that will help both the adults and children involved be as emotionally healthy as they were before the divorce. The book especially provides helpful information for couples in which "staying together for the sake of the children" is not a viable option.

★★★ *Helping Your Kids Cope with Divorce* (1998) by M. Gary Neuman with Patricia Romanowski. New York: Times Books.

This parents' book on divorce through a child's eyes explains how children think and feel about divorce and, more importantly, how they interpret what has happened. The central concept is that, more often than not, the child is thinking differently than the parent thinks. The result is that children blame themselves and make distorted attributions about why it happened, what their role was, and what will happen to them now. Activities teach parents how to stop reasoning and to start communicating by knowing how to find out what the child thinks and feels through art, play, activities, and simply asking different questions. One chapter each is devoted to age-specific information on the infant and toddler to the 17-year-old. Other topics include fighting, the first day of the divorce, moving, custody and visitation, and divorce-related changes (e.g., finances, home, changing schools, child care).

★★★ *For Better or for Worse: Divorce Reconsidered* (2002) by E. Mavis Hetherington and John Kelly. New York: Norton.

Hetherington and Kelly paint a very different picture of divorce than Judith Wallerstein in *The Unexpected Legacy of Divorce* (reviewed above) and *Second Chances* (reviewed below). Based on Hetherington's extensive research on more than 1,400 families over three decades, the authors argue that although divorce can be destructive in the short-term, it can also be positive, creating new opportunities for long-term growth. Readers are taken through the stages of divorce, single parenthood, remarriage, and stepfamily life, and given many recommendations for how to cope with the stress involved. Excellent strategies are provided for both adults and children. Many excerpts from cases in Hetherington's study are provided to illustrate various aspects of divorce.

★★★ *Second Chances: Men, Women, and Children a Decade after Divorce* (revised ed., 1996) by Judith S. Wallerstein and Sandra Blakeslee. Boston: Houghton Mifflin.

Based on a long-term study of divorced couples and their children, Wallerstein and associates examined how 60 families fared five years after divorce. In *Second Chances*, Wallerstein and Blakeslee describe the reevaluation of 90% of the original 60 families 10 years after divorce, with some analysis of their lives at the 15-year mark. Additional commentary is included about divorced families seen at the California clinic Wallerstein directs. The authors argue that divorce is emotionally painful and psychologically devastating for a large proportion of children. In their view, divorced parents who are struggling to meet their own needs often fail to meet their children's needs; through their own instability and continuing conflict with each other, divorced parents add to the psychological burdens of their children. Interview excerpts are interwoven with clinical interpretations and research findings to tell the emotionally difficult story of the long-term negative effects of divorce on children. The book, though recommended, is a sober read for many divorcing parents.

★★★ *The Divorce Book* (2001) by Matthew McKay, Joan Blades, Richard Gosse, and Peter Rogers. Oakland, CA: New Harbinger.

The authors—psychologists and lawyers—combined their expertise to help adults negotiate the painful legal and emotional hurdles of divorce. Their book distinctively provides information about the legal aspects of ending a marriage, including conflict resolution, divorce mediation, and custody arrangements.

★★★ *The Parents' Book about Divorce* (revised ed., 1991) by Richard Gardner. New York: Bantam.

Gardner, a leading expert on divorce, provides helpful information about the psychological and emotional aspects of divorce. He takes parents through a chronological time table of the circumstances involving divorce, telling parents how and when to tell children about an impending separation, strategies for informing friends and teachers, and providing guidelines for adapting to new homes and stepfamilies. Although rated favorably in our national studies, this book pales in comparison to the exceptional ratings accorded to Gardner's *The Boys and Girls Book about Divorce* (reviewed above).

★★★ *Creative Divorce* (1973) by Mel Krantzler. New York: Signet.

This book, anchored in the 1970s, is about divorced individuals' opportunities for personal growth. When he was 50 years of age, Krantzler and his wife separated after 24 years of marriage. He describes his ordeal—self-pity, guilt, loneliness, and helplessness—and how it helped him grow as a person. The author also draws on the experiences of his male and female clients. Krantzler considers divorce the death of a relationship, requiring a mourning period followed by reflective self-evaluation and planning. The self-destructive patterns that many divorced adults engage in are portrayed, such as when men say they want companionship but pursue women as sexual objects. The book was a best-seller in the 1970s, but its popularity has declined since then, and many readers may regard it as both dated and too optimistic.

Diamond in the Rough

◆ *Dumped: A Survival Guide for the Woman Who's Been Left by the Man She Loved* (1999) by Sally Warren and Andrea Thompson. New York: HarperCollins.

Sally Warren, left by her husband after a 19-year marriage, collaborates with freelance writer Thompson on this survival guide. Research for the book included interviews with 108 women who had been abandoned by their partners. The book includes tips about what is happening and explains what is happening to oneself and others, the emotional stages passed through, ways to avoid destructive actions, and the path to healing and new relationships. The stages of being dumped are addressed with humor, candor, and respect. Validation, reassurance, and reality testing for women are big pluses for this book, which, along with the recent publication date, is why this well-researched book earned its Diamond in the Rough status.

Not Recommended

★ *Mars and Venus Starting Over* (1998) by John Gray. New York: HarperCollins.

FILMS

Strongly Recommended

★★★★ *Kramer vs. Kramer* (1979) directed by Robert Benton. PG rating. 105 minutes.

Wife leaves marriage; husband assumes care of their five-year-old son; father discovers the responsibilities and joys of parenting; wife returns and fights for custody of son. The ensuing legal proceedings are bitter and cruel, resulting in a decision favoring the mother and ordering the father to relinquish custody. But then the Kramers negotiate a mature arrangement on their own that attends to the needs of the child and themselves. A powerful film, recipient of five Academy Awards, it vividly demonstrates multiple realities of marriage, divorce, and custody: adult self-involvement with work (the father), search for identity (the mother), avoiding heartrending custody battles, attending to the child's needs during custody, the pain of nasty legal battles, and, ultimately, the superiority of working cooperatively.

★★★★ *An Unmarried Woman* (1978) directed by Paul Mazursky. R rating. 124 minutes.

An affluent Manhattan lawyer suddenly informs his steadfast wife that he doesn't love her and is leaving their 20-year marriage. The wife, accustomed to defining herself in terms of her husband, makes the difficult transition to being an unmarried woman, developing a mature identity, and learning to love without losing herself. One of the earliest and still best films that realistically depict women redefining their postdivorce identities. The film also beautifully explores the loving relationship between a mother and her teenage daughter.

Recommended

★★★   *The Four Seasons* (1981) directed by Alan Alda. PG rating. 107 minutes.

Three middle-aged couples are lifelong friends and vacation together until one of the men decides to divorce his wife. He brings his young girlfriend on their next vacation, a cruise around the Virgin Islands, and the other two couples are both disturbed and envious of the couple's romantic relationship. The divorced wife subsequently accuses her lifelong friends of deserting her, and the three couples continue to support one another, adapt, and struggle through the travails of life and marriage. The film uses Vivaldi's *Four Seasons* as a metaphor for the development and inevitable changes in the couples' lives and marriages. Useful for illustrating the interpersonal ramifications of divorce and accepting changes in friends.

★★★   *The Good Mother* (1989) directed by Leonard Nimoy. R rating. 104 minutes.

A divorced mother falls in love with a man who naively allows the woman's young daughter to touch his penis, resulting in the divorced father's filing a suit for custody. Although the psychologists conclude that the child has suffered no harm and that she is securely attached to the mother, the lawyer convinces the mother to make her boyfriend the scapegoat in order to maintain the relationship with her daughter. This provocative and sad film shows the challenges of intimacy for single parents and the charge of sexual molestation being used as a weapon by a former spouse.

★★★   *Husbands and Wives* (1992) directed by Woody Allen. R rating. 107 minutes.

A film in which art imitated life. Woody Allen and Mia Farrow endured a public battle over Allen's affair with Farrow's adopted daughter. A few months later, Allen released this film, starring himself and Farrow acting out a virtually identical plot: An unhappy marriage crumbles when the husband strays with a much younger woman (in this case, a student). In the film, a friend of Allen's character discards his longtime wife for an aerobics instructor, shocking their friends and planting seeds of marital dissolution all around. *Husbands and Wives* is a lacerating comedy, an honest look at conflicts that beset many marriages. It is a story about the fragility of relationships and the foolishness of older men seeking to recapture their youth with younger women.

★★★   *Starting Over* (1979) directed by Alan J. Pakula. R rating. 105 minutes.

This honest film casts Burt Reynolds as a newly divorced man struggling to adjust to single life in the late 1970s. Reynolds plays an unsuccessful writer torn between his neurotic girlfriend (Jill Clayburgh) and his flighty, sexy ex-wife (Candice Bergen). The man is vulnerable, indecisive, and confused—at one point suffering a hilarious anxiety attack in public. Wonderfully acted (the female leads were nominated for Oscars) and quirkily entertaining, *Starting Over* only disappoints with an abrupt ending. A valuable self-help resource for sharing ambivalent feelings about an ex-spouse and about the indecision of reconciliation. The film is also useful for it depiction of coping with single life and dating again.

★★★ *Mrs. Doubtfire* (1994) directed by Chris Columbus. PG-13 rating. 119 minutes.

An idealistic and fun-loving father clashes with a sensible and sedate mother in marriage and then in divorce, when the mother is awarded custody of their three children. The father transforms himself into an elderly English nanny, Mrs. Doubtfire, and is hired to care for the children. That's when the high jinks begin. Nicely demonstrates the genuine pain and loss of divorce, parental devotion to children despite the end of a marriage, and the realistic struggles to accommodate everyone's needs in postdivorce families.

★★★ *Bye Bye Love* (1995) directed by Sam Weisman. PG-13 rating. 106 minutes.

Three divorced California fathers attempt to juggle their children's and their own needs over a weekend. There are no enviable role models here, but the film will trigger discussion of the difficult postdivorce adjustment and balancing multiple needs in limited time.

Not Recommended

★ *The First Wives Club* (1996) directed by Hugh Wilson. PG rating. 102 minutes.

Strongly Not Recommended

† *The War of the Roses* (1990) directed by Danny DeVito. R rating. 116 minutes.

INTERNET RESOURCES

Metasites

★★★★ *Divorce Magazine* http://www.divorcemag.com

This is the printed magazine's online commercial site, with articles and links to all kinds of sites. There is much repetition, puffery, and irrelevancy here, but there are many excellent resources for those willing to examine the links with a goal in mind.

Psychoeducational Materials for Clients and Families

So much information is available online for this topic that we review the most valuable sites under four subtopics: General Sites; Separating; Legal Aspects; and Kids and Custody.

General Sites

★★★★★ *Divorce Central* http://www.divorcecentral.com

Complete and supportive, this site provides materials on legal, financial, parental, and personal aspects of divorce. Resources can be found by state. The frequently asked questions in the Resource Guide contain solid and complete information, and Laws by State contains much information that is not available elsewhere.

★★★★ *Divorceinfo.com* http://www.divorceinfo.com

This site claims that more than 100,000 documents are available though it. Simple and plain, it addresses all the issues with good, if short, readings, all cross-linked. This might be a good site to recommend to those needing a lot of orienting information that they can comfortably explore.

★★★★ *Divorce Support* http://www.divorcesupport.com

This site offers lots of readings, chats, information links, and other resources. Somewhat commercialized (mainly selling books) and busy, it covers every aspect of divorce from laws to men's issues and affairs to insurance. This might be a good site to recommend to those who need a lot of information.

★★★★ *Divorce Online* http://www.divorceonline.com

In the text, click on Psychological Effects to reach about 25 professionally written articles taken mainly from books for sale. Although we have not read them all, they seem impressive and appear to be a fine survey and introduction to all the aspects of divorce.

Separating

★★★★ *Frequently Asked Questions on Surviving the Emotional Trauma of Divorce* by Mitchell A. Baris, PhD
http://www.divorcecentral.com/lifeline/life_ans.html#notsaved

A 10-page FAQ that is well-done and complete. A good starting place for looking at the likely consequences of a divorce.

★★★ *Guidelines for Separating Parents* http://home.clara.net/spig/guidline.htm

Only three pages, but solid, sensitive, and inclusive directions.

★★★ *The Relationship and Personal Development Center*
http://www.relationshipjourney.com/growth.html

Five, good-quality articles on divorce by Dawn Lipthrott, LCSW, among other articles on relationships.

★★★ *Bill Ferguson's How to Divorce as Friends* http://www.divorceasfriends.com

Ferguson combines legal and relationship advice in brief selections from his book.

★★★ *Divorce Ceremonies* http://www.globalideasbank.org/1993/1993-35.HTML

Based on a book, this site offers a few ideas for a ceremony marking the end of a marriage. This might be useful for anyone divorcing, because our culture does not have a ceremony for marking the end of a marriage and going on.

Legal Aspects

★★★★★ *Divorce Helpline: Tools to Keep You Out of Court*
              http://www.divorcehelp.com/index.html

Although this is a commercial site designed to sell books and make referrals, the brief articles in the Reading Room are educational, both legally and emotionally. The Short Divorce Course is an alternative to the courts and should certainly be considered.

★★★★ *Nolo Press* http://www.nolo.com/encyclopedia/mlt_ency.html

The site of Nolo Press sells high-quality, do-it-yourself legal guides. Their Legal Encyclopedia offers about 30 complete and well-written readings on legal aspects of divorce.

★★★★ *Annulment* http://marriage.about.com/msubanul.htm?pid=2817&cob=home

At this site are links to a dozen other sites with all the information one might need for seeking an annulment.

★★★★ *Flying Solo* http://www.lifemanagement.com/flyingsolo/

Click on Divorce Separation in the text or the left column. Here are perhaps 100 articles primarily on the legal and financial side of divorce, taxes, some tips, FAQs, and so on. Some are difficult to read, but most are to the point and some are unique. A fine site for those who can read a lot and need much information on multiple aspects of divorce. Click on Mediation for several good introductions to mediation and its benefits.

★★★ *DivorceNet* http://www.DivorceNet.com

"The Net's largest divorce resource since May 1995" includes chat and by-state information. The site is legally oriented and searchable.

Kids and Custody

★★★★ *Helping Children Understand Divorce* by Sara Gable and Kelly Cole
              http://muextension.missouri.edu/xplor/hesguide/humanrel/gh6600.htm

In about nine pages, this guide discusses the stresses on kids and their likely reactions.

★★★★ *Coping with Separation and Divorce: A Parenting Seminar* by Judy Branch, MS,
              and Lawrence G. Shelton, PhD
              http://www.nnfr.org/curriculum/topics/sep_div.html

Covers all the issues in about 45 pages of a handbook and curriculum guide.

★★★★ *Child Custody and Access—US Legislation*
              http://home.clara.net/spig/us-law/detail-1.htm#top

If you want to understand the laws of most states, this nine-page site explains them in ordinary English.

★★★ *Child Custody and Divorce Resources State by State*
   http://www.custodysource.com/state.htm

The lists of links and resources under each state are a mixed bag of commercial sites, support groups, and public organizations. However, those seeking information or referral can likely find something of value here.

★★★ *Breaking the News* http://www.fsbassociates.com/fsg/whydivorce.html#excerpt

Part of a book chapter, this site gives clear rules on how to tell and not to tell the kids about a divorce.

★★★ *Your Parents' Divorce* http://www.couns.uiuc.edu/brochures/divorce.htm

A brief but good pamphlet from a university counseling service.

★★★ *Learning to "Get Along" for the Best Interest of the Child* by Hedy Schleifer, MA
   http://www.hedyyumi.org/child.html

A four-page essay suitable as a handout to explain the value of counseling for kids after a divorce. Parts of it push Imago Relationship Therapy.

NATIONAL SUPPORT GROUPS

ACES (Association for Children for Enforcement of Support)
2260 Upton Avenue
Toledo, OH 43606
Phone: 800-739-2237

Children's Rights Council
6200 Editors Park Drive, Suite 103
Hyattsville, MD 20782
Phone: 301-559-3120
http://www.gocrc.com
   Concerned parents provide education and advocacy for reform of the legal system regarding child custody.

Joint Custody Association
10606 Wilkins Avenue
Los Angeles, CA 90024
Phone: 310-475-5352
http://www.jointcustody.org

North American Conference of Separated and Divorced Catholics
PO Box 360
Richland, OR 97870
Phone: 541-893-6089
E-mail: krista@nacsdc.org
http://www.nacsdc.org

See also Child Development and Parenting (Chapter 13), Families and Stepfamilies (Chapter 20), and Marriage (Chapter 23).

CHAPTER 19

Eating Disorders

We are a nation obsessed with food, spending an extraordinary amount of time thinking about it, gobbling it, and avoiding it. Eating disorders include compulsive overeating, anorexia nervosa (the relentless pursuit of thinness through starvation), bulimia (a binge-and-purge eating pattern), and a general obsession with weight and body image. Eating disorders are far more common in women than in men, the most extreme case being anorexia nervosa, in which about 95% of cases are female.

In this chapter, we critically review self-help books, autobiographies, films, and Internet resources on eating disorders. Chapter 35 on Weight Management covers overlapping materials as well. Both chapters conclude with a listing of national support groups on these topics.

SELF-HELP BOOKS

Strongly Recommended

★★★★ *Dying to Be Thin: Understanding and Defeating Anorexia Nervosa and Bulimia* (updated ed., 2001) by Ira M. Sacker and Marc A. Zimmer. New York: Warner Books.

This book is about the secrets and private worlds of anorexics and bulimics. The authors have included sections on personal histories; information for the person with an eating disorder and their families, friends, and teachers; and resources. By reading this book, you will see how people can carry dangerous secrets for a long time before they admit that the secret has taken control of their lives. For persons who may think or know they suffer from an eating disorder, or those connected with someone with an eating disorder, this book provides insight, motivation, and knowledge about the complexity of eating disorders. The highest rated self-help book for eating disorders in our national studies.

RECOMMENDATION HIGHLIGHTS

Self-Help Books

- For a research-supported treatment of binge eating:
  - ★★★ *Overcoming Binge Eating* by Christopher G. Fairburn

- For the practical treatment of eating disorders:
  - ★★★★ *Dying to Be Thin* by Ira M. Sacker and Marc A. Zimmer

- For transitioning from compulsive eating to a healthy lifestyle:
  - ★★★ *The Hunger Within* by Marilyn Ann Migliore with Philip Ross
  - ★★★ *Healing the Hungry Self* by Deirdre Price

- For sociocultural and familial roots of eating disorders:
  - ★★★ *Bulimia/Anorexia* by Marlene Boskind-White and William White, Jr.
  - ★★★ *The Golden Cage* by Hilde Bruch

Autobiographies

- On the development and treatment of anorexia:
  - ★★★ *Am I Still Visible?* by Sandra Harvey Heater

- On the harsh realities of anorexia and bulimia:
  - ★★★ *Starving for Attention* by Cherry B. O'Neill

Films

- On the familial origins and drastic consequences of anorexia:
  - ★★★★★ *The Karen Carpenter Story*
  - ★★★★ *Best Little Girl in the World*

- On women and food:
  - ★★★★ *Eating*

Internet Resources

- For factual and well-organized sites for therapist and client alike:
  - ★★★★★ *Something Fishy* http://www.something-fishy.org
  - ★★★★ *Anorexia Nervosa and Related Eating Disorders* http://www.anred.com
  - ★★★★ *Close to You Family Resource Network: The Eating Disorders Site* http://closetoyou.org/eatingdisorders/index.htm

- For an excellent source of educational materials:
  - ★★★★ *National Eating Disorders Association* http://www.nationaleatingdisorders.org/p.asp?WebPage_ID=294

Recommended

★★★   *The Hunger Within: A Twelve-Week Guided Journey from Compulsive Eating to Recovery* (1998) by Marilyn Ann Migliore with Philip Ross. New York: Main Street.

This book shows the on-and-off dieter how his or her individual struggle with eating is a response to feelings of emotional deprivation established in childhood. It provides a step-by-step program that explores the core reasons for overeating, identifies triggers that precipitate bingeing, and shows how to break the cycle of yo-yo dieting. The book includes motivational sayings, guided weekly sessions, exercises to help stay on track, a hunger awareness diary, a vicious cycle worksheet, and weekly food for thought programs. A person who eats compulsively is enacting an emotional script, and the script is what has to be changed. This is a 12-week program with three stages. For people who have ridden the roller coaster of dieting, this book may prove to be helpful. A favorably evaluated book that, probably due to its recent publication, is not yet known by many mental health professionals.

★★★   *Healing the Hungry Self: The Diet-Free Solution to Lifelong Weight Management* (1998) by Deirdre Price. New York: Plume.

This book provides a comprehensive program for healthy eating using a variety of physical, mental, emotional, and spiritual concepts. The author addresses the difference between physical and emotional hunger, the importance of three meals a day, recognizing danger zones, alternatives to food in coping with emotions, and sensible exercise programs. There are case studies, self-help tests, charts to monitor progress, checklists, and a six-week plan. Adults or adolescents wishing to modify their dietary lifestyles will find practical and useful advice in this three-star resource.

★★★   *Overcoming Binge Eating* (1995) by Christopher G. Fairburn. New York: Guilford Press.

Fairburn is a well-known authority on eating disorders. His book has two main parts. The first part reviews the current scientific literature about binge eating, and the second offers a structured cognitive-behavioral self-help manual to treat binge eating problems. Given the reluctance of people with eating disorders to reveal their problem to anyone, the book could be a safe and helpful first step in accepting help and beginning treatment. The author advises friends and therapists on how they can use this book most effectively. Had this book been more frequently rated in our studies, it would have probably reached a four-star status. In any case, *Overcoming Binge Eating* is an exceptional resource with research-supported treatment strategies.

★★★   *The Golden Cage* (reprinted ed., 2001) by Hilde Bruch. Cambridge, MA: Harvard University Press.

The Golden Cage symbolizes the high expectations many anorexic women feel. They feel like a sparrow, a very ordinary bird, who is meant to fly free, not be viewed as an exotic, beautiful bird in a cage. Psychiatrist Bruch originally wrote the book 20 years ago; it has been periodically reprinted. She describes the profile of many of the youngsters with whom she worked who grew up in high-socioeconomic-status families and for whom there were high expectations and rigid parental control. The core characteristics of anorexia are viewed as fear of failure to live up to expectations, not being good enough, and being disappointing. The resulting self-concept is that they are not deserving of what they have been given materially at the sacrifice of the family. The youngsters become prideful about self-deprivation and self-discipline; in fact, they come to view the hunger state as rewarding. Bruch believes that most medication, behavioral modification, and psychoanalytic approaches miss the mark. The effective treatment plan is one in which self-concept and self-valuing are primary treatment goals. Although many mental health experts agree with Bruch's major points, they also believe that the book is somewhat dated and neglects the research-supported effectiveness of CBT and some medications.

★★★ *Bulimia/Anorexia* (3rd ed., 2000) by Marlene Boskind-White and William C. White, Jr. New York: Norton.

This third edition of this book, first published in 1993, reflects the continuing phenomenon of girls and women in body-image crisis and self-concept despair. The evolving process of an eating disorder is traced from childhood to teen years, in which self-concept is determined largely by social interaction skills, and acceptance begins to suffer with pressure to conform. The college years for this population also reflect pressure to conform, use of food as a coping mechanism, and a struggle between total control and no control. Treatment myths about bulimia are described. Psychotherapy for bulimia focuses on decision making, conformity, and movement away from self-sabatoge. Psychotherapy for anorexia addresses relationship with therapist, consciousness raising, changing the ways one thinks, and anger control. The negative sociocultural roots of anorexia and the treatment of eating disorders within managed care are significant additions to the new edition.

★★★ *The Twelve Steps and Twelve Traditions of Overeaters Anonymous* (1995). Rio Rancho, NM: Overeaters Anonymous.

This book is devoted to detailed discussions of the Twelve Steps and Twelve Traditions used in Overeaters Anonymous (OA), a program of physical, emotional, and spiritual recovery based on the original Alcoholics Anonymous principles. The often-moving writing explains how OA's principles help members recover and how the fellowship functions. The common bonds shared by OA members are the disease of compulsive eating from which all have suffered, and the solutions found in the principles embodied in the 12 steps. This book, in concert with an OA group and probably therapy, will prove helpful to people who find the spiritual emphasis of 12-step programs congenial.

★★★ *Fat Is a Family Affair* (1996) by Judi Hollis. Cedar City, MN: Hazelden.

This book covers a number of eating disorders, including the bingeing and vomiting of bulimia, the starvation of anorexia nervosa, and compulsive overeating. Hollis recommends a 12-step program as the best treatment for eating disorders. The book is divided into two main parts: Part I, The Weigh In, and Part II, The Weigh Out. The Weigh In discusses how eating disorders evolve and provides a self-test to determine whether you have an eating disorder. Hollis believes that most people with eating disorders are surrounded by 10 or 12 codependent people who, for reasons of their own, are enmeshed in trying to help or change the eating disorder but instead only perpetuate it. Hollis includes many success stories of people who have followed her advice. Special attention is given to the family's role in eating disorders. This three-star book promotes OA, which has helped many individuals learn to change their eating habits. But critics didn't like the preachy tone of the book and the codependency explanations.

★★★   *Why Weight? A Guide to Ending Compulsive Eating* (1989, reissued 1993) by Geneen Roth. New York: Plume.

Geneen Roth founded the Breaking Free workshops that help people cope with eating disorders. She overcame her own compulsive overeating several years ago. First, she put an end to constant dieting that inevitably led to weight gain. She eliminated her compulsive overeating by developing seven eating guidelines that form the core of her Breaking Free program:

- Eat only when you are hungry.
- Eat only when sitting down.
- Eat without distractions.
- Eat only what you want.
- Eat until you are satisfied.
- Eat in full view of others.
- Eat with enjoyment.

The 16 chapters include written exercises that help compulsive overeaters become aware of what they are doing and information on the emotional basis of overeating, how it would feel to be thin, how it really felt to diet and binge all those years, and how the overeater can learn to eat only when physically hungry. Each chapter also contains charts and lists that focus on what is eaten, why, and when, and feelings associated with food. The three-star book is full of helpful exercises for overeaters, is free of psychobabble, and provides insights about the nature of eating problems.

★★★   *When Food Is Love* (1991) by Geneen Roth. New York: Dutton.

This book explores the relation between eating disorders and close relationships. It was written by Geneen Roth, the author of *Why Weight?* (reviewed above). The book focuses on how family-of-origin experiences contribute to the development of eating disorders. Roth reveals her own childhood abuse, which led to compulsive overeating in adulthood and prevented her from having a successful intimate relationship with a man. According to Roth, similar patterns are found in people who are compulsive overeaters and lack intimacy in their life: excessive fantasizing, wanting what is forbidden, creating drama, needing to be in control, and the "one wrong move syndrome" (placing too much importance on doing the absolutely correct thing at this moment). This three-star book does a good job of explaining how inadequate close relationships and eating disorders are linked. Critics say that Roth does not adequately consider biological and sociocultural factors that determine eating disorders.

★★★ *Food for Thought* (1980) by the Hazelden Foundation. New York: Harper & Row.

Subtitled *Daily Meditations for Dieters*, this book presents a spiritually based approach to eating disorders. The Hazelden Foundation, based near Minneapolis, is known primarily for its alcohol treatment program. Through short daily meditations, *Food for Thought* offers encouragement to anyone who has ever tried to diet, to people who overeat or have an eating disorder, and to members of Overeaters Anonymous. Each day's brief reading addresses the concerns of people with eating disorders. The book is especially designed for use by individuals who go to OA meetings and will have special appeal to individuals who want a spiritual approach to eating problems.

Diamond in the Rough

◆ *Anatomy of Anorexia* (2000) by Steven Levenkron. New York: Norton.

The intrusive dominance of anorexia in the lives of girls and their families is the central concept of this sensitive book. Levenkron discusses milestones in the development of the disease, including the effects on the family system, importance of evaluating readiness for college, treatment formats, transferential dynamics, an authoritative/nurturing therapeutic alliance, and the effects of incest on anorexia development. The etiology of anorexia is explained as a failure by the family system to engender trust, healthy dependency, and a positive attachment to the parent figure. The subsequent development of perfectionism, mistrust, and emotional insecurity as preludes to anorexia are poignantly described. Each chapter features case vignettes that demonstrate the powerful effect of anorexia. This book is written for mental health professionals to help them identify anorexia before it is too late. The author's earlier book, *The Best Little Girl in the World* (1978), was made into a movie by the same name and is reviewed later in this chapter.

Not Recommended

★★ *You Can't Quit Eating until You Know What's Eating You* (1990) by Donna LeBlanc. Deerfield Beach, FL: Health Communications.

★★ *Weight Watchers Stop Stuffing Yourself* (1999) by Weight Watchers. New York: Weight Watchers.

★ *Love Hunger: Recovery from Food Addiction* (1990) by Frank Minirth, Paul Meier, Robert Helmfelt, Sharon Sneed, and Don Hawkins. Nashville, TN: Thomas Nelson.

Strongly Not Recommended

† *The Love-Powered Diet* (1992) by Victoria Moran. San Rafael, CA: New World Library.

AUTOBIOGRAPHIES

Recommended

★★★ *Am I Still Visible? A Woman's Triumph over Anorexia Nervosa* (1983) by Sandra Harvey Heater. White Hall, VT: Betterway.

The author, who teaches preschool reading, describes the development and treatment of her anorexia. She also provides a history of the disorder and theories, and describes treatment options. The book is out of print and not easy to obtain.

★★★ *Starving for Attention* (1995) by Cherry Boone O'Neill. Center City, MN: Hazelden Foundation.

The daughter of singer and TV personality Pat Boone gives a frank, first-person account of her eating disorders, including the lies and deceptions that accompanied them. She suffered from both anorexia and bulimia. This book confronts the reader with the harsh realities and twisted perceptions of body image in both conditions, as well as the health problems due to being underweight in anorexia and the binge–purge cycle of bulimia. There is also a detailed discussion of the author's personal life, career, and religious faith, which she believes helped her to overcome the eating disorders.

Diamond in the Rough

♦ *Good Enough: When Losing Is Winning, Perfection Becomes Obsession, and Thin Enough Can Never Be Achieved* (1998) by Cynthia N. Bitter. Penfield, NY: HopeLines.

The author grew up in a difficult family situation. Her father had a bipolar disorder, and her mother was in denial about it. At age 14, she developed anorexia, binge–purge type, which almost resulted in her death; this condition ended when she was 39. The book describes the numerous medical complications of the disorder, the self-destructive behaviors, the food obsessions, and the benefits of therapy, both inpatient and outpatient, that helped her finally overcome her disorder. Favorably but infrequently rated, probably owing to its recent publication, this book is designated a Diamond in the Rough.

FILMS

Strongly Recommended

★★★★★ *The Karen Carpenter Story* (1989, made for TV) directed by Richard Carpenter III and Joseph Sargent. Not rated. 100 minutes.

Anorexia is portrayed as a family-based disorder that led singer Karen Carpenter to have little sense of control, except over the food she ate. Her brother Richard was designated the talented one of the family, and when Karen's voice overshadowed Richard's, she felt she had betrayed her parents' dream. The complexity and power of eating disorders come through effectively and accurately. This five-star film biography of a contemporary pop star may serve as a valuable model for adolescent girls.

★★★★ *Best Little Girl in the World* (1981, made for TV) directed by Sam O'Steen. Not rated.

Being the second daughter and following a troublesome older sister sets Casey up for unrealistically high expectations of herself that place her on a trajectory toward self-starvation. When hospitalized, Casey meets two people, a fellow patient and a psycho-therapist, who give her hope, support, and motivation. This story portrays the road to recovery and the need to confront long-standing familial conflicts.

★★★★ *Eating* (1990) directed by Henry Jaglom. R rating. 110 minutes.

A birthday party attended by women friends sets the stage for candid self-disclosures about relationships, food, money, food, loneliness, food, men, and food. In other words, many aspects of women's lives are revealed and shared, particularly women's love–hate relationship with eating. The characters are familiar and real people—people who make the subject seem ordinary, natural, and at times very funny. Subtitled *A Very Serious Comedy about Women and Food,* this movie is also rated under Women's Issues (Chapter 36).

Recommended

★★★ *For the Love of Nancy* (1994, made for TV) directed by Paul Scheider.

Nancy is a very anxious high school graduate whose social isolation, constant exercising, and sudden temper tantrums were clear signs of an addictive behavioral cycle, but no one heard. The familiar pattern of family attempts to force eating, resulting in further restraint from food, is well illuminated. The story poignantly reveals that the family must experience healing and positive change before anorexia can be treated. This is a touching story with an overarching message that, in many cases, the family is the patient.

INTERNET RESOURCES

Metasites

★★★★★ *Something Fishy* http://www.something-fishy.org

In this rich site, well worth exploring, every therapist will learn something, and if a client reads even half the materials, he or she will understand the disorders very well. Old Fashioned Ideas is an excellent corrective to inaccuracies about eating disorders and sufferers. The Eating Disorders Links list is superb and enormous.

★★★★ *Anorexia Nervosa and Related Eating Disorders* http://www.anred.com

The factual materials here are numerous, detailed, and organized. They can be edited into handouts. They also deal with rarely addressed issues and disorders.

★★★★ *Close to You Family Resource Network: The Eating Disorders Site*
      http://www.closetoyou.org/eatingdisorders/index.htm

The column on the left, What Are They?, opens five diagnoses with very comprehensive but brief descriptions. Click on Medical Info for information on Medical Complications, Caffeine, Why Our Bodies Need Fats, Dehydration, Nutrition, Vitamin Deficiencies, Normal Eating, OTC Drug Use, Diet Drugs, and more. Click on Reading Materials and then Articles to Read for about two dozen links to articles on the net.

★★★★ *The Mining Company* http://eatingdisorders.miningco.com/cs/eat

The Mining Company editors have found and evaluated hundreds of sites and keep them updated. Cultural Influences and Body Hatred are especially good.

Psychoeducational Materials for Clients and Families

★★★★ *National Eating Disorders Association*
      http://www.nationaleatingdisorders.org/p.asp?WebPage_ID=294

Among the best educational materials, with clear explanations of dynamics and causative factors, focused materials for families, information to use in school settings, and criteria for evaluating a treatment option.

★★★★ *Mirror, Mirror* http://www.mirror-mirror.org/eatdis.htm

Relapse prevention does not use the Marlatt model, but the Relapse Prevention Plan is a fill-in form that may be clinically useful. The Relapse Warning Signs is a good list.

★★★★ *Eating Disorders* http://www.mentalhealth.com/book/p45-eat1.html

This eight-page brochure from the National Institute of Mental Health is complete and straightforward.

★★★★ *Eating Disorder Referral and Information Center* http://www.edreferral.com

Besides the two dozen buttons that lead to lots of information, the site offers referrals to local support groups, practitioners, treatment facilities, and guidelines for choosing a therapist and evaluating your first visit.

★★★ *Is Food a Problem? (Eating Disorders)*
      http://www.utexas.edu/student/cmhc/booklets/eating/eating.html

There are three factual brochures here, each well-written and for college students, but more widely usable.

★★★ *Peace, Love, and Hope*
      http://www.healthyplace.com/communities/eating_disorders/peacelovehope

Many aspects are covered. Click on Body Views to access body dysmorphic disorder; this seems to be the only site with this information.

★★★ *Tips for Doctors* http://www.something-fishy.org

Under "Doctors and Patients," this site offers well-articulated fears of patients. It can sensitize health care providers.

★★★ *Vomiting and Emetophobia (fear of vomiting)*
http://www.gut-reaction.freeserve.co.uk

Although not well known, emetophobia is now listed as the sixth most common phobia in both the United Kingdom and the United States. This site has research, treatments, support, and all else one might need for patient education.

★★★ *The Road to an Eating Disorder Is Paved with Diet Rules*
http://closetoyou.org/eatingdisorders/more/road.htm

Simple and hard-hitting.

★★★ *Eating Disorder Self-Test and Perfectionism Scale*
http://closetoyou.org/eatingdisorders/more/selftest.htm

Useful, simple questionnaires.

★★★ *How You Can Help Someone with an Eating Disorder*
http://closetoyou.org/eatingdisorders/more/familyhelp.htm

Four pages of good ideas and advice for relatives and friends.

★★★ *15 Styles of Distorted Thinking*
http://closetoyou.org/eatingdisorders/more/disthink.htm

Each style is explained well in the eight pages. A good reference for cognitive therapy.

Other Resources

★★★★★ *The Gurze Bookstore* http://www.gurze.com

Hundreds of books about eating disorders, with brief reviews and ways to order online.

NATIONAL SUPPORT GROUPS

Compulsive Eaters Anonymous
550 East Atherton Street, Suite 227-B
Long Beach, CA 90815-4017
Phone: 562-342-9344
http://www.ceahow.org

A 12-step recovery program.

Food Addicts Anonymous
4623 Forest Hill Boulevard, Suite 109-4
West Palm Beach, FL 33415-9120
Phone: 561-967-3871
E-mail: info@foodaddictsanonymous. org
http://www.foodaddictsanonymous.org

To find a local group, visit the website or call the World Service Office.

National Association of Anorexia Nervosa and Associated Disorders
PO Box 7
Highland Park, IL 60035
Phone: 847-831-3438
E-mail: anad20@aol.com
http://www.anad.org

For persons with eating disorders.

National Eating Disorders Association
603 Stewart Street, Suite 803
Seattle, WA 98101
Phone: 206-382-3587 or 800-931-2237;
  fax: 206-829-8501
E-mail: info@NationalEatingDisorders.
  org
http://nationaleatingdisorders.org

For persons with eating disorders, their families, and friends.

Overeaters Anonymous (OA)
PO Box 44020
Rio Rancho, NM 87174-4020
Phone: 505-891-2664
E-mail: info@overeatersanonymous.org
http://www.overeatersanonymous.org

A 12-step, self-help fellowship. Free local and online meetings are listed on the website.

We Insist on Natural Shapes (WINS)
PO Box 19938
Sacramento, CA 95819
Phone: 800-600-WINS
E-mail: winsnews@aol.com
http://www.winsnews.org

A nonprofit organization dedicated to educating adults and children about what comprises normal, healthy shapes.

See also Weight Management (Chapter 35) and Women's Issues (Chapter 36).

CHAPTER 20

Families and Stepfamilies

"A friend loves you for your intelligence, a mistress for your charm, but your family's love is unreasoning; you were born into it and are of its flesh and blood. Nevertheless, it can irritate you more than any group in the world," observed French philosopher André Maurois. Families that do not function well together often foster maladjusted behavior on the part of one or more members.

In this chapter, we limit our evaluation to general books on families and stepfamilies, especially those that examine how families or blending families can be a source of distress. Other chapters cover the family's role in a number of specific areas, such as abuse (Chapter 2), addictive disorders (Chapter 3), child development (Chapter 13), divorce (Chapter 18), love and intimacy (Chapter 22), marriage (Chapter 23), and teenagers (Chapter 34).

Children born in the United States today have a 40% chance of living at least part of their lives in a stepfamily before they are 18 years of age. Stepfamilies are a heterogeneous group—about 70% are stepfather families, about 20% are stepmother families, and about 10% are so-called blended families to which both partners bring children from previous marriages. And many stepfamilies produce children of their own. We review a number of self-help resources directed specifically at stepfamilies and blended families.

Following our summary of recommended self-help resources, we consider in detail books, films, and Internet resources related to families and stepfamilies. A list of national support groups rounds out the chapter.

SELF-HELP BOOKS

Strongly Recommended

★★★★★ *Old Loyalties, New Ties: Therapeutic Strategies with Step-Families* (1988) by Emily Visher and John Visher. New York: Brunner/Mazel.

This book is designed to help stepfamilies cope more effectively. Visher and Visher argue that remarried families are not imperfect copies of nuclear families but are rather family systems created from the integration of old loyalties and new ties. They outline

RECOMMENDATION HIGHLIGHTS

Self-Help Books

- For a family systems therapy approach to solving family problems:

    ★★★★ *The Family Crucible* by Augustus Napier and Carl Whitaker

- For a wide variety of family and stepfamily circumstances:

    ★★★★ *Old Loyalties, New Ties* by Emily Visher and John Visher

    ★★★ *The Shelter of Each Other* by Mary Pipher

- For stepfathers:

    ★★★★ *Step-Fathering* by Mark Rosin

- For blended families:

    ★★★★ *Step by Step-Parenting* by James D. Eckler

    ★★★ *Stepfamilies* by James H. Bray and John Kelly

- For creating two stable and happy homes for children of divorce:

    ★★★ *Mom's House, Dad's House* by Isolina Ricci

Films

- On surviving victimization and wanting more for our children:

    ★★★★★ *The Joy Luck Club*

- On finishing life tasks and reconnecting with family:

    ★★★★★ *Life as a House*

- On familial bonding and moral growth in caring for family members:

    ★★★★ *Rain Man*

    ★★★★ *What's Eating Gilbert Grape*

- On the enduring value of flawed love in mother–daughter relationships:

    ★★★★ *Terms of Endearment*

- On the costs, struggles, and possibilities of remarriage:

    ★★★★ *Stepmom*

- On healing a strained parental relationship by helping others:

    ★★★★ *Fly Away Home*

- On second chances and choosing a family:

    ★★★★ *The Family Man*

Internet Resources

- For single parents:

    ★★★★★ *Fathering Magazine* http://www.fathermag.com

    ★★★★ *Flying Solo* http://www.lifemanagement.com/flyingsolo/

- For foster parents, adoptive parents, and grandparents:

    ★★★★ *Foster Parent Community* http://www.fosterparents.com

- For stepfamilies:

    ★★★★★ *Stepfamily in Formation*
    http://www.stepfamilyinfo.org/site/map.htm

    ★★★★ *Wicked Stepmothers, Fact or Fiction?*
    http://www.siskiyous.edu/class/engl12/stepmom.htm

- For information on infertility and adoption:

    ★★★★ *Shared Journey* http://www.sharedjourney.com

special therapeutic strategies they believe are most effective with stepfamilies—such as helping stepfamily members enhance their self-esteem, reducing a sense of helplessness, teaching negotiation, and encouraging mutually rewarding dyadic relationships—all designed to achieve greater integration and stability in the stepfamily. Concrete ways in which therapists can help stepfamilies with specific types of problems are also described. Among them are how to deal with the many changes and losses in their lives, identify realistic beliefs so that expectations are manageable, resolve loyalty conflicts, develop adequate boundaries, cope with life-cycle discrepancies and complexities, and create a more equal distribution of power. Many case study examples illustrate the authors' therapy strategies. This is a very good book about remarried families, but it was written primarily for a professional audience rather than a self-help audience. Nonetheless, it is well-written, and the self-help reader can gain considerable insight into the dynamics of remarried families and therapy strategies.

★★★★ *The Family Crucible* (1978) by Augustus Napier and Carl Whitaker. New York: Harper & Row.

This book presents a family systems approach to solving family problems. In family systems therapy, the family unit is viewed as a system of interacting individuals with different subsystems (husband–wife, sibling–sibling, mother–daughter, father–sibling–sibling, and so on). A basic theme is that most problems that seem to be the property of a single individual evolved from relationships within the family. Therefore, the best way to solve problems is to work with the family rather than the individual. Napier and Whitaker say that problem families have in common certain general patterns: acute interpersonal or intrapersonal stress, polarization (family members at odds with each other) and escalation (the conflict intensifies), triangulation (one member is the scapegoat for other members who are in conflict but pretend not to be), diffusion of identity (no one is free to be autonomous), and fear of immobility, which Napier and Whitaker equate with fear of death (of the family). The authors describe in considerable detail how they used family systems therapy with a particular family—an angry adolescent and other equally distressed family members. This book is widely considered to be one of the classics in family systems therapy. However, it is written mainly for a professional audience and is somewhat dated.

★★★★ *Step by Step-Parenting: A Guide to Successful Living with a Blended Family* (2nd ed., 1993) by James D. Eckler. White Hall, VA: Betterway.

This book, as is evident from its title, is about blended families, families to which each adult has brought children from a previous marriage. The book reflects both the adjustments that made author James Eckler's blended family a successful one and his years of experience as a minister and pastoral counselor. A wide array of issues are covered, including the games stepchildren play, the rights of the stepparent, name changes, the pros and cons of adoption, discipline, stepsibling rivalries, marital communication, grandparents, and dealing with children at different developmental levels (preschool, elementary school, and adolescence). Our mental health experts considered this a good self-help book for blended families; it presents a balanced approach and includes detailed discussions of blended families' stressful experiences, and wise strategies for successful living in a blended family.

★★★★ *Step-Fathering* (1987) by Mark Rosin. New York: Simon & Schuster.

This was among the first self-help books to describe the stepfather family from the stepfather's perspective. Rosin draws on his own experiences as a stepfather and in-depth interviews with more than 50 stepfathers to help men cope effectively in a stepfather family. Chapters take stepfathers through such topics as the adjustment involved in becoming a stepfather, the problems of combining families, how to handle discipline and authority, communication with the wife/mother, dealing with the other father, money matters, adolescent stepchildren, and the rewards of stepfathering. The expert consensus is that this is a fine self-help book for stepfathers. It is well-written and includes insightful examples to which most stepfathers will relate.

Recommended

★★★ *Families: Applications of Social Learning to Family Life* (revised ed., 1975) by Gerald Patterson. Champaign, IL: Research Press.

This volume presents a behavioral approach to improving children's behavior. To begin, Patterson explains some important behavioral concepts such as social reinforcers, aversive stimuli, and accidental training. Time-out procedures and behavioral contracts are integrated into a step-by-step reinforcement management program for parents to implement with their children. Behavioral management strategies are also tailored to children with specific problems. This book was very favorably evaluated by our mental health experts, but by only 12 of them, thus leading to a lower rating. Mental health professionals of a behavioral persuasion described this book as exceptionally good for parents who want to improve a child's behavior, especially if the child is aggressive.

★★★ *The Shelter of Each Other: Rebuilding Our Families* (1996) by Mary Pipher. New York: Grosset/Putnam.

This is not a how-to book but a how-to-think book that sensitively exposes the breadth of family struggles. Psychologist Pipher brings us face-to-face with a culture in which parents sell Girl Scout cookies to colleagues because Girl Scouts can't go door to door anymore, and with an electronic revolution that has resulted in making media personalities more recognizable than neighbors. Pipher organizes the stories of families around the three central themes of character, will, and commitment. Through these themes, she brings hope that we as families and as a community can shelter each other and decide the future and the culture we want, now that we see what we have become. This book was highly rated in our national study but was evaluated by only 14 experts, thus receiving a modest three-star designation.

★★★ *Mom's House, Dad's House* (1997) by Isolina Ricci. New York: Fireside.

Written by Isolina Ricci, a family therapist who directs the Family Court services for the California judicial branch, this fine book provides guidance for creating two happy, stable homes for children of divorce. Legal, emotional, and practical aspects of the circumstances are examined. Advice includes how to talk to a former mate, steps to building a positive coparenting relationship, and when to use mediation. Self-tests, checklists, strategies, and extensive examples are included. Had this book been more frequently rated in our studies, it would have been a four- or five-star resource.

★★★ *Stepfamilies* (1999) by James Bray and John Kelly. New York: Broadway.

The results of a nine-year project on the development of stepfamilies are presented clearly through the three types of stepfamilies and the identification of cycles through which they move. This book provides good advice for easing the conflicts of stepfamily life and coping with the stress of divorce. The authors includes many emotionally laden stories of stepfamilies to illustrate how not to cope and how to cope effectively with life in a stepfamily. The ups and downs of different types of stepfamilies are described. Special focus is given to important aspects of the stepfamily structure, such as bridging the insider–outsider gap, the stepmother, the nonresidential parent, and adolescence. This is a splendid book for stepfamilies.

★★★ *Back to the Family* (1990) by Ray Guarendi. New York: Basic Books.

Subtitled *How to Encourage Traditional Values in Complicated Times,* this book is the result of a study sponsored by the Children's Hospital in Akron, Ohio, to identify the characteristics of healthy, adaptive families. One hundred happy families were nominated by award-winning educators in the National/State Teachers of the Year organization. Guarendi distilled information from interviews with the families and developed a how-to manual for parents who want to build a happy home. The interviews reveal how families can mature through good and bad times, and how parents in happy, competent families sifted through various types of child-rearing advice to arrive at the way they reared their own children. At times, the book is inspirational, but families frequently need more than a pep talk to solve their problems.

★★★   *The Second Time Around: Why Some Second Marriages Fail* (1991) by Louis Janda and Ellen MacCormack. New York: Carol.

Janda and MacCormack's study of more than 100 people in second marriages furnished much of the material in this book. Readers learn that a majority of individuals in stepfamilies find the adjustment to be more difficult than they anticipated. The authors believe that many people expect too much when they enter a stepfamily. And they say that stepchildren make any second marriage a challenge. The book received a three-star rating because it was positively reviewed, but by only 10 respondents. The few mental health professionals who knew about it said that it includes a number of good examples of stepfamily problems and how to solve them effectively.

★★★   *Love in the Blended Family: Stepfamilies* (1991) by Angela Clubb. Deerfield Beach, FL: Health Communications.

This self-help resource concerns stepmother families, not blended families in the accepted sense of the term. At the beginning of the book, Clubb tells readers that what they are reading is biased, because it is written by a stepmother and second wife. Her husband brought two children to the newly formed stepmother family, and the Clubbs subsequently had two children of their own. Thus, the book is primarily about relationships and experiences in one stepmother family, although Clubb does occasionally bring in mental health experts' views on stepfamily issues. This three-star effort clearly shows Clubb's professional background as a writer; the book reads in places like a finely tuned novel. Many of the problems and issues Clubb has experienced in her stepmother family are those that any stepmother has to face.

★★★   *Strengthening Your Stepfamily* (1986) by Elizabeth Einstein and Linda Albert. Circle Pines, MN: American Guidance.

This 133-page book contains five comprehensive chapters. Chapter 1 describes stepfamily structure and how it is different from previous family structure. The authors discuss common stepfamily myths and unrealistic expectations. Chapter 2 focuses on the couple relationship and how to communicate more effectively and share feelings. Chapter 3 examines strategies for creating positive relationships between stepparents and stepchildren. Chapter 4 explores children's feelings and behaviors in stepfamilies, along with guidelines for helping children cope more effectively. Chapter 5 discusses making a stepfamily function well, along with hints for dealing with issues that range from daily routines to holiday celebrations. The book was positively but infrequently rated in our national studies. This is an easy-to-read overview of stepfamily problems and ways to solve them.

★★★   *Blending Families: A Guide for Parents, Stepparents, Grandparents, and Everyone Building a Successful New Family* (1999) by Elaine F. Shimberg. New York: Berkley.

This self-help resource takes a unique approach in viewing stepfamily dynamics. Interviews, surveys, and discussion groups were conducted, and the resulting information is distilled in the book, presented in a practical fashion, with ideas and perspectives offered directly by stepfamily members about what worked for them and what strengthened their families. The book contains reflective quotes from adult children of stepfamilies looking back on their experiences, as well as contemporary quotes by stepfamily members. The author intended the book to be a practical guide based on actual successes and shortcomings of people who have lived in a stepfamily system. The content of the book is directed not only at stepparents but also at stepchildren and extended family members.

★★★ *Adult Children: The Secrets of Dysfunctional Families* (1988) by John Friel and Linda Friel. Deerfield Beach, FL: Health Communications.

This book is primarily intended for adults who grew up in dysfunctional families and suggests what they can do to improve their lives. Modeled after the Twelve-Step program of Alcoholics Anonymous, it tries to shed light on why adults who grew up in dysfunctional families developed problems as adults—problems such as addiction, depression, compulsion, unhealthy dependency, stress disorders, and unsatisfying relationships. Five sections discuss (1) who adult children are and what their symptoms are, (2) family systems and how dysfunctional families get off track, (3) how the dysfunctional family affects the child, (4) a model of codependency, and (5) recovery. *Adult Children* barely received a three-star rating; many mental health experts frown on the codependency approach of the authors.

Not Recommended

★★ *Bradshaw on the Family* (1988) by John Bradshaw. Deerfield Beach, FL: Health Communications.

FILMS

Strongly Recommended

★★★★★ *The Joy Luck Club* (1994) directed by Wayne Wang. R rating. 138 minutes.

This is a film about neither joy nor luck, but about hope and triumph of the will. When one of a group of four Chinese immigrant women dies, the event prompts the recollections of great hardships, despair, and loss and, most importantly, the effect these experiences had on their relationships with their own daughters. Two of the dominant themes are the effects of feelings of self-worthlessness on women's lives and mothers' desire for a better life for their children. This heartwarming five-star film transcends culture, race, and generations.

★★★★★ *Life as a House* (2001) directed by Irwin Winkler. R rating. 125 minutes

Kevin Kline, an architect who learns he will soon die, tries to finish his life's tasks: reconnecting with his 16-year-old, drug-using, and suicide-chasing son; making amends with his ex-wife who has her own marital troubles; and turning the shack he inherited from his father into a house. Although veering into the maudlin, the movie reminds us that we can neither erase our pasts nor ignore how we repeat our family dynamics. This superbly acted film underscores the centrality and urgency of attending to family relationships while we can.

★★★★ *The Family Man* (2000) directed by Brett Ratner. PG-13 rating. 125 minutes.

In a milder remake of *Its a Wonderful Life*, Nicholas Cage plays a successful and talented businessman. He is happily living his single life until he magically awakens on Christmas morning, married to the girlfriend (Téa Leoni) he abandoned 13 years earlier. He now has a house in New Jersey, two adorable kids, a minivan (instead of his Ferrari), and a job selling tires for his father-in-law. He struggles with wanting his old life back but slowly recognizes the pleasures of domestic bliss. The film's strongest points are that it is a *marital* love story and that any life is a mixture of pleasure and pain. It may be superficial at times, but it contains a core of genuine warmth and could help with marital reconciliation.

★★★★ *Terms of Endearment* (1983) directed by James L. Brooks. PG rating. 130 minutes.

This film dominated the Academy Awards in 1983, but its popular acclaim should not overshadow its therapeutic value and portrayal of characters who struggle with enmeshment, marital infidelity, and loss in a poignant and heartwrenching way. The mother, Aurora, is overprotective, dominant, and consumed by running her daughter's life, while the daughter is overattached and dependent. A midlife relationship changes Aurora, while infidelity and sickness change her daughter. The film's enduring messages are the value of (flawed) love, strength in (flawed) relationships, and familial survival through pain.

★★★★ *Rain Man* (1988) directed by Barry Levinson. R rating. 130 minutes.

Twenty-something, self-centered Charlie, disinherited by his deceased father, discovers that he has an autistic older brother, Raymond, who has inherited the father's $3 million. The real story, however, is about Charlie's learned selflessness, the brothers' fraternal bonding, and Charlie's moral growth as he learns to care for Raymond. Raymond is tragic and funny, a survivor, and yet fragile; he has built a life of required predictability that Charlie can penetrate only momentarily. This film realistically portrays mental illness and what it means to the life of a family. *Rain Man* deservedly garnered four Academy Awards in 1988, including Best Picture.

★★★★ *Fly Away Home* (1996) directed by Carroll Ballard. PG rating. 107 minutes.

Adolescent Amy loses her mother in an auto accident and must move from her home in New Zealand to Canada to live with her father, with whom she has a strained relationship. When Amy finds a gaggle of geese that follow her around and will not fly on their own, she and her father join forces to nurture the geese and teach them how to fly. This is a classic story of the healer who is healed through caring for others. Amy and her father find common ground and common values in assisting others and in identifying with the desire to fly free.

★★★★   *What's Eating Gilbert Grape* (1994) directed by Lasse Hallström. PG-13 rating. 118 minutes.

The energy, the relationships, and the purpose of life for the members of the Grape family are driven by disabilities. The father committed suicide; the mother subsequently ballooned to 500 pounds and developed mild agoraphobia; and one son has severe mental retardation. The mother places herself squarely in the lives of the family, while the breadwinning son becomes responsible for all family members. This story is about family loyalty, community caring, fraternal caretaking, a mother's letting go, and most of all, the power of internal strength.

★★★★   *Stepmom* (1998) directed by Chris Columbus. PG-13 rating. 123 minutes.

This film has much to offer about the costs, struggles, and possibilities of remarriage—if you can ignore the unrealistic aspects of finances, relatives, and the mother's (Susan Sarandon) terminal illness. *Stepmom* realistically shows how the kids may suffer. Twelve-year-old Anna's brattishness is so annoying, yet so clearly an expression of the conflicts of a child who loves both her divorced parents. The film shows how a successful professional woman, the stepmom (Julia Roberts), feels limited by the new responsibilities of children not her own. She does all that might be expected of a stepmom but loves her work and won't give it up. The birth mother is a paragon who places her children's needs above her own and cannot understand the stepmom's "neglect." In the end, the birth mother's impending death resolves the kids' divided loyalties and the conflicts between herself and the stepmom. The struggles of all are realistically portrayed, but viewers should be cautioned that the Hollywood solution of killing off the birth mother is an unrealistic cop-out to complicated relationships.

★★★★   *Radio Flyer* (1992) directed by Richard Donner. PG-13 rating. 120 minutes.

Life becomes horrific for Mike and Bobby when their mother marries an alcoholic man who physically and verbally abuses them. They escape into their own world as they dream of turning their Radio Flyer wagon into an airplane in order to fly away. The film reveals the pain of physical abuse, living with substance abuse, the denial of the mother about what is happening, and the valiant attempts of young children to insulate their mother from pain. This is a story for everyone who has walked this path and for people who have experienced the resilience of children in an abusive home. Also reviewed in Abuse (Chapter 2).

Recommended

★★★   *The Father of the Bride* (1991) directed by Charles Shyer. PG rating. 114 minutes.

George and Nina are the parents of a daughter who has grown up when they weren't looking. The daughter has distressed her father by announcing her engagement. The film continues with the antics of wedding plans, costs, and invitations, but underneath is the story of a father who sees himself losing his little girl and fighting it by complaining about expense, potential flaws in the fiancé, and the bossiness of the wedding coordinator. The film is touching and funny and speaks to all families moving through adult–child transitions.

INTERNET RESOURCES

Psychoeducational Materials for Clients and Families

Families (General)

★★★★★   *Fathering Magazine*   http://www.fathermag.com

Hundreds of articles are available online. The site might be ideal for expanding and validating a father's view of his role.

★★★★   *Flying Solo*   http://www.lifemanagement.com/flyingsolo

A fine site dedicated to families and single parenting. Click on Divorce and Separation on the left or in the text, and then on Remarriage and Stepfamilies. The 25 articles cover finances, law, prenuptial agreements, and research. SAA Article and Research Findings about Stepchildren leads to two articles for kids. This site could be a useful addition to a more focused set of readings.

★★★★   *Family Life Library*
       http://www.oznet.ksu.edu/library/famlf2/

Numerous articles suitable as handouts and brochures from a Kansas State University program that have to be downloaded and opened in Adobe's Acrobat Reader.

Blended Families/Stepfamilies

★★★★★   *Stepfamily in Formation*   http://www.stepfamilyinfo.org/site/map.htm

There are about 700 pages of information and ideas here, covering almost every family topic. It is a lot to read, but it is clearly written and well-arrayed. It does not espouse any exclusive perspective and is of use in any kind of family structure. Use the left column headings to navigate, but it will take a while to grasp the site's organization and to identify the valuable pages. Thank you, Peter Gerlach, MSW.

★★★★   *Supporting Stepfamilies: What Do the Children Feel?*
       http://www.ianr.unl.edu/pubs/family/nf223.htm

Focuses on the emotions of children during blending or combining families.

★★★★   *Divorce and the Family in America* by Christopher Lasch
       http://www.TheAtlantic.com/politics/family/divorce.htm

For those needing a historical perspective on family and divorce, this is superb, despite being from 1966. College education may be needed to understand the material.

★★★★   *Wicked Stepmothers, Fact or Fiction?*
       http://www.siskiyous.edu/class/engl12/stepmom.htm

A seven-page paper that details the pervasiveness and harm done by culturally transmitted stereotypes of stepmothers. Thought-provoking materials for counseling. See also

The Evil Stepmother by Maureen F. McHugh at http://www.en.com/users/mcq/step-mother.html.

★★★   *Ten Steps for Steps* http://www.stepfamily.org/tensteps.html#forstepfath

Actually 80 steps because there are guidelines for all roles and relatives. These might be useful handouts to focus discussions on issues and practices.

★★★   *Blended Families* by Willard F. Harley, Jr., PhD
         http://www.pastornet.net.au/jmm/afre/afre0448.htm

About 10 pages of advice addressing conflicts and problems.

★★★   *Stepfamily Information* http://www.positive-way.com/step.htm

This site has four sections: an Introduction with 11 good suggestions, Tips for Stepfa-thers, Tips for Stepmothers, and Tips for Remarried Parents. They are all brief and use-ful.

★★★   *Stepfamilies on Television* by Marie Van Dam
         http://www.msu.edu/course/mc/111/journal/STEPFAMS.html

Only two pages, but the site may help people differentiate media portrayals from reality.

★★★   *How to Succeed as a Stepfather* by Barbara F. Meltz
         http://www.boston.com/globe/columns/meltz/061898.htm

Only four pages, but the site deals with important issues: discipline, closeness, rejection.

★★★   *Stepfamily Association of America* http://www.saafamilies.org

Under the button Facts & FAQs are fact sheets, a longer FAQ, and eight research arti-cles suitable for handouts and introduction to the issues.

★★★   *The Second Wives Club* http://www.secondwivesclub.com/

Although a commercial site, it offers readings on just about all aspects of being a step-parent.

Single-Parent Families

★★★   *Single Rose: Article Database* http://www.singlerose.com/articles/

About 60 articles on many aspects of being a single mom, such as Arts and Crafts, Child Development, Education, Family Concerns, Home Maintenance, and Time Manage-ment. A smaller place to start exploring than the metasites.

★★★   *Parents World* http://www.parentsworld.com/articles.html

About 20 casual, short pieces on simple techniques for dealing some of the stresses of single parenting. The menu at left has many more resources and links.

★★★ *Facts about Single Parent Families*
      http://www.parentswithoutpartners.org/support1.htm

A two-page list of surprising facts; possibly useful for overcoming stereotypes and media illusions.

★★★ *Practical Parenting . . . Tips to Grow On*
      http://www.parentswithoutpartners.org/support2.htm

A six-page listing of practical advice on topics such as Coping and Grieving, Talking to Children, Child Discipline, Visitation, and Never-Married Parents. A useful, quick guide for beginning discussions of single parenthood.

Adoption

★★★★ *Shared Journey* http://www.sharedjourney.com

This site offer materials on infertility and adoption. There is a minitextbook on infertility's medical aspects. Just keep clicking for a full education. The Adoption button leads to some basic readings.

★★★★ *Adoption Library* http://www.adoptionlibrary.com

There are hundreds of articles on this complex process and its outcomes. A fine resource for client education.

★★★ *The Adopted Child* http://www.aacap.org/publications/factsfam/adopted.htm

A brief essay on telling a child about his or her adoption.

NATIONAL SUPPORT GROUPS

Concerned United Birthparents (CUB)
PO Box 230457
Encinitas, CA 92023
Phone: 800-822-2777
E-mail: group@cubirthparents.org
http://www.cubirthparents.org

  For adoption-affected people.

Families Anonymous
PO Box 3475
Culver City, CA 90231
Phone: 800-736-9805
E-mail: famanon@familiesanonymous.org
http://www.familiesanonymous.org

  Twelve-step fellowship for relatives and friends concerned about substance abuse and behavioral problems.

National Foster Parent Association
7512 Stanich Avenue, Suite 6
Gig Harbor, WA 98335
Phone: 253-853-4000 or 800-557-5238
E-mail: info@nfpainc.org
http://www.nfpainc.org

  Support, education, and advocacy for foster parents and their children. Advocates for child support enforcement and collection.

Parents without Partners
1650 South Dixie Highway, Suite 510
Boca Raton, FL 33432
Phone: 561-391-8833
E-mail: pwppr@parentswithoutpartners.
   org
http://www.parentswithoutpartners.org

Stepfamily Association of America
650 J Street, Suite 205
Lincoln, NE 68508-1814
E-mail: saa@saafamilies.org
Phone: 800-735-0329

Information and advocacy for stepfamilies.

See also Child Development and Parenting (Chapter 13), Divorce (Chapter 18), and Teenagers and Parenting (Chapter 34).

CHAPTER 21

Infant Development and Parenting

In this chapter, we evaluate self-help resources that focus on parenting infants. In other chapters, we examine parenting and other periods of development: pregnancy in Chapter 27, childhood in Chapter 13, and adolescence in Chapter 34.

Infancy is a special period of growth and development, requiring extensive time and support by caregivers. Unlike the newborn of some species (the newborn wildebeest runs with the herd moments after birth!), the human newborn requires considerable care. Good parenting requires long hours, interpersonal skills, and emotional commitment. Many parents learn parenting practices and baby care from their parents—some of which they accept, some of which they discard. Unfortunately, when parenting practices and baby care are passed on from one generation to the next, both desirable and undesirable practices are perpetuated.

Many parents eagerly, perhaps anxiously, want to know the answer to such questions as: How should I respond to the baby's crying? Is there a point at which I can spoil the baby? What are normal developmental milestones for my child? How should I stimulate my young child intellectually? What discipline methods are most effective, yet most humane? Many parents turn to self-help resources on parenting for answers and advice on the best way to handle their children. And those who do find no shortage of written and Internet resources.

Here are the clinician-recommended self-help books and Internet resources on infant development and parenting.

RECOMMENDATION HIGHLIGHTS

Self-Help Books

- For sound general advice on parenting infants:

  ★★★★★ *Infants and Mothers* by T. Berry Brazelton

  ★★★★★ *What Every Baby Knows* by T. Berry Brazelton

  ★★★★★ *Dr. Spock's Baby and Child Care* by Benjamin Spock and Steven J. Parker

- For month-to-month descriptions of infant development and care:

  ★★★★★ *What to Expect the First Year* by Arlene Eisenberg and Associates

  ★★★★★ *What to Expect: The Toddler Years* by Arlene Eisenberg et al.

  ★★★★★ *Your Baby and Child* by Penelope Leach

- For a broad-based nonmedical approach to parenting infants:

  ★★★★★ *The First Three Years of Life* by Burton White

  ★★★★★ *The First Twelve Months of Life* by Frank Caplan

Internet Resources

- For comprehensive sources of parenting information:

  ★★★★★ *Zero to Three, National Center for Infants*
  http://www.zerotothree.org/index.htm

  ★★★★★ *Infant and Toddler Care*
  http://www.nncc.org/InfantToddler/inftod.page.html

  ★★★★★ *BabyCenter* http://www.babycenter.com/rcindex.html

- For excellent sites on bonding, brain development, and no spanking:

  ★★★★★ *The Natural Child Project* http://www.naturalchild.com/home

  ★★★★★ *Project NoSpank* http://www.nospank.net/toc.htm

  ★★★★ *Brain Wonders*
  http://www.zerotothree.org/brainwonders/index.html

SELF-HELP BOOKS

Strongly Recommended

★★★★★ *What to Expect: The Toddler Years* (1996) by Arlene Eisenberg, Heidi E. Murkoff, and Sandee E. Hathaway. New York: Workman.

It is unimaginable that there is a question that could be asked that is not answered in this book. As is the case for its predecessor *What to Expect the First Year* by the same authors (reviewed in this chapter), this book has an encyclopedic level of information that is well organized and understandable. Each chapter is subheaded "What your toddler may be doing now," "What you may be concerned about," "What it's important to know," and "What it's important for your toddler to know." Each chapter highlights a particular month in the two-year span, and final chapters address safety, feeding, toilet learning, injuries, special needs, toddlers with siblings, and child care. Descriptions are conversational and inviting, as though one were sitting down with the authors over a cup of coffee. The authoritative, practical, and engaging presentation ensures continued high appeal for this series of books.

★★★★★ *Infants and Mothers* (revised ed., 1983) by T. Berry Brazelton. New York: Delta.

This book concerns the infant's temperament, developmental milestones in the first year of life, and the parents' (especially the mother's) role in the infant's development. Author T. Berry Brazelton, a pediatrician, has recently been crowned America's baby doctor, a title once reserved for Benjamin Spock. Brazelton describes three different temperamental or behavioral styles: active baby, average baby, and quiet baby. He takes readers through the developmental milestones of these three different types of babies from birth to age 12 months. Most of the chapters are titled with the babies' ages: The Second Month, The Third Month, and so on. In every chapter, Brazelton tells mothers the best way to parent the different types of babies. He advises the mother to be a sensitive observer of her baby's temperament and behavior, believing that this strategy will help the mother chart the best course for meeting the infant's needs. This five-star book is now considered a classic. Brazelton's approach is well-informed, warm, and personal.

★★★★★ *What Every Baby Knows* (1987) by T. Berry Brazelton. Reading, MA: Addison-Wesley.

This self-help book is based on the Lifetime cable television series that Brazelton hosts and, like the series, is a broad approach to parenting infants that is organized according to the experiences of five different families. Brazelton presents in-depth analyses of the families and their child-rearing concerns, such as how to handle crying, how to discipline, how to deal with the infant's fears, sibling rivalry, separation and divorce, hyperactivity, birth order, and the child's developing sense of self. The descriptions of each family include the circumstances of the family's visits to Dr. Brazelton and lengthy excerpts of pediatrician–parent dialogues, interspersed with brief explanatory notes. Each family also is portrayed two years later, to see how they resolved their child-rearing difficulties and where they are at that point. In this five-star book, Brazelton dispenses wise advice to parents. He does an excellent job of helping parents become more sensitive to their infants' needs and of providing them with sage recommendations on how to handle a host of problems that may arise.

★★★★★ *Dr. Spock's Baby and Child Care* (7th ed., 1998) by Benjamin Spock and Steven J. Parker. New York: Pocket Books.

Initially published in 1945, this is one of the classics of self-help literature. Author Benjamin Spock was considered America's baby doctor for decades, and this book was perceived by many to be the bible of self-help books for parents of infants and young children. *Dr. Spock's Baby and Child Care* is a broad approach to infant and child development. It not only has more medical advice than most of the other books in the infant and parenting category but it also includes a number of chapters of child-rearing advice. Most of the material in earlier editions has been carried forward into the 1998 edition, which includes advice on feeding, daily care, illnesses, first aid, nutrition, and a myriad of other topics. The revision gives more attention to adolescence, single-parent families, stepparenting, and the role of fathers in the child's development. An expanded section on breastfeeding for mothers who work outside the home appears in the newer editions. The book has retained its political flavor. The authors fervently state that children should not play with toy guns or watch cowboy movies, advocate a nuclear freeze, and argue for abolishing competitiveness in our society. Across almost five decades, more than 30 million copies of this book have been sold, placing it second on the nation's overall best-seller list (after the Bible). The book's enthusiasts say that it is extremely well-organized and serves as a handy guide for parents to consult when they run into problems with their infant or child. The medical advice is outstanding. However, some critics maintain that Spock's approach to discipline is still too permissive.

★★★★★ *The First Three Years of Life* (20th ed., 1995) by Burton White. New York: Fireside.

This book presents a broad-based, age-related approach to parenting infants and young children. White strongly believes that most parents in the United States fail to provide an adequate intellectual and social foundation for their children's development, especially between the ages of eight months and three years. White provides in-depth discussion of motor, sensory, emotional, sociability, and language milestones. He divides the first three years into stages. For each of the seven stages, White describes the general behavior and educational development of the young child, and parental practices that he does and does not recommended. His goal is to provide parents with the tools to help every child reach his or her maximum level of competence by structuring early experiences. White presents advice about child-rearing topics such as sibling rivalry, spacing children, types of discipline, and detection of disabilities. Appropriate toys and materials are listed, and how to obtain professional testing of a child is outlined. His recommendations about which toys parents should and should not buy, how to handle sibling rivalry, and how to discipline children are also excellent. This five-star book has been a very popular self-help book; however, White has been criticized in the past because he essentially does not think mothers should work outside the home during the child's early years. Critics say White's view places an unnecessary burden of guilt on the high percentage of working mothers with infants.

★★★★★ *What to Expect the First Year* (1996) by Arlene Eisenberg, Heidi Murkoff, and Sandee Hathaway. New York: Workman.

This is an encyclopedic (almost 700 pages) volume of facts and practical tips on how babies develop, how to become a better parent, and how to deal with problems as they arise. The authors give chatty answers to hypothetical questions arranged in a month-by-month format. The book is full of questions commonly asked by parents. What to buy for a newborn, first aid, recipes, adoption, low-birth-weight babies, and the father's role also are discussed. Some of the book's enthusiasts called it the best source on the market for parents of infants in their first year of life. The volume covers an enormous array of topics that concern parents and generally provides sound advice.

★★★★★ *Your Baby and Child: From Birth to Age Five* (revised ed., 1997) by Penelope Leach. New York: Knopf.

This book describes normal child development from birth to 5 years of age and provides suggestions for parents about how to cope with typical problems at different ages in infancy and the early childhood years. Leach describes the basics of what parents need to know about feeding, sleeping, eliminating, teething, bathing, and dressing at each period of early development—during the first 6 months, from 6 to 12 months, from 1 to 2½ years, and 2½ to 5 years. Nontechnical graphs of growth rates are easy to interpret. Leach also explores the young child's emotional world, telling parents what children are feeling and experiencing in different periods of development. Despite describing normal development in different periods, Leach carefully points out individual variations in growth and development. She concludes that when parents have a decision to make about their child, their best choice is usually to go "by the baby"—their sensitive reading of the child's needs—rather than "by the book" or what is generally prescribed for the average child. The index in *Your Baby and Child* cleverly doubles as a glossary of terms. The final pages of the book are a handy illustrated guide to first aid, accidents, safety, infectious diseases, and nursing. Leach's extensive experience with children comes through in her sensitive, five-star suggestions on handling children in the early years of life. The material is extensive, well-organized, and packed with more than 650 well-executed charts, drawings, and photographs.

★★★★★ *The First Twelve Months of Life* (revised ed., 1995) by Frank Caplan. New York: Bantam.

This is a broad-based, developmental milestone approach to the infant's development in the first year of life. A month-by-month assessment of normal infant development is provided. The time tables in the book are presented in a rather rigid way. The author does warn the reader not to use them that way but rather as indicators of appropriate sequences of growth. Feeding, sleeping, language, physical skills, guidance, parental emotions, and learning stimulation are among the topics covered in depth. Each chapter contains a detailed developmental chart outlining the appropriate sensory, motor, language, mental, and social developmental milestones for that month. The book also includes 150 photographs. This five-star book is well organized, well written, and easy to follow. Although Caplan warns readers not to take the time tables for developmental milestones as gospel, it's almost impossible not to do so, because that is the way the book is organized.

Recommended

★★★ *The Baby Book* (2003) by William Sears and Martha Sears. Boston: Little, Brown.

A unique theme of this book is attachment parenting. Five attachment tools are introduced: connecting with your baby early, reading and responding to baby's cues, breastfeeding your baby, carrying the baby, and sharing sleep with the baby. Frequently asked questions about this approach are discussed. The 28 chapters thoroughly discuss stages of the first two years of life. Specific features of child care are presented, including parenting a colicky baby, postpartum adjustments, baby's sleep difficulties, twins, the adopted baby, toilet training, mild medical emergency needs, and day care. This book thoroughly addresses the key components of child rearing in early years; *The Baby Book* is written for parents and those working in collaboration with parents.

★★★   *The Father's Almanac* (2nd ed., 1992) by S. Adams Sullivan. Garden City, NY: Doubleday.

The Father's Almanac, a guide for the day-to-day care of children, is written primarily for fathers. It begins before the child is born and includes a discussion of childbirth classes. The father's role at birth and infancy is chronicled, as is his relationship with the child during the preschool years. The traditional role of the father is emphasized by Sullivan. For example, one chapter devoted to "Daddy's Work" describes how business travel or commuting cuts into the time available to the father to spend with his children. Another chapter stresses the importance of the father's being supportive of the mother. Other chapters focus on the father's play with children, building things with them, learning with them, and hints about photographing the family. This three-star resource includes a great deal of practical advice for helping fathers interact with their young children effectively.

INTERNET RESOURCES

There are dozens upon dozens of websites about parenting infants, almost all of them commercial. They are essentially magazines with advertisements and are generally avoided in the following list.

Metasites

★★★★★   *Zero to Three, National Center for Infants*
http://www.zerotothree.org/index.htm

Vast amount of information on development, child care, and special needs is available for parents and professionals. The Magic of Everyday Moments is an age-graded set of booklets designed to help parents "gain ideas for how to use simple, everyday moments to promote your child's social, emotional, and intellectual development." The site is ideal for those seeking more quality time with their kids. The section on Choosing Quality Child Care is extensive and principle-based. Those parents concerned about possible delays in development should visit New Visions for Parents and read about assessments, terms, means, and so on. Parents wanting to promote their child's literacy can read much more in the Early Literacy section with excellent questions and answers, tips, book lists, and activities.

★★★★★   *Infant and Toddler Care*
http://www.nncc.org/InfantToddler/inftod.page.html

About 50 links to papers (fact sheets, articles, newsletters) and a few sites under the following major headings: Growth and Development; Health and Safety; Nutrition; Infant/Toddler Concerns; and Resources. Just about all that is known about development is here.

★★★★ *BabyCenter* http://www.babycenter.com/rcindex.html

A truly enormous site! Although very commercial, it has thousands of pages of information: from before pregnancy to the end of toddlerhood. A good site to start with when parents are unsure just what they want to learn.

Psychoeducational Materials for Clients and Families

★★★★★ *The Natural Child Project* http://www.naturalchild.com/home

The aim of this site seems to be to encourage simple and close-bonding parenting. It offers perhaps a hundred of the very best articles by experts under these topic headings: Attachment, Parenting, Babies, Breast-Feeding, Child Advocacy, Learning, Living with Children, and Sleeping. If an intelligent and interested parent wants to enlarge his or her perspective on children, this is the place to go.

★★★★★ *Today's Parent Online* http://www.todaysparent.com

For lots of high-quality information on each developmental stage, go to Step and Stages, select an age (from 0 to 12), use the pop-up menus to choose an article, then click on Go.

★★★★★ *Project NoSpank* http://www.nospank.net/toc.htm

A superb site for those who wish to campaign against paddling in the schools and the like. Lots of research, cases, links, and logic. Numbers 3 and 6 are of direct use in protecting one's children. For those partial to James Dobson's views, see section 47.

★★★★ *ParenthoodWeb* http://www.parenthood.com

A magazine with all kinds of information and advice focusing on the early years.

★★★★ *National Center for Fathering* http://www.fathers.com

Under Fathering Tips, about 30 practical tips, are hundreds of brief and sometimes sappy essays on stages, roles, responsibilities, and functions. The site is best as a source of beginning ideas or for expanding some men's ideas of what it could mean to be a father.

★★★★ *Building Baby's Intelligence: Why Infant Stimulation Is Important*
        http://www.envisagedesign.com/ohbaby/smart.html

A simple page of explanation and advice, with links to a dozen popular but quality readings.

★★★★ *Parenting the First Year*
        http://www.uwex.edu/ces/flp/parenting/pfylinks.html

Under each month are about a dozen links to articles about concerns, development, parenting, health, and the like. All sites have been reviewed by developmental specialists.

Because they are not organized by topic but by age, this site is perhaps best used as an introduction to family life.

★★★★ *Parenting and Marriage* by Kalman Heller, PhD
        http://www.drheller.com/index.html

Here are about 10 short but very well-written and authoritative essays (under Preschool) by an obviously experienced psychologist.

★★★★ *Brain Wonders* http://www.zerotothree.org/brainwonders/index.html

A site that explains brain development from zero to three years. It is a large project. Clicking on Parents leads to an introduction and then a choice of one of eight ages. That leads to an introduction, then What Is Going On and What You Can Do sections. Different materials are presented for child care providers and for professionals. The site is large, requires at least high school reading skills, and is based on solid research.

★★★★ *Parenting the Preschooler* http://www.uwex.edu/ces/flp/pp

In this site, you will find 6 to 12 brief, nicely printed newsletters on specific topics: Development; Discipline; Feeding/Nutrition; Financial; Health/Safety; Nurturing/Love; Parent Support; Play Activities; and Social Interactions. These newsletters developed by University of Wisconsin staff are aimed at low-skilled readers and available for free distribution.

★★★★ *Parenting* http://www.uwex.edu/ces/flp/parenting

Here are eight-page, age-paced monthly newsletters that have been shown to improve parenting. They cover the child's first three years, are available in Spanish, are written at the fifth-grade reading level, and are developed by the University of Wisconsin. They are for sale here, as well for use in a marketing or public educational campaign.

★★★ *Growing Together: Infant Development*
        http://www.nncc.org/Child.Dev/grow.infant.html

These seven pages of solid, basic information and perhaps a good handout for those who need to learn what to expect.

See also Pregnancy (Chapter 27) and Child Development and Parenting (Chapter 13).

CHAPTER 22

Love and Intimacy

For centuries, philosophers, songwriters, and poets have been intrigued by love. Only recently, though, have psychologists turned their attention to love and offered recommendations on how to improve your love life and your intimacy.

Love is a vast and complex territory of human behavior. Much of romantic love and physical intimacy has traditionally occurred in the context of marriage, a topic to which we devote the next chapter (Chapter 23). In this chapter, we cover self-help books, films, and Internet resources devoted to love and intimacy that, admittedly, overlaps with the following chapter. Indeed, simply because of the immense pool of resources, we chose not to review the hundreds of autobiographies touching on the subject.

SELF-HELP BOOKS

Strongly Recommended

★★★★★ *Love Is Never Enough* (1988) by Aaron Beck. New York: Harper & Row.

This volume presents a cognitive therapy approach to love from one of the founders of cognitive therapy. Beck tells couples how to overcome misunderstandings, resolve conflicts, and improve their relationship by following cognitive therapy strategies. He first helps partners understand the specific self-defeating attitudes that plague troubled relationships. Then, he applies his cognitive therapy to what he labels the most common marital problems:

- How negative perceptions can overwhelm the positive aspects of marriage.
- The swing from idealization to disillusionment.
- The clash of differing perspectives.
- The imposition of rigid expectations and rules.
- How partners fail to hear what is said and often hear things that are not said.

RECOMMENDATION HIGHLIGHTS

Self-Help Books

- On improving relationships with communication and cognitive therapy:

  ★★★★★ *Love Is Never Enough* by Aaron Beck

  ★★★★ *The Relationship Cure* by John Gottman and Joan DeClaire

- On the nature and the forms of love:

  ★★★★ *The Art of Loving* by Erich Fromm

  ★★★★ *The Triangle of Love* by Robert Sternberg

- On improving relationships by understanding yourself and relationships:

  ★★★★ *The Dance of Intimacy* by Harriet Lerner

  ★★★★ *The Dance of Connection* by Harriet Lerner

  ♦ *In the Meantime* by Iyanla Vanzant

- On improving relationships by learning effective communication:

  ★★★★ *I Only Say This Because I Love You* by Deborah Tannen

- On seeking partners and maintaining a loving relationship:

  ★★★★ *Keeping the Love You Find* by Harville Hendrix

- On improving gay and lesbian relationships:

  ♦ *Permanent Partners* by Betty Berzon

Films

- On changing romantic partners as couples grow old together:

  ★★★ *The Four Seasons*

- On the complexity and challenge of heterosexual relationships:

  ★★★ *When Harry Met Sally*

Internet Resources

- On understanding love:

  ★★★★ *Love Is Great* http://loveisgreat.com

  ★★★★ *The Nature of Attraction and Love*
  http://mentalhelp.net/psyhelp/chap10/chap10d.htm

- On dating:

  ★★★★★ *One Straight Male's Thoughts and Advice on Successful Use of Internet Personals* by Dean Esmay
  http://www.deanesmay.com/straight-faq.html

  ★★★★ *Singlescoach* http://www.singlescoach.com/resources.html

- On talking and flirting:
  - ★★★★★ *Erotic Talk for Lovers and Performers*
    http://www.sexuality.org/talk.html
  - ★★★★ *SIRC Guide to Flirting* http://www.sirc.org/publik/flirt.html

---

- How automatic negative thinking leads to conflict.
- How partners cognitively distort a relationship, which drives couples apart.

In the last half of the book, Beck presents a number of different cognitive methods to fit the specific needs of couples. The book was written primarily as a self-help guide to improve love relationships, and it remains the highest-rated book in its category. Practical, inspiring, and clear.

★★★★ *The Relationship Cure* (2002) by John Gottman and Joan DeClaire. New York: Crown.

Leading researcher John Gottman describes how happiness is based on everyday communication that involves emotion. He says that this happiness depends on "bids" and how other people respond, or fail to respond, to such approaches. Gottman puts forth a five-step program to show readers how to become a master "bidder" in the emotional communications. Numerous case studies, sample dialogues, and self-assessments are included. A superb, research-supported book that would probably have reached five-star status had more psychologists in our studies rated it.

★★★★ *The Dance of Intimacy: A Woman's Guide to Courageous Acts of Change in Key Relationships* (1989) by Harriet Lerner. New York: Harper Perennial.

Written for women and about women's intimate relationships, *The Dance of Intimacy* weaves a portrait of the current self and relationships that Lerner believes is derived from long-standing relationships with mothers, fathers, and siblings. Drawing on a combination of psychoanalytic and family systems theories, Lerner tells women that, if they are having problems in intimate relationships, they need to explore their upbringing to find clues to the current difficulties. Women learn how to avoid distancing themselves from their families of origin and overreacting to problems. Lerner intelligently tells women that they should balance the *I* and the *we* in their lives, and be neither too self-absorbed nor too other-oriented. To explore unhealthy patterns that have been passed down from one generation to the next, Lerner helps women create a "genogram," a family diagram that goes back to the grandparents or earlier. This is an outstanding self-help book on understanding why close relationships are problematic and how to change them in positive ways. It does not give simple, quick-fix strategies. Lerner accurately avows that change is difficult, but she shows that it is possible.

★★★★ *The Dance of Connection* (2002) by Harriet Lerner. New York: HarperCollins.

Continuing the themes of *The Dance of Intimacy* (reviewed above), psychologist Lerner describes the importance of positively connecting with the people who matter most to us in life. She analyzes the most stressful problems people face when others hurt them and tells readers how to take a conversation to a more positive level when they feel desperate. Individuals learn when to let things go, as well as the steps to take when they face betrayals and inequities in relationships.

★★★★ *Keeping the Love You Find* (1993) by Harville Hendrix. New York: Pocket Books.

Hendrix describes a self-help program for singles who seek a loving, rewarding romantic relationship. He especially focuses on how to maintain a positive relationship with someone you love over the long term. Although the book's title and the writing may appear a little slick, the mental health professionals in our studies consistently rate this book positively.

★★★★ *The Art of Loving* (1956, reissued 2002) by Erich Fromm. New York: Harper & Row.

This philosophical and psychological treatise on the nature of love, penned by Erich Fromm, a well-known psychoanalyst and social philosopher, describes love in general, as well as different forms of love. In Fromm's view, love is an attitude that determines the relatedness of the person to the whole world, not just toward one love object. Love is an act of faith, a commitment, a complete giving of oneself. There are no quick fixes for developing love; rather Fromm argues that learning to love is a long and difficult process requiring discipline, patience, sensitivity to self, and the productive use of skills. He stresses that although the principle underlying capitalistic society and the principle of love are incompatible, love is the only sane and satisfactory solution to the human condition. As such, this book is very different from most of the books evaluated in our national studies; it doesn't include the usual exercises, case histories, and clinical examples. Rather, *The Art of Loving* tackles the complex question of what love is and how society can benefit if people learn how to love more effectively. Widely regarded as a classic, this intellectually challenging piece is not written as clearly as most self-help books.

★★★★ *I Only Say This Because I Love You* (2001) by Deborah Tannen. New York: Random House.

Tannen explains how individuals can avoid or redirect conversations and circumstances with their loved ones that are rapidly becoming destructive. She provides many examples of conversations that have gone sour and discusses numerous strategies for communicating more effectively with people you love. A fine self-help book with interesting examples.

★★★★ *The Triangle of Love* (1987) by Robert Sternberg. New York: Basic Books.

The three sides of love's triangle are the fire of sexual and romantic passion, the close emotional sharing of intimacy, and the enduring bond of commitment. The type and quality of a relationship depend on the strength of each side of the triangle in each partner and how closely the partners' triangles match. Sternberg argues that each side has its own time table. For example, passion dominates the early part of a love relationship, whereas intimacy and commitment play more important roles as relationships progress. In the author's view, the ultimate form of love combines passion, intimacy, and commitment. Sternberg gives specific guidelines for improving love relationships and includes a love scale for measuring one's own love. An insightful perspective on the nature of love, this book gives good advice about how to achieve perfect love, but it includes more academic discussion than is typical of self-help books. Nonetheless, Sternberg's analysis of love's nature is much easier reading than Fromm's *The Art of Loving*.

Recommended

★★★   *Fear of Intimacy* (2001) by Robert Firestone and Joyce Catlett. Washington, DC: American Psychological Association.

Based on their extensive clinical experience, the authors argue that relationships fail not for commonly given reasons but rather because psychological defenses formed in childhood act as barriers to closeness in adulthood. Numerous case studies illustrate the childhood precursors of adult relationship problems. It is a bit academic for a self-help book but was favorably rated by mental health experts familiar with it; in fact, had it been more widely known, it would have probably obtained a four-star designation.

★★★   *Obsessive Love: When It Hurts Too Much to Let Go* (2002) by Susan Forward and Craig Buck. New York: Bantam.

This book is for people who are obsessive lovers and their targets. Obsessive love is not really love at all, according to Forward and Buck, but rather a pathological compulsion. They believe that obsessive love is caused by rejecting parents or separation problems in childhood. According to the authors, obsessive love occurs about equally in women and men and takes different forms: worshiping someone from afar, fantasizing about saving a troubled partner, or refusing to let go of a lover who has broken off a relationship. The authors intelligently tell obsessive lovers who are violence-prone to see a therapist immediately rather than simply relying on her self-help book. For obsessive lovers who are not violence-prone, they recommend detailed logging of emotions, a two-week vacation from contact with the target, and a probing self-evaluation in which obsessors ask themselves tough questions about whether anything in the relationship can be salvaged.

★★★   *Do I Have to Give Up Me to Be Loved by You?* (1983) by Jordan Paul and Margaret Paul. Minneapolis: CompCare.

This best-selling self-help book advocates probing and understanding the unspoken motivations behind what we do to solve our relationship problems. Using their intention therapy as a base, the authors tell readers how to become aware of self-created obstacles and develop more intimate relationships. A number of exercises help couples work on their power struggles, sexual expectations, and many other marital problems.

★★★   *Soul Mates: Honoring the Mysteries of Love and Relationship* (1994) by Thomas Moore. New York: HarperCollins.

Moore, a former Catholic monk turned best-selling author, reawakens the reader to discernment and nurturance of the soul in an effort to cultivate loving relationships. He looks at relationships from a position of mystery, religion, and theology, believing it is a mistake to talk authoritatively about mysteries. Moore's objective is to help individuals change well-entrenched ideas of what it means to love and be one with others in friendship, marriage, and community. This three-star book would probably be best received by religiously and spiritually oriented readers.

★★★ *Creating Love: The Next Great Stage of Growth* (1992) by John Bradshaw. New York: Bantam.

This best-selling author writes on the many dimensions of love and demystifies the belief that love is easy and a given among blood relatives. To paraphrase Bradshaw, love is difficult and requires hard work and honesty. The reader is forced to evaluate and perhaps surrender counterfeit love in exchange for the soul-building work of real love. Bradshaw addresses how to create love in various relationships (e.g., with God, parents, children, friends, spouses, work, and self). This three-star book brings to the surface the mystical, spiritual, and soulful characteristics of love and will probably be useful to people who have struggled with uncertainty about love.

★★★ *A Return to Love* (1992) by Marianne Williamson. New York: HarperCollins.

This book is a spiritual journey back to our natural tendency to love. Best-selling author Williamson argues that we have frequently been taught to detach, to compete, and to dislike ourselves. Through her psychological, emotional, and spiritual approach, she encourages us to relinquish our social fears and accept back into our hearts the love we have been denying. It is a book about the practical application of love and its daily practice. An inspiring book for the spiritually minded and for those seeking a life based on the practice of love.

★★★ *Going the Distance: Secrets of Lifelong Love* (1991) by Lonnie Barbach and David Geisinger. New York: Plume.

The advice in *Going the Distance* is appropriate for a wide range of couples, from people just embarking on a close intimate relationship to those who want to renew their commitment to marital partners. According to Barbach and Geisinger, we bring the scars of old psychic wounds to any new relationship; a good close relationship is a healing one; and even individuals with a long history of troubled relationships can learn the skills needed to make a marriage work. The authors stress the importance of chemistry, courtship, trust, respect, acceptance, and shared values. They also suggest methods for overcoming commitment phobias, strategies to resolve power conflicts for control, and ways to improve a couple's sex life. A 50-item compatibility questionnaire helps couples evaluate how well-suited they are. Solid advice and well-written, even if standard fare for relationship books.

★★★ *Women Who Love Too Much* (1985) by Robin Norwood. New York: Pocket Books.

This volume was one of many best-selling self-help books in the 1980s that blame most of women's problems on a male-dominated society. Among the characteristics of a woman who loves too much are a childhood in which her emotional needs were not met, willingness to assume the majority of blame for a relationship's problems, low self-esteem, and a belief that she has no right to be happy. Such women choose men who need help, inevitably causing their marriage to become troubled. These women are addicted to pain, says Norwood, just as an alcoholic is addicted to liquor. The first step to a woman's recovery from a relationship addiction is to back off from the partner—quit nagging and stop making demands—and start focusing on her own problems. Norwood advocates finding a support group and leaving the relationship if necessary. *Women Who Love Too Much* headed the *New York Times* best-seller list for 37 weeks. It can inspire women who are trapped in bad relationships to evaluate their situations and chart better courses for their lives. On the other hand, critics say that it attributes women's problems disproportionately to men and doesn't adequately deal with what happens to a woman once she "recovers."

Diamonds in the Rough

♦ *In the Meantime: Finding Yourself and the Love That You Want* (1998) by Iyanla Vanzant. New York: Simon & Schuster.

The author focuses on the vision and purpose humans need to find their way through life. Vanzant asks, as you are working to achieve a state of love, what do you do in the meantime? Mental housekeeping is the answer—for example, repairing past hurts, addressing fears, and correcting inaccurate information that stand in the way of finding true love. Vanzant states that love will come to us, but most of us won't recognize it, because love rarely shows up in the place we expect or looks the way we expect it to look. She reinforces the point that true self-love needs to be in place in order to find the love that we want. Taking each experience and learning more about oneself is part of what to do in the meantime. But it's not easy. Reflection, evaluation, and unlearning require a willingness to do the grunge work. A highly but infrequently rated book for adults trying to understand themselves and willing to learn in the meantime.

♦ *Permanent Partners: Building Gay and Lesbian Relationships* (1988) by Betty Berzon. New York: Dutton.

This book was written from the personal and professional experiences of the author, a psychotherapist. Her purposes are to help homosexual couples see the relationship stressors that may inhibit growth and to develop new options for dealing with those stressors. The wide-ranging topics include establishing compatibility, learning to understand the underlying issues, identifying the effects of internalized homophobia, improving communication with partners, negotiating out of power struggles, fighting constructively, dealing with sexual issues and financial arrangements, having children, and dealing with change in the partnership. Among the obstacles explored are the lack of visible, long-term same-sex couples as role models, absence of support from society, and the guidance gap that has not provided adequate advice on effectively building a life with another man or another woman. This book was written explicitly for gay and lesbian couples. Highly but infrequently rated in two of our national studies, thus meriting a Diamond in the Rough designation.

Not Recommended

★★ *Relationship Rescue: A Seven-Step Strategy for Reconnecting with Your Partner* (2000) by Philip McGraw. New York: Hyperion.

★★ *Loving Each Other* (1984) by Leo Buscaglia. Thorofare, NJ: Slack.

★★ *Men Who Hate Women and the Women Who Love Them* (1986) by Susan Forward. New York: Bantam.

★★ *Men Who Can't Love: When a Man's Fear Makes Him Run from Commitment* (1987) by Steven Carter. New York: Evans.

★ *When Someone You Love Is Someone You Hate* (1988, reprinted 1996) by Stephen Arterburn and David Stoop. Dallas: Word.

★ *What Smart Women Know* (1990) by Steven Carter and Julia Sokol. New York: Evans.

Strongly Not Recommended

† *Mars and Venus in the Bedroom: A Guide to Lasting Romance and Passion* (1995) by John Gray. New York: HarperCollins.

† *Women Men Love, Women Men Leave* (1987) by Connell Cowan and Melvyn Kinder. New York: Clarkson N. Potter.

† *What Every Woman Should Know about Men* (1981) by Joyce Brothers. New York: Simon & Schuster.

FILMS

Recommended

★★★ *The Four Seasons* (1982) directed by Alan Alda. PG rating. 107 minutes.

This film provides a realistic view of small-group dynamics—that is, the group members' relationship to each other and also the subset relationships of each person to his or her partner. Three couples have taken their vacations together for many years when one couple suddenly divorces. The man brings his new wife to the group's holiday, thereby challenging the nature of their relationships and the meaning of love. The film highlights the foibles of growing up and older together in very funny scenarios, while also capturing the spirit of lifetime romantic changes. Also reviewed in Chapter 18 on divorce.

★★★ *When Harry Met Sally* (1990) directed by Rob Reiner. R rating. 95 minutes.

Harry and Sally run into each other every five years or so and find themselves at differing points in their romantic relationships. They repeatedly discuss the possibility of being friends, but Harry proclaims that men and women can't be friends because of the inevitability of sex. The uncertainty of their relationship and their commitment and caring for each other are the themes of this story. The complexity and challenge of contemporary relationships between men and women is revealed in funny, yet poignant ways.

★★★ *The Way We Were* (1973) directed by Sydney Pollack. PG rating. 118 minutes.

Tearjerker in which a man and woman meet and fall in love years after their friendship in college. They find themselves with very different political and ideological perspectives that eventually drive them apart. The movie demonstrates the challenges of love and the difficulties of holding on to one's beliefs while accepting differences in a partner. The story is energetic, sad, and hopeful; in the end, it chronicles coping with interpersonal loss based on principles.

★★★   *The Story of Us* (1999) directed by Rob Reiner. R rating. 96 minutes.

Bruce Willis and Michelle Pfeiffer have been married 15 years and seem to get along for the sake of their wonderful children. After the kids leave for summer camp, they start a trial separation. The movie focuses on how they cope with the separation and understand their marriage. He is a disorganized and laid-back comedy writer who finds her too rigid; she is a crossword puzzle writer who finds him irresponsible. The marriage is told in a series of flashbacks, including some high points, endless screaming fights, and times of bland distance. While any married person will find several things to relate to and will appreciate the marital therapy sessions, the couple shows little growth or insight. In the end, the couple decides to remain married, but this is a sobering, non-romantic picture of a struggling marriage.

★★★   *Sleepless in Seattle* (1994) directed by Nora Ephron. PG rating. 100 minutes.

The despair over a spouse's death and the search for a soulmate drive this heartwarming and funny story. Sam's wife died, leaving Sam and son Jonah adrift. Sam's initial abdication of a love life and his awkward attempts to console his son are realistic portrayals of a family in turmoil. Holding out for the real thing, so that love conquers all, and the irrepressibility of a child's mission to make his family complete are the dual lessons of this story.

Not Recommended

★★   *Pretty in Pink* (1987) directed by Howard Deutch. PG-13 rating. 96 minutes.

★   *Serendipity* (2001) directed by Peter Chelsom. PG-13 rating. 90 minutes.

Strongly Not Recommended

†   *9½ Weeks* (1987) directed by Adrian Lyne. R rating. 113 minutes.

INTERNET RESOURCES

We review websites devoted to love and romance in general, dating, and specialized topics.

Love and Romance

★★★★★   *Erotic Talk for Lovers and Performers*   http://www.sexuality.org/talk.html

An unusual site: 46 pages of the best from seven books on how to talk sexy. This handout prepared for a workshop is quite detailed, sex-positive, and, toward the end, instructive about setting up a phone sex-for-profit operation (so warn those you refer to this site). Ideal for the shy but eager client.

★★★★   *The Nature of Attraction and Love*
         http://mentalhelp.net/psyhelp/chap10/chap10d.htm

Romantic and companionate love are different and must be understood. This is a wide-ranging introduction in eight pages.

★★★★ *SIRC Guide to Flirting* http://www.sirc.org/publik/flirt.html

Thirty pages on what behavioral science tells us about flirting and how to do it. Everything about beginning relationships based on the research. Ideal for the overly ideational but socially inexperienced, college-educated reader or others with social anxiety who need specific guidance.

★★★★ *Love Is Great* http://loveisgreat.com

There are thousands of sites about love and relationships. This is the most useful we have found about love: finding love, understanding and keeping love, and providing ways to show love. Lots of activities and ideas for those beginning to think about love and romance.

★★★ *Types of Love* http://dataguru.org/love/fehrtyp.asp

The term *love* is packed with multiple meanings, yet we cling to it and use it frequently. In this site, it has been separated into several types, and the material here may help clarify the thinking of the naive or confused.

★★★ *Some Great Advice on Reading Female Nonverbal Signals*
       http://www.dataguru.org/love/misc/signals9706.asp

A useful essay for straight guys who seem to get rejected regularly.

★★★ *How to Kiss* http://www.kissingbooth.com/kiss.htm

Two pages on how to kiss.

★★★ *Romantic Ideas* http://www.lovingyou.com/romance101/ideas.shtml

This site indicates that there are 1,161 romantic ideas (actually messages posted to a online group), so it might be useful for those baffled by what the term *romantic* means these days.

★★★ *Rekindle Romance* http://www.positive-way.com/rekindle.htm

A very nice list of 14 brief and practical suggestions. Part of a larger marital communication project.

★★★ *Advice on Flirting* http://www.sexuality.org/flirtadv.html

A five-page collection of tips from a discussion group and a book on flirting.

Dating: In Person and Online

★★★★★ *The Straight FAQ: One Straight Male's Thoughts and Advice on Successful Use of Internet Personals* by Dean Esmay
       http://www.deanesmay.com/straight-faq.html

Here are the best, most complete advice and examples available. Anyone can read this and learn what to do and not do. For gay men, a companion FAQ is at http://www.deanesmay.com/nssf.html

★★★★★ *The Rebuttal from Uranus* http://ourworld.compuserve.com/homepages/women_rebuttal_from_uranus

John Gray's *Men Are from Mars, Women Are from Venus* and subsequent books have been popular. This site offers intelligent and devastating critiques. Thank you, Susan Hamson.

★★★★ *Singlescoach* http://www.singlescoach.com/resources.html

Although this is a commercial site, 80 columns written by psychotherapist Nina Atwood contain usable, nonrigid suggestions. The site is even searchable. An acceptable starting place for those seeking relationships.

★★★ *Web-Based Matchmaking Services* http://www.sexuality.org/personal.html

A brief essay on the nature and uses of online personals ads.

★★★ *The Dating Doctor* http://www.datingdoctor.com

Although this is a commercial site, the FAQ could be useful to those with minor problems because it shows that others have the same kinds of problems. The advice is pretty solid and responsible.

★★★ *Guys Guide to Girls* by Philip Ovalsen http://www.philipov.com/guys1.htm

About 20 pages of musings on love, shyness, writing letters, and other social skills. The first four essays are gently written and supportive; the last two give good advice on using the Internet and finding a Russian woman as a mate. Useful as a starting point.

★★★ *Out of the Cave: Exploring Gray's Anatomy* by Kathleen Trigiani
http://web2.airmail.net/ktrig246/out_of_cave

"This series of five essays takes a macroscopic look at the Mars and Venus phenomenon and concludes that we don't have to settle for Gray's worldview. This site is ideal for people who are interested in gender issues but don't have time to read the major literature."

Specialized Sites

★★★★ *HeartBeat—Relationship Advice with Flava!*
http://www.askheartbeat.com/home.html

"Oriented towards the relationship issues of women of color." There are lots of advice sites; this one is both specialized and full of intelligent, usable, specific advice.

★★★★ *The Backrubs FAQ* http://www.kjartan.org/backrubfaq

Lots of information, maybe too much, on how to do it.

★★ *Short Persons Support* http://www.shortsupport.org/index.html

Solid information on all aspects of shortness, including dating. Highly recommended.

See also Marriage (Chapter 23) and Sexuality (Chapter 30).

Marriage

The changes in American marital patterns have been revolutionary, not evolutionary. Just 50 years ago, people married in their teens and early 20s, had children, and stayed together for the rest of their lives. Men worked outside the home and were the breadwinners; women worked inside the home and cared for the children. In today's world, many people marry later or not at all. When they do get married, many couples postpone having children until both partners have developed their careers, or they choose to remain childless. Divorce captures 40% of all first marriages and 50% of subsequent marriages. Couples want their relationship to be deep and loving, and if it isn't, they increasingly see a psychologist or marriage counselor or consult a self-help resource to improve their marital relationship.

In this chapter, we present the evaluative ratings and narrative descriptions of self-help resources on marriage. The content of this chapter obviously overlaps with the preceding chapter on love and intimacy, but if the thrust of the resource is marriage or couplehood, we placed it here.

SELF-HELP BOOKS

Strongly Recommended

★★★★★ *Why Marriages Succeed or Fail* (1994) by John Gottman. New York: Simon & Schuster.

Based on research conducted over a number of years with hundreds of couples, the principles presented in this book diagnose, interpret, and predict the success or failure of a marriage with a high degree of accuracy. Psychologist Gottman, an internationally known researcher, effectively and systematically describes the three types of marriage styles and how healthy or unhealthy each may be depending on the interaction. The four warning signs that a marriage is spiraling downward are described (criticism, con-

---

RECOMMENDATION HIGHLIGHTS

Self-Help Books

- On healthy and unhealthy marriage styles:

  ★★★★★ *Why Marriages Succeed or Fail* by John Gottman

- On solving marital problems and improving the relationship:

  ★★★★★ *The Seven Principles for Making Marriages Work* by John Gottman and Nan Silver

  ★★★★ *Intimate Partners* by Maggie Scarf

  ★★★★ *Divorce Busting* by Michele Weiner-Davis

  ★★★ *Fighting for Your Marriage* by Howard Markman et al.

  ★★★ *Reconcilable Differences* by Andrew Christensen and Neil Jacobson

- On pastoral marital counseling:

  ◆ *Love for a Lifetime* by James Dobson

Internet Resources

- On improving your marriage:

  ★★★★★ *Relationship Information for Couples* http://www.positive-way.com/relation.htm

  ★★★★ *Parenting and Marriage Articles* http://www.drheller.com

  ★★★★ *Marriage Mythology* http://researchmag.asu.edu/articles/marriage.html

- On rebuilding relationships after extramarital affairs:

  ★★★★★ *The Other Woman* http://www.gloryb.com

  ★★★★ *Marriage Builders* http://www.marriagebuilders.com/graphic/mbi5525_qa.html

---

tempt, defensiveness, and stonewalling), and in concluding chapters, four keys to improving a marriage and reversing the spiral are discussed. Gottman's advice is logical, clear, and research-based. Quizzes allow couples to self-identify the status of their marriages. According to our mental health experts, this a very valuable and research-based self-help book.

★★★★★ *The Seven Principles for Making Marriages Work* (2000) by John Gottman and Nan Silver. New York: Crown.

This outstanding self-help book received very high ratings. Written by leading marriage researcher John Gottman (who also wrote *Why Marriages Succeed or Fail*, reviewed above) and based on his extensive observations, this book provides a number of positive strategies for helping couples to understand their problems and make their relationship work. Gottman's principles for making a marriage work include establishing love maps, turning toward each other instead of away, letting your partner influence you, solving solvable conflicts, overcoming gridlock, and creating shared meaning. Extensive examples and self-assessments are included. His two books received the highest ratings for this category in our national studies.

★★★★ *Intimate Partners: Patterns in Love and Marriage* (1986, reprinted 1996) by Maggie Scarf. New York: Ballantine.

This book tells readers how to solve their marital problems, especially by understanding the stages of development and the family of origin. Scarf charts the lives of five married couples in depth, categorizing them according to their life stage: idealization, disenchantment, child-rearing and career-building, child-launching, and the retirement years. She starts with relative newlyweds and ends with a couple who have finished rearing their children and are free to focus on each other once again. Interviews with 32 couples are woven through the book. Scarf emphasizes the importance of a couple's birth families, configurations, and genograms (diagrams of lines of attachment between marital partners and their parents, grandparents, and siblings) to illuminate how people often repeat the past. Unfulfilled needs are powerful, unconscious forces that shape a marriage from the beginning and continue to dominate it throughout the marriage stages. Scarf does an excellent job of encouraging partners to examine their stages of marriage and their families of origin.

★★★★ *Getting the Love You Want* (1988) by Harville Hendrix. New York: Henry Holt.

This book is based on workshop techniques that Hendrix has developed to help couples construct a conscious marriage—a relationship based on awareness of the unresolved childhood conflicts that cause individuals to select particular spouses. The author tells readers how to conduct a 10-week course in marital therapy in the privacy of their homes. In a stepwise fashion, he teaches readers how to communicate more clearly and sensitively, to eliminate self-defeating behaviors, and to focus attention on meeting their partners' needs. Hendrix's goal is to transform the downward spiral of the power struggle into a mutually beneficial relationship of emotional growth. This four-star book is superb for marital partners engulfed in conflict. Hendrix does an excellent job of helping the reader become aware of long-standing family influences on current close relationships.

★★★★ *Divorce Busting* (1992) by Michele Weiner-Davis. New York: Summit.

This book advocates a brief, solution-oriented approach to keeping a marriage together. Author Weiner-Davis says that divorce is not the answer to an unhappy marriage. She says she came to this conclusion after observing that former spouses often continue to be unhappy after the divorce. Weiner-Davis's approach focuses on the present and the future, and on actions rather than feelings. It is accomplished in brief rather than lengthy therapy or problem-solving sessions. (In her practice, she sees most couples for only four to five sessions.) *Divorce Busting* offers step-by-step strategies that couples can follow to make their marriage loving again. Brief case histories show how couples have successfully used Weiner-Davis's approach to solve their marital difficulties. The steps can be followed alone or with a spouse. The therapeutic techniques are well translated into everyday language that the reader will easily comprehend.

Recommended

★★★ *Fighting for Your Marriage* (revised ed., 2001) by Howard Markman, Scott Stanley, and Susan Blumberg. New York: Wiley.

Based on the Prevention and Relationship Enhancement Program (PREP), this book provides couples with strategies for handling conflict more constructively, protecting happiness, and reducing the chances of breaking up. Howard Markman is a leading figure in the study of marital relationships. A research-based and practical self-help book.

★★★ *Reconcilable Differences* (2000) by Andrew Christensen and Neil Jacobson. New York: Guilford Press.

Two leading researchers in couple and marital therapy describe why couples have the same fights over and over again and how to reconcile their differences. Couples learn how to defuse arguments, accept differences, and change for the better. The authors describe concrete steps for individuals to develop compassionate acceptance of some of their partner's behaviors. Numerous case studies provide insights about differences and how to deal with them. Each chapter concludes with relevant couple exercises. As is the case in *Fighting for Your Marriage* (above), this is a research-based, practical self-help book.

★★★ *I Love You, Let's Work It Out* (1987) by David Viscott. New York: Simon & Schuster.

The cycle of working it out in Viscott's model begins with commitment and communication. The central focus of the book is a model for diagnosing and interpreting what couples argue about, how they argue, and what their individual and joint styles of interacting reveal about how to successfully work out problems. Protective styles (i.e., dependent, controlling, and competitive) are analyzed in relationship to couple styles, and an interaction is predicted and described for each. Working it out successfully means that once the dynamics and interactions that maintain conflict are understood, couples can break the cycle and make different choices. This volume presents an interactive, organized system for understanding conflict patterns and lends itself to cognitive approaches toward solutions.

★★★ *Husbands and Wives: Exploring Marital Myths* (1989) by Melvyn Kinder and Connell Cowan. New York: Clarkson N. Potter.

The major problem in most marriages, the authors maintain, is that each partner tries to change the other instead of focusing on improving his or her own behavior. Kinder and Cowan call their approach self-directed marriage; it emphasizes the importance of each partner's taking responsibility for his or her own happiness and replacing other-directed blame with acceptance. The authors tell marital partners to accept their differences, become friends, and rediscover the enjoyment of marital life. *Husbands and Wives* barely received a three-star rating in the national study.

★★★ *Getting Together and Staying Together* (2000) by William Glasser and Carleen Glasser. New York: HarperCollins.

Why some marriages make it and others fail is examined. Based on William Glasser's "choice theory," partners learn how to create loving, long-lasting relationships. Another self-help book that barely made it into the Recommended category.

Diamonds in the Rough

♦ *We Love Each Other but . . .* (1999) by Ellen Wachtel. New York: Golden.

Intimate relationships are most often lost because of failure in basic, daily interactions, not because of major events. This self-help resource directs the reader to just those basics and tells how to regain the fundamental elements of the relationship that brought the two people together in the first place. There are no exercises, activities, or artificial interventions. Instead, Wachtel suggests how to think and act differently toward problems so that both partners will be heard and understood. She offers four basic truths about being in relationships and identifies seven areas of conflict that have emerged as most common in her work with couples. Very doable solutions are offered for each problem, accompanied by numerous examples from the author's experience with couples who successfully enhanced their relationships. Highly rated in two of our studies but not yet well-known. A wise and comforting book.

♦ *Marital Myths Revisited* (2001) by Arnold A. Lazarus. San Luis Obispo, CA: Impact.

In this self-help book, prominent psychologist Arnold Lazarus takes "A Fresh Look at Two Dozen Mistaken Beliefs About Marriage," as the subtitle puts it. Lazarus identifies and dispels 24 myths that disrupt marriages, such as husbands and wives should be best friends, romantic love makes the best marriages, and opposites attract and complement each other. The book is lively, focused, and practical, laced with compelling examples and a fine sense of humor. The 24 myths are followed by brief sections on what can be done to alter the marital myths and Lazarus's top eight tips for a successful marriage. The first edition of this book was released just before one of our earlier studies and was thus not widely known at the time of the study; this new or revisited edition will, we predict, be more widely and favorably received.

♦ *Love for a Lifetime* (1998) by James Dobson. Sisters, OR: Multnomah.

James Dobson, a psychologist widely known for his many books on marriage and parenting, has written this book for adult singles, engaged couples, and those married less than 10 years. The author's objectives are to identify the major pitfalls that undermine a relationship and to make suggestions on how to avoid them. Christian principles frame the narrative, and his perspectives on relationships, money, sex, and family are consistent with Christian teachings. Topics addressed are controversial either in Christian teaching or in the general society, such as premarital sex, divorce, homosexuality, and gender differences. The teachings of this book will be helpful to people looking for guidance in relationship building within conventional Christian beliefs. Diamond in the Rough status is given to this book because of its moderately high but infrequent ratings in two of our studies.

INTERNET RESOURCES

Psychoeducational Materials for Clients and Families

★★★★★   *Relationship Information for Couples*
          http://www.positive-way.com/relation.htm

This site has 15 short and practical sections on improving a relationship, with good ideas about issues such as Warning Signs, Hidden Issues and Expectations, Expressing Your Feelings, Who's The Boss, How to Love Your Mate, Rekindle Romance, Relate to Create Happiness, Men, Housework, Better Sex, and Problem Solving. Each section has guidelines and suggestions, and often questionnaires, all of which seem eminently useful. This might be a good site to orient stuck couples.

★★★★   *Parenting and Marriage Articles* by Kalman Heller, PhD
         http://www.drheller.com/index.html

About a hundred very well-written, one-page articles on various aspects of married life, like conflict, gender, marital therapy, fair fighting, and so on.

★★★★   *Marriage Mythology* by Tara Blanc
         http://researchmag.asu.edu/articles/marriage.html

"When the reality of marriage doesn't meet our expectations, we tend to blame reality." Good for introducing marital therapy.

★★★★   *Marriage—A Many-Splendored, Sometimes Splintered, Thing* by Daniel Wayne
         Matthews, PhD   http://www.ces.ncsu.edu/depts/fcs/pub/marriage.html

In only six pages, Matthews presents the challenges couples face when they marry, myths, financial and in-law issues, and more. An excellent premarital orientation.

★★★★   *About.com Marriage*   http://www.marriage.about.com

The contents keep changing, but some readings will always be of use to some individuals, for example, those under Stages of Marriage, Difficult Times, Love and Romance, and so on.

★★★★   *Intentional Dialogue: A Process for Dissolving Conflict* by Dawn Lipthrott, MSW
         http://www.relationshipjourney.com

Click on Marriage & Relationships and then on this title. A handout of about seven pages describing how to use this tool.

★★★   *When the Answer Is "Not Tonight"* by Marlene M. Maheu, PhD
        http://shpm.com/articles/sex/sex.html

Maheu offers five possible causes and some interventions. This might be suitable for opening up discussions of this part of a couple's relationship.

★★★ *Marriage Support—Couples Place* http://www.marriagesupport.com

Marriage therapist David E. Stanford and his wife Joyce offer courses in relationship skills.

★★★ *Traditional Family Values* by Peter McWilliams
http://www.mcwilliams.com/books/aint/404.htm

Debunks the myths of perfect families of the 1950s. Useful to clear out assumptions of what marriage was and should be.

Affairs/Infidelity

★★★★★ *The Other Woman* http://www.gloryb.com/index.html

This is a support and informational site for the partner of the married person having an affair. It presents all sides, offers personal stories, and provides a large FAQ. The MM to English Dictionary is a painful read.

★★★★ *Marriage Builders* by Willard F. Harley, Jr., PhD
http://www.marriagebuilders.com/graphic/mbi5525_qa.html

Harley is clearly against affairs but writes well about the emotional issues. Here are about a dozen articles he wrote in response to letters. All of these may be useful to people who need to see all sides of an affair.

★★★★ *Marital Infidelity* by Robin Truhe http://www.umkc.edu/sites/hsw/affairs

In about eight pages (and lots of good links), almost all aspects are presented. This might be an excellent introductory handout.

★★★★ *Articles about Affairs* http://www.vaughan-vaughan.com/affairsmenu.html

Peggy Vaughn, author of a book on affairs, offers good but brief essays on about 30 aspects of affairs. A very good orientation.

★★★ *Possible Good from an Affair?*
http://www.divorcesource.com/info/affairs/good.shtml

A very brief list of six benefits—mainly knowing the truth. This might be useful to someone who has just discovered a spouse's affair.

Alternatives to Marriage

★★★★ *Alternatives to Marriage Project* http://www.atmp.org/homepage.html

The FAQ of just five pages is enlightening and assertive about voluntary singlehood. The Resources list is very helpful. This is a wonderful site for those struggling to affirm the positives of relationships outside of marriage.

Other Resources

Marriage Encounter http://marriage-encounter.org

"National Marriage Encounter is a Judeo/Christian Based Ministry and Support Organization for Married Couples." It has programs all over the country and in every kind of church. It's purpose is to examine attitudes and improve good marriages.

PAIRS http://www.pairs.com

This is the home page of a marital communication training program. The site might be useful to clients even if you do not use the PAIRS model to stimulate their thinking about their relationship's qualities and patterns.

Retrouvaille http://www.retrouvaille.org

Another marriage improvement program with a few articles to read. Oriented toward Roman Catholics.

NATIONAL SUPPORT GROUPS

Association for Couples in Marriage Enrichment
PO Box 10596
Winston-Salem, NC 27108
Phone: 800-634-8325
E-mail: acme@bettermarriages.org
http://www.bettermarriages.org

No Kidding!
PO Box 2802
Vancouver, BC, Canada V6B 3X2
Phone: 604-538-7736
E-mail: info@nokidding.net
http://www.nokidding.net

Mutual support and social activities for married and single people who either have decided not to have children, are postponing parenthood, or are unable to have children.

Smart Marriages' Directory of Marriage Education Programs
http://www.smartmarriages.com/
directory_browse.html

This is a searchable listing of about 150 local and national programs, with annotations and complete addresses.

See also Families and Stepfamilies (Chapter 20), Love and Intimacy (Chapter 22), and Sexuality (Chapter 30).

CHAPTER 24

Men's Issues

The male of the human species—what is he really like? What does he truly want and need? At no other point in human history have males and females been placed under a psychological microscope the way they have been in the last 25 years. It began with the emergence of the women's movement and its attack on male bias and discrimination against women. As a result of the movement, women have been encouraged to value sensitive feelings and connectedness with others, to develop their own identity, and to resist men's attempts to dominate them.

In response to women's efforts to change themselves and to change men, men developed their own movement. The men's movement has not been as political or as activist as the women's movement. Rather, it has been more of an emotional, spiritual movement that reasserts the importance of masculinity and urges men to resist women's efforts to turn them into "soft" males. Or it has been a psychological movement that recognizes that men need to be less violent and more nurturant but still retain their masculine identity. Many disciples of the men's movement argue that society's evolving gender arena has led men to question what being a man really means.

Self-help resources on men's issues traverse a large and heterogeneous group of materials. The early men's movement books broadly focused on coping with fluctuating gender roles, while men's movement books in the early 1990s relied on mythological and spiritual accounts of man's recapturing his true identity. The more recent self-help resources are emphasizing liberation from societal myths and reconstructing the definition of masculinity. In what follows, we critically review self-help books, films, and Internet resources on this expansive topic of men's issues.

RECOMMENDATION HIGHLIGHTS

Self-Help Books

- On rescuing sons from the destructive myths of boyhood:

    ★★★★ *Real Boys* by William Pollack

- On understanding the stages and transitions of men's life cycles:

    ★★★★ *Seasons of a Man's Life* by Daniel J. Levinson

- On improving the quality of men's identity and life:

    ★★★ *Being a Man* by Patrick Fanning and Matthew McKay

    ★★★ *Masculinity Reconsidered* by Ronald Levant and Gini Kopecky

Films

- On male identity development and father–son rapprochement:

    ★★★★★ *Billy Elliot*

    ★★★★★ *October Sky*

- On caring for an aging father and dissolving lifelong distance:

    ★★★★★ *I Never Sang for My Father*

    ★★★ *Nothing in Common*

- On the magic of baseball for men and recapturing youth:

    ★★★★ *Field of Dreams*

- On male competitiveness and pressure in the business world:

    ★★★ *Glengarry Glen Ross*

Internet Resources

- On the men's movement:

    ★★★ *Men's Stuff* http://www.menstuff.org

- On domestic violence:

    ★★★ *Domestic Violence Resources* http://www.silcom.com/~paladin/madv

- On fathers coping with divorce and custody:

    ★★★★★ *Fathers Rights to Custody* http://www.deltabravo.net/custody

- On men's health issues:

    ★★★★ *Prostate Cancer Program*
    http://www.cancer.med.umich.edu/prostcan/prostcan.html

SELF-HELP BOOKS

Strongly Recommended

★★★★　*Real Boys: Rescuing Our Sons from the Myths of Boyhood* (1998) by William Pollack. New York: Henry Holt.

The author explores this generation of boys' feelings of sadness, loneliness, and confusion while they try to appear tough, cheerful, and confident. Pollack takes the reader through the stages of childhood and adolescent development, ferreting out truth from myth, and recognizing the cultural and relational influences on male sexuality and behavior. He discusses how to let real boys be real men by revising the "Boys' Code" and still feeling connected. Pollack writes about what boys are like, how to help them, and what happens if they aren't helped. Negative influences include early and harsh disconnection from family, mixed messages, and outdated models, rules, and assumptions that are making boys sick. Parents, teachers, and professionals actively connected with boys will find this book valuable and revealing. *Real Boys* was very favorably evaluated by our mental health experts and received the highest ratings of any book in this category. (Also reviewed in Violent Youth, Chapter 37.)

★★★★　*Seasons of a Man's Life* (1978) by Daniel J. Levinson. New York: Ballantine.

This national bestseller is reviewed in Chapter 4 (Adult Development) but merits a brief mention here. It outlines a number of stages men pass through, including the midlife crisis. Levinson describes the stages and transitions in the male life cycle from 17 to 65 years of age.

Recommended

★★★　*Being a Man: A Guide to the New Masculinity* (1993) by Patrick Fanning and Matthew McKay. Oakland, CA: New Harbinger.

This is a practical book written for men and what they can do to improve the quality and length of their lives. Filled with assurance, assistance, and information, the book addresses multiple topics, such as appreciating gender differences, relating to one's father, clarifying and acting on values, finding meaningful work, making male friends, and raising children. The authors convincingly argue that identity is strongly determined by whether an individual was born a boy or girl and who the person's parents were. A man can't change these circumstances, but he can understand them better. For any man who wishes to evaluate the quality and context of his life, and for the woman wishing to understand man in context, this is an interesting and practical book. Indeed, its three-star rating underestimates its value according to the psychologists who evaluated it highly; had more known of it, this would surely be a four- or perhaps five-star resource.

★★★　*Man Enough: Fathers, Sons and the Search for Masculinity* (1993) by Frank S. Pittman. New York: Putnam.

In this book, masculinity is conceptualized as a group activity, as a cultural concept. Masculinity is different for each generation. It is supposed to be passed on from father to son. If a boy does not have men in his family, his need for mentors begins early. When children try to get close to their fathers, the practice of masculinity frequently gets in the way. Psychiatrist Pittman writes tellingly of the plight of men who didn't get the fathering they needed to make them comfortable with their masculinity and of the healing of men who have rediscovered the forgotten profession of fatherhood. This book was rated favorably but relatively infrequently, resulting in its relegation to the three-star category. It is an enlightening and helpful resource for adult males at any stage of their development.

★★★ *The Hazards of Being Male* (1976) by Herb Goldberg. New York: Signet.

Published in 1976, this was the first self-help book for men to come out after the woman's movement began to take hold. Goldberg became a central figure in the early development of the men's movement in the 1970s and early 1980s, mainly as a result of his writing about men's rights in *The Hazards of Being Male* and *The New Male*. Goldberg argues that a critical difference between men and women creates a precipitous gulf between them: Women can sense and articulate their feelings and problems; men—because of their masculine conditioning—can't. The result in men is an armor of masculinity that is defensive and powerfully maintains self-destructive patterns. Goldberg says that most men have been effective work machines and performers, but that about everything else in their lives suffers. Goldberg believes that millions of men are killing themselves by striving to be "true" men, a heavy price to pay for masculine privilege and power. Goldberg encourages men to

- Recognize the suicidal success syndrome and evade it.
- Understand that occasional impotence is nothing serious.
- Become aware of their real desires and get in touch with their own bodies.
- Elude the binds of masculine role playing.
- Relate to women as equals rather than serving as women's guilty servant or hostile enemy.
- Develop male friendships.

This three-star book is definitely dated, but it still delivers important messages to men.

★★★ *Masculinity Reconstructed* (1995) by Ronald Levant and Gini Kopecky. New York: Dutton/Plume.

One of psychology's leading experts on masculinity and men's relationships, Ronald Levant considers American men to be in a crisis because of their inability to establish positive relationships, especially with women. He believes this crisis has developed because men lack adequate emotional empathy and tend to act rather than feel. The authors provide a number of strategies to help men develop insights into the emotional aspects of their lives and establish more positive relationships with women.

★★★ *The New Male: From Self-Destruction to Self-Care* (1980) by Herb Goldberg. New York: Signet.

The themes of Goldberg's second book on men's issues are similar to the first (reviewed above). In Part I, He, Goldberg evaluates the traditional male role and its entrapments, and in Part II, He and She, he explores the traditional relationship between men and women. Part III, He and Her Changes, analyzes how the changes in roles of women brought about by the women's movement have affected men. Part IV, He and His Changes, provides hope for men by elaborating on how men can combine some of the strengths of traditional masculinity—such as assertiveness and independence—with increased exploration of the inner self, greater awareness of emotions, and more healthy, close relationships with others to become more complete men. Dated in content and examples, this three-star book expresses the timeless message of challenging men to explore their inner selves, get in touch with their feelings, and pay more attention to developing meaningful relationships.

★★★ *Chicken Soup for the Father's Soul* (2001) by Jack Canfield, Mark Donnelly, Jeff Aubery, and Mark Hansen. Deerfield Beach, FL: Health Communications.

Contributions about the nature of fatherhood are provided by famous fathers, including Bill Cosby. Moments of pride and fulfillment are described in a series of stories about fathers. Little direct advice or assistance, but much inspiration.

★★★ *Fire in the Belly* (1991) by Sam Keen. New York: Bantam.

While Goldberg's books were the men's movement bibles in the 1970s and 1980s, two authors ushered in a renewed interest in the men's movement in the 1990s—Sam Keen and Robert Bly. (Bly's book, *Iron John*, is listed in the Not Recommended category.) Keen's theme is that every man is on a spiritual journey to attain the grail of manhood. He strives to provide a road map for the journey, advising men on ways to avoid the dead ends of combative machismo and the blind alleys of romantic obsession. Keen says that he wrote *Fire in the Belly* because men have lost their vision of what masculinity is. Keen's answer is that men's true identity is fire in the belly and passion in the heart. Although this book was a *New York Times* best-seller, it received only a three-star rating in our national studies. Virtually all books on men's issues—and women's issues—are controversial and stir up inflammatory feelings in the opposite sex. On the positive side, our experts applauded Keen's efforts to get men to reexamine their male identity, to incorporate more empathy into their relationships, and to reduce their hostility. On the other side, Keen's critics, especially female critics, didn't like his trashing of androgyny, his exaggeration of gender differences, and the mysticism that permeate the book. Keen adopts a Jungian perspective on man's inner journey to find himself, a perspective that is filled with symbols and metaphors that are not always clearly presented.

Diamond in the Rough

◆ *FatherLoss: How Our Sons of All Ages Come to Terms with the Death of Their Dads* (2001) by N. Chethik. New York: Hyperion.

This book analyzes men's anxieties about the deaths of their fathers. It especially tackles the cultural expectation that men are supposed to respond to loss with emotional strength and not grieve openly, which places them at risk for not adequately coping with death. Descriptions of how John F. Kennedy, Jr., Ernest Hemingway, and other well-known men coped with the death of their fathers are provided. The author gives strategies for preparing for the loss of a father, coping immediately after his death, grieving, and preparing a son for a father's own death. Favorably but infrequently rated in our latest national study, leading to the Diamond in the Rough designation.

Not Recommended

★★ *Straight Talk to Men* (2000) by James Dobson. New York: W Publishing Group.

★★ *Iron John: Straight Talk about Men* (1990) by Robert Bly. New York: Vintage.

★ *Why Men Don't Get Enough Sex and Women Don't Get Enough Love* (1990) by Jonathan Kramer and Diane Dunaway. New York: Pocket Books.

Strongly Not Recommended

† *What Men Really Want: Straight Talk from Men about Sex* (1990, reprinted 1991) by Susan Bakos. New York: St. Martin's Press.

† *Ten Stupid Things Men Do to Mess Up Their Lives* (1997) by Laura Schlessinger. New York: Cliff Street.

FILMS

Strongly Recommended

★★★★★ *I Never Sang for My Father* (1969) directed by Gilbert Cates. PG rating. 92 minutes.

A son tries to care for an aging father, accepting his father's eccentricities and changing the quality of their relationship before its too late. The difficulties of disclosure, of admitting lifelong hurt, and of finding a way to dissolve the distance between them are the universal tasks undertaken by the father and son. The moving story is a realistic glimpse into the complexity and the fundamental challenges of father–son relationships. This five-star resource is one of the most favorably rated of all films in our national studies.

★★★★★ *Billy Elliot* (2000) directed by Stephen Daldry. PG-13 rating. 110 minutes.

Set in a harsh northern England mining town, this is the uplifting story of 11-year-old Billy's (Jamie Bell) struggle to find his way and be true to himself against his family's and his community's homophobia and anticultural attitudes. Billy is forced to take boxing lessons at great cost to his poor family to toughen him, but accidentally discovers that his real talent lies in ballet dancing. Although encouraged by the dance teacher, he and she know that the others will see this as unmanly, if not homosexual, in their unremittingly macho world. Billy tries to keep his secret, but reveals himself and copes with his father, whose love eventually overpowers his archaic beliefs. The dancing is absolutely wonderful, as is the music and the happy ending earned by the father's and son's courage. Deservedly rated a five-star movie.

★★★★★ *October Sky* (1999) directed by Joe Johnston. PG rating. 108 minutes.

An exhilarating story of the power of the human spirit conveyed through a young West Virginia boy, whose life in the coal fields stands in stark contrast to his goal of launching a rocket. The boy's dream represents escape and triumph for the coal miners, whose lives are painfully and realistically portrayed. They rally around the boy and support his science achievements and his attempt to go to the national science fair, but the father, who loves his son, does not believe science is a realistic way out. The eventual success of the boy and his father's change of heart are characterized in this true story. The boy grew up to become a NASA scientist, as portrayed in his book *Rocket Boys*. This is a wonderful film for adolescents struggling with identity and for the approval of their fathers.

★★★★ *Field of Dreams* (1989) directed by Phil Alden Robinson. PG rating. 106 minutes.

Reminiscence about the glory days of baseball is its secondary theme, but the real story is the magic of baseball for boys and men. For them, baseball was another world, a cherished world. An Iowa farmer, Ray, builds a magical field in his cornfield, and the ghosts of professional ballplayers show up and compete in games. This is a warm and poignant film about men who connect to other men (and Ray to his father) through the special love of baseball.

Recommended

★★★ *Glengarry Glen Ross* (1992) directed by James Foley. R rating. 100 minutes.

The four salesmen in a real estate office (Jack Lemmon, Alan Arkin, Ed Harris, and Al Pacino) are forced into a sales contest by their big bosses downtown. The pressure is immense, the sales leads are worthless, and, in desperation, they commit a stupid robbery that makes things even worse. Their desperation is palpable and pitiful. The film keenly displays the pressure and competitiveness experienced by many men in the business world. If someone does not understand what male workers feel, this film will explain it.

★★★ *Nothing in Common* (1986) directed by Garry Marshall. PG rating. 118 minutes.

David is in his mid-30s and has been estranged from his critical, cynical father for many years. Suddenly, he learns that his mother is leaving his father. His father, scared but belligerent, lonely but angry, needs him. Resentment, reconciliation, acceptance, and dealing with old pain are all part of the dynamics between David and his father. David learns that his unresolved problems with his father have to be faced in order to begin healing.

★★★ *Disney's The Kid* (2000) directed by Jon Turtletaub. PG rating. 101 minutes.

An angry, alone, and empty "image consultant" is revisited by his eight-year-old self and together they revisit their pasts, especially a playground defeat. They revise the past by having the man teach the boy fighting skills and standing up for his rights. Unfortunately, the movie suggests that the solution for interpersonal conflict is fighting skills rather than cooperation and compromise. Nonetheless, the movie does show with some humor and tenderness a man and a boy trying to help each other improve themselves. A sweet "inner child" story.

★★★ *American Beauty* (1999) directed by Sam Mendes. R rating. 122 minutes.

Kevin Spacey has lived a life lost. He loses his pointless job, his wife is chronically irritable and having an affair, his daughter is disaffected and distant, and then he falls in lust with his daughter's girlfriend. These events lead him to alter his life radically, running wild in sheer freedom. This Academy Award winning best film is, at once, a compelling satire of suburban life and a hopeful tale of how a man might recapture his life, gain the confidence to rebel, and reestablish dignity.

★★★ *City Slickers* (1992) directed by Ron Underwood. PG-13 rating. 110 minutes.

Three urban men, friends since adolescence, take a cattle-drive vacation in the midst of their various midlife crises. Billy Crystal is approaching his 40th birthday and reevaluating his life and masculinity. This funny film is best at demonstrating the bonds among male friends, revealing their middle-age complaints and choices, and acknowledging male perseverance when "the chips are down."

★★★ *Tootsie* (1983) directed by Sydney Pollack. PG rating. 116 minutes.

Michael, an out-of-work actor, takes on the identity of a female character, Dorothy, and wins a part in a daytime soap opera. He meets Julie on the set and they become women friends, although Michael has strong romantic feelings for Julie. Living the life of Dorothy and having relationships as a female dramatically transforms Michael's perspective about women, men, and himself. This is a touching and funny story of gender roles and subsequent insights into the subtle but significant differences in how we relate as men and women.

★★★ *The Rape of Richard Beck* (1985, made for TV) directed by Karen Arthur. Not rated.

Richard Beck (Richard Crenna) is a big-city cop who is insensitive and uncaring, particularly to women. He rejects the trauma and violation of rape until he himself is raped. He is thrown into the same experience of humiliation and rage as the women he has known who have been victims of sexual assault. Although flawed, this film is one of the few that depicts the rape of a man; the reversal of a familiar story is eye-opening. The film conveys compassion and caring for all victims of sexual assault.

INTERNET RESOURCES

As is the case with Women's Issues in Chapter 36, the list of Internet sites on men's issues is long and heterogeneous. Thus, this section has more than the usual number of sites and subsections.

Metasites

★★★★ *Men's Stuff: The National Men's Resource* http://www.menstuff.org

"A free international resource covering all six major segments of the men's movement (men's rights, mythopoetic, pro-feminist, recovery, re-evaluation counseling, and religious) with over 40 megs of information on over 100 men's issues." Under the Issues link on the left are about 25 essays and bibliographies, some of which are valuable: Divorce and Custody; Fathers, Feelings, and Homophobia; among others. Under the Re-sources link on the left are a great number of organizations that involve positive change in male roles and relationships.

★★★ *The Men's Issues Page* http://www.menweb.org/throop

Although there is much of value here, many sites are one-sided rants. We would not of-fer the whole site to a male client, but for someone seeking some support and direction, there are perspectives unique to this site.

Psychoeducational Materials for Clients and Families

★★★ *Menweb—Men's Voices Magazine* http://www.menweb.org/page1.htm

There are a dozen articles, some brief audiotapes, suggested books, advice on house husbanding, ideas about male violence, and so on. A good start toward enlightenment.

★★★ *Domestic Violence Resources* http://www.silcom.com/~paladin/madv

A good set of links to informative materials and readings, agency sites with more mate-rials, and helplines.

★★★ *Slowlane: The Online Resource for Stay at Home Dads* http://www.slowlane.com

Not exactly self-help, but the 50 or so articles and columns are often funny, touching, and can help men understand what mothers' lives are like.

★★★ *Single African American Fathers' Exchange*   http://saafe.com/saafe/ issuesaroundthehouse.htm#black%20fathers,%20invisible%20men

Several articles on male roles and single-parent adoption.

Health and Sexuality

★★★★ *Prostate Cancer Program*
       http://www.cancer.med.umich.edu/prostcan/prostcan.html

A medical site, but some of the articles are useful for background or current interpreta-tions. Start with Staging Information.

★★★ *Online Sexual Disorders Screening for Men*
       http://www.med.nyu.edu/Psych/screens/sdsm.html

A 10-item, interactive test on male sexual disorders.

Fathers and Child Support

These sites were created mainly to assert fathers' rights against the perceived over-emphasis on mothers' rights and their political and legal manifestations. The sites tend to be hostile toward mainstream legal proceedings and mental health practices.

★★★★★ *Fathers Rights to Custody: Information to Assist Fathers in Gaining Custody*
http://www.deltabravo.net/custody

Here you can read a very complete *Guide to the Parenting Evaluation Process* and dozens of articles on coping with the divorce and custody processes, as well as download many materials to help make a case for father custody. High-quality and very complete.

★★★★ *American Coalition for Fathers and Children* http://www.acfc.org

This is a large site for political action and education. The Studies and Reports include many research articles on issues such as custody, divorce, gender bias, posttraumatic stress disorder, and "parental alienation syndrome," so it can be a source of solid information. The Reading Room offers hundreds of (unfortunately unannotated) popular articles that can be thought provoking.

★★★★ *Separated Parenting Access and Resource Center* http://www.deltabravo.net

The FAQs and Articles Archive contain perhaps 100 articles of solid information to support and defend a father's position in a divorce or custody conflict.

★★★★ *Children's Justice* http://childrens-justice.org

Hostile to the current system (which is well-explained in their Facts and Myths and FAQ), the site offers a set of position papers, legislative agendas, and model child support formulas that would fix the system.

Men's Rights/Backlash

★★★★ *The Men's Defense Association* http://www.mensdefense.org

Downloadable readings of the Men's Manifesto, Father Custody, and fact sheets. Designed to counter antimale discrimination, especially in divorce.

★★★★ *National Coalition of Free Men* http://www.ncfm.org/readroom.htm
About 20 articles to read and many links.

★★ *The Fathers' Rights and Equality Exchange* http://dadsrights.org
The Legislation section is strong.

Pornography

★★★★ *Pornography Issues*
http://dir.yahoo.com/society_and_culture/sexuality/pornography_issues/

Not everyone against pornography is an archconservative or religiously motivated. Porn can be addictive, support abuse, and distort relationships. If you suspect this applies in your life, these sites are a starting place.

★★★★ *Linnea's Playboy Site* http://www.talkintrash.com/playboy

About 30 pages that offer insightful and well-articulated paragraphs about the roles of pornography in lives and development. An excellent start to giving up pornography.

NATIONAL SUPPORT GROUPS

Several of these entries are based on a list by David R. Throop (throop@vix.com) and posted to the *World Wide Web Virtual Library* as Men's Organizations.

Coalition for the Preservation of Fatherhood
PO Box 700
Milford, MA 01757
Phone: 617-723-3237
http://www.fatherhoodcoalition.org

Fathers behind Bars
525 Superior Street
Niles, MI 49120

This group publishes a book and serves as a support group for incarcerated fathers.

Fathers' Resource Center
PO Box 50052
One Main Place Station
Dallas, TX 75250-0052
Phone: 214-953-2233
E-mail: mail@fathering.org
http://www.fathers4kids.org

They publish *Father Times* and have a gopher.

Joint Custody Association
10606 Wilkins Avenue
Los Angeles, CA 90024
Phone: 310-475-5352
http://www.jointcustody.org

Male Survivors: National Organization of Male Sexual Victomization
5505 Connecticut Avenue, NW
Washington, DC 20015-2601
Phone: 800-738-4181
E-mail: male@malesurvivor.org
http://www.malesurvivor.org

They publish a newsletter for male sexual abuse survivors.

Men's Defense Association
17854 Lyons Street
Forest Lake, MN 55025-8107
Phone: 651-464-7887
E-mail: info@mensdefense.org
http://www.mensdefense.org

Book distributors, nationwide attorney referral, and newsletter publishing.

The National Center for Men
PO Box 555
Old Bethpage, NY 11804
Phone: 516-942-2020; activism/message line: 503-727-3686; office: 516-938-8329
E-mail: menscenter@aol.com

Offers nationwide phone counseling on men's issues from a male-positive perspective.

National Organization for Men
30 Vesey Street, Room 1400
New York, NY 10007
Phone: 212-766-4030
http://www.tnom.com

For men seeking equal rights divorce, custody, property, and visitation laws.

National Men's Resource Center
PO Box 800
San Anselmo, CA 94979-0800
E-mail: menstuff@menstuff.org
http://www.menstuff.org

Promise Keepers
PO Box 1003001
Denver, CO 80250-3001
Phone: 800-888-7595
http://www.promisekeepers.org

Born-again Christian men's movement.

Real Men
3701 O Street, Suite B5
Lincoln, NE 68510
Phone: 402-474-7325
E-mail: pomeroy@realmen.org
http://www.realmen.org

Strongly profeminist.

See also Child Development and Parenting (Chapter 13), Divorce (Chapter 18), and Sexuality (Chapter 30).

CHAPTER 25

Obsessive–Compulsive Disorder

An obsession is a persistent thought or image. A compulsion is a repetitive or ritualistic behavior. When frequent and severe, they form obsessive–compulsive disorder (OCD). OCD is an anxiety disorder that afflicts about 2% of the population.

In severe form, OCD presents in mainly two subdivisions of ritualistic behavior. Washers, the largest group, are people who feel contaminated when exposed to certain stimuli, such as dirt, sex, and bodily secretions. In turn, they avoid the contaminants at all costs or engage in the compulsive behavior of excessive cleaning. Checkers are people who repetitively check, count, or perform stereotyped actions to avoid a future "disaster."

About 10–15% of the population suffers from some OCD features. Some of these people suffer from obsessive–compulsive personality, in which they are preoccupied with orderliness, perfectionism, and control. Some are consumed with ruminations, a word whose first meaning is "chewing the cud." Ruminant animals, such as cattle and goats, chew a cud composed of regurgitated, partially digested food—not a very appealing image of what people who ruminate do with their thoughts, but an exceedingly apt one.

Fortunately, in recent years, we have seen considerable advances in our understanding of OCD and the development of highly effective treatments for it. The most popular treatments are behavioral (or cognitive-behavioral) therapies and medications, typically the antidepressant and antianxiety medications.

In this chapter, we review expert opinions on the value of dozens of self-help books, autobiographies, films, and Internet sites on OCD. But first, our Recommendation Highlights.

RECOMMENDATION HIGHLIGHTS

Self-Help Books

- For top-notch, cognitive-behavioral programs for treating OCD:

  ★★★★★ *S.T.O.P. Obsessing* by Edna B. Foa and Reid Wilson

  ★★★★ *Overcoming Obsessive–Compulsive Disorder* by Gail Steketee

- For balanced and comprehensive approaches to OCD:

  ★★★★ *Obsessive–Compulsive Disorders* by Steven Levenkron

  ◆ *Obsessive–Compulsive Disorders* by Fred Penzel

Autobiographies

- For a humorous and acerbic recounting of OCD and phobias:

  ★★★ *Memoirs of an Amnesiac* by Oscar Levant

Films

- For a humorous film on OCD and its interpersonal impact:

  ★★★★ *As Good As It Gets*

Internet Resources

- For excellent overviews and introductions to OCD:

  ★★★★★ *Again and Again: Obsessive–Compulsive Disorder Web Sites*
  http://www.geonius.com/ocd

  ★★★★ *About OCD* http://www.ocfoundation.org

- For expert consensus on treatments:

  ★★★★★ *Expert Consensus Treatment Guidelines for OCD*
  http://www.psychguides.com/oche.html

SELF-HELP BOOKS

Strongly Recommended

★★★★★ *S.T.O.P. Obsessing: How to Overcome Your Obsessions and Compulsions* (1991) by Edna B. Foa and Reid Wilson. New York: Bantam.

Two authorities on the treatment of anxiety disorders present a cognitive-behavioral approach. The book begins with a questionnaire to understand and analyze the severity of obsessions and compulsions. Included is a self-help program to overcome the milder symptoms and a more intensive three-week program for severe symptoms. Guidelines to help determine whether a person needs professional help are presented with clarity and practicability. Our mental health experts consistently agree that this book is very useful for people suffering from obsessions and compulsions.

★★★★ *Overcoming Obsessive–Compulsive Disorder: A Behavioral and Cognitive Protocol for the Treatment of OCD* (1999) by Gail Steketee. Oakland, CA: New Harbinger.

Prolific researcher Steketee offers a step-by-step, session-by-session treatment plan for OCD. The book includes worksheets, homework assignments, in-session exercises, and didactic material. As the subtitle states, it is a research-based, cognitive-behavioral treatment that relies heavily on exposure and cognitive therapy. Steketee also provides a relapse prevention program to maintain treatment gains. An appendix features a number of individual and family symptom inventories. This book and *S.T.O.P. Obsessing* (reviewed above) are the cream of the self-help crop according to the mental health experts in our national studies.

★★★★ *Obsessive–Compulsive Disorders* (1992) by Steven Levenkron. New York: Warner Books.

Levenkron believes OCD is the personality's attempt to reduce anxiety, which may stem from a painful childhood or a genetic tendency toward anxiousness. Levenkron believes that people can reduce their obsessions and compulsions if they follow four basic steps: (1) rely on a family member or a therapist for support and comfort, (2) unmask their rituals, (3) talk in depth to trusted family members or a therapist, and (4) control their anxiety. A useful, balanced self-help book.

Recommended

★★★ *Brain Lock* (1996) by Jeffrey M. Schwartz and Beverly Beyette. New York: Regan.

The authors present a four-step method to defeat irrational impulses by a process of relabeling, reattributing, refocusing, and reevaluating. The same treatment methods can be applied to overeating, substance abuse, pathological gambling, and compulsive sexual behavior. Each chapter features a nice summary of key points, and the book provides a useful OCD Patient Diary. Had the book been rated by more reviewers in our national studies, it would probably have earned a four-star evaluation.

Diamonds in the Rough

♦ *Obsessive–Compulsive Disorder: The Facts* (2nd ed., 1998) by Padmal de Silva and Stanley Rachman. New York: Oxford University Press.

A sensible and straightforward book both for individuals suffering from OCD and their family members. Written by two clinical psychologists known for their work in anxiety disorders, the book comprehensively covers the causes, symptoms, diagnosis, and treatment of OCD. In this second edition, the authors also cover compulsive hoarding and obsessive–compulsive behavior in children. This valuable self-help resource is classified as a Diamond in the Rough because it was favorably but infrequently rated in our studies.

♦ *Obsessive–Compulsive Disorders: A Complete Guide to Getting Well and Staying Well* (2000) by Fred Penzel. New York: Oxford University Press.

This book has been described as "near-encyclopedic" for the sufferers of obsessive–compulsive spectrum disorders. Penzel addresses the broad spectrum of these disorders, from obsessive–compulsive to body dysmorphic disorder to trichotillomania (compulsive hair pulling). He details the cognitive-behavioral treatments, the leading medications, and the family advice. An effective self-help resource for professionals and laypersons, this book was highly rated but not frequently by our mental health experts, thus receiving the designation of Diamond in the Rough.

AUTOBIOGRAPHIES

Recommended

★★★　*Memoirs of an Amnesiac* (1990) by Oscar Levant. Hollywood, CA: Samuel French Trade Books.

A famed pianist recounts a life with many mental and physical disorders. In a humorous and acerbic style, Levant describes his OCD, phobias, and addiction to barbiturates. Chapter titles include "Total Recoil," "My Bed of Nails," and "Stand Up and Faint." Levant was treated with an enormous number of different drugs and underwent psychotherapy, several hospitalizations, and electroconvulsive therapy. Levant was a better pianist and writer than he was a client, because he lacked the motivation to get well. Hopefully, writing the book had cathartic value. Also reviewed in Chapter 7, Anxiety Disorders.

FILMS

Strongly Recommended

★★★★　*As Good As It Gets* (1997) directed by James L. Brooks. PG-13 rating. 138 minutes.

Jack Nicholson's portrayal of a nasty, selfish bigot with a mix of anxiety symptoms (compulsions and phobias) won him an Oscar because of the humanizing experiences with his neighbor and the only waitress he can trust. Probably useful to show that even a person crippled by symptoms can find the courage to reach out and improve (if not cure) his relationships, especially with the help of caring others (Helen Hunt, who won a Oscar as the waitress; an ugly dog; and Jack's suffering neighbor).

INTERNET RESOURCES

Metasites

★★★★★　*Again and Again: Obsessive–Compulsive Disorder Web Sites*
　　　　http://www.geonius.com/ocd

This site is absolutely comprehensive, from diagnostic criteria and treatment guidelines, thorough materials, links to bulletin boards, humor, music, religion and scrupulosity.

Psychoeducational Materials for Clients and Families

★★★★★　*Expert Consensus Treatment Guidelines for Obsessive–Compulsive Disorder: A Guide for Patients and Families* http://www.psychguides.com/oche.html

Based on *The Expert Consensus Guideline Series: Treatment of Obsessive–Compulsive Disorder* by John S. March, MD, Allen Frances, MD, Daniel Carpenter, PhD, and David A. Kahn,

MD (available at http://www.psychguides.com/ocgl.html), this site tells almost everything about treatment in 16 pages. It leans heavily on behavior therapy and medications.

★★★★ *National Institute of Mental Health's Library*
http://www.nimh.nih.gov/anxiety/anxietymenu.cfm

NIMH offers six booklets on anxiety disorders and their treatment. They can be read online or ordered (call 1-888-8-ANXIETY). Authoritative and very well done.

★★★★ *Obsessive–Compulsive Disorder (OCD)*
http://lexington-on-line.com/naf.ocd.2.html

A good but brief (five-page) explanation.

★★★★ *About OCD* http://www.ocfoundation.org (top of left side of page)

Here are brochures offering a very good quality and appropriately full presentation of the nature of OCD and its treatment (cognitive-behavior therapy and medications for adults and children) and a screening test. Overall, somewhat heavier on pills, but each article has solid information in about 10–12 pages.

★★★★ *Obsessive–Compulsive Disorder* http://www.mayoclinic.com

Search for "obsessive-complusive disorder" and select the March 27, 2003, article. About 10 pages from the Mayo Clinic with solid information.

★★★ *Guidelines for Families Coping with OCD* Adapted from *Over and Over Again* by Nesiroglu and Yaryura-Tobias http://www.ocdhope.com/gdlines.htm

A very good list for families.

★★★ *Out Damn Spot: The Nature and Treatment of Contamination Fears* by Dean McKay, PhD http://www.ocdonline.com/articlesmckay.htm

A 10-page presentation on the contamination anxiety of OCD.

★★★ *Obsessive–Compulsive Personality Disorder: A Defect of Philosophy, not Anxiety* by Steven Phillipson, PhD http://www.ocdonline.com/articlephillipson6.htm

A 14-page discussion of OC personality disorder in a folksy style by a cognitive-behavioral therapist with his own point of view.

NATIONAL SUPPORT GROUPS

Anxiety Disorders Association of America (ADAA)
8730 Georgia Avenue, Suite 100
Silver Spring, MD 20910
Phone: 240-485-1001
http://www.adaa.org

Their bookstore is excellent for its prices and the wide range of books.

Obsessive–Compulsive Foundation
337 Notch Hill Road
North Branford, CT 06471
Phone: 203-315-2190
E-mail: info@ocfoundation.org
http://www.ocfoundation.org

Their Internet site is very broad, with research, book reviews, chat, newsletters, and conferences.

Obsessive–Compulsive Anonymous
PO Box 215
New Hyde Park, NY 11040
Phone: 516-739-0662
http://hometown.aol.com/west24th

Twelve-step, self-help group for people with OCD.

Shoplifters Anonymous
PO Box 55
New York, NY 10276
E-mail: tobbit@juno.com

Twelve-step group for individuals who wish to stop their compulsive stealing.

Trichotillomania Learning Center
303 Potrero #51
Santa Cruz, CA 95060
Phone: 831-457-1004
E-mail: info@trich.org
http://www.trich.org

Information and support for the families of and those afflicted with trichotillomania (compulsive hair pulling).

See also Anxiety Disorders (Chapter 7) and Stress Management and Relaxation (Chapter 32).

CHAPTER 26

Posttraumatic Stress Disorder

Posttraumatic stress disorder, or PTSD, is a complex and serious anxiety condition that affects approximately 2–5% of the American population. As the name suggests, PTSD follows exposure to a traumatic stressor involving actual or threatened death or serious injury, witnessing an event that involves death or injury, or learning about such a trauma experienced by a family member or friend. Typical traumatic stressors are military combat, sexual assault, abduction, terrorist attack, incarceration, natural disasters, and severe accidents.

PTSD symptoms include reexperiencing the traumatic event, avoidance of situations associated with the trauma, and increased arousal. The traumatic event can be reexperienced in various ways, such as recurrent nightmares or flashbacks. Triggering events, such as anniversaries of the trauma, can lead to intense psychological distress or physical symptoms. The PTSD victim may make deliberate efforts to avoid thinking or talking about the event and will avoid activities, situations, or people who provoke recollections of it.

In this chapter, we feature professionals' ratings on self-help books, autobiographies, films, and Internet resources regarding PTSD. The self-help resources cover the assessment and treatment of PTSD, the core experiences of trauma survivors, survival guilt, and PTSD as a result of rape, childhood abuse, and physical attacks. We conclude the chapter with a listing of self-help and support groups.

SELF-HELP BOOKS

Strongly Recommended

★★★★★ *Trauma and Recovery* (1997) by Judith Lewis Herman. New York: Basic Books.

Truth telling and secrecy are the "twin imperatives" that define psychological trauma and form the basis of the recovery model described in this book. Herman thoughtfully

RECOMMENDATION HIGHLIGHTS

Self-Help Books

- For survivors of trauma:

  ★★★★★   *Trauma and Recovery* by Judith Lewis Herman

  ★★★★   *I Can't Get Over It* by Aphrodite Matsakis

  ★★★   *Life after Trauma* by Dena Rosenbloom and Mary Beth Williams

  ★★★   *The PTSD Workbook* by Mary Beth Williams and Soili Poijula

- For rape victims:

  ★★★   *Reclaiming Your Life after Rape* by Barbara Olasov Rothbaum and Edna B. Foa

Autobiographies

- For recovering from rape:

  ♦   *Telling: A Memoir of Rape and Recovery* by Patricia Weaver Francisco

Films

- On rape's torment and the judicial system's insensitivity:

  ★★★★   *The Accused*

- On war-related PTSD:

  ★★★   *Born on the Fourth of July*

  ★★★   *Full Metal Jacket*

  ★★★   *The Deer Hunter*

- On recovery from PTSD:

  ★★★   *Fearless*

Internet Resources

- For comprehensive information on traumatic experiences:

  ★★★★★   *David Baldwin's Trauma Information Pages*
  http://www.trauma-pages.com

  ★★★★   *National Center for PTSD*   http://www.ncptsd.org/index.html

  ★★★★   *Psychology in Daily Life: Traumatic Stress*
  http://helping.apa.org/daily/traumaticstress.html

- For more specific traumas:

  ★★★★★   *Sexual Abuse*
  http://incestabuse.miningco.com

  ★★★★   *Terrorism Fear*   http://www.lexington-on-line.com/naf.html

describes the dialectic of the comfort of denial and the indomitable need to speak. Fundamental commonalties are identified between those who survive domestic and sexual violence (the traditional sphere of trauma for women) and those who survive war and political imprisonment (the traditional sphere of trauma for men). The stages of recovery—establishing safety; reconstructing the trauma story; reuniting survivors with their communities, significant others, and with themselves—are described and set the stage for a conceptual framework for psychotherapy and more accurate diagnoses. The core experiences of trauma, disempowerment, and disconnection are key therapeutic components of the recovery model and are treated as healing properties in the survivors' re-entry. An excellent resource, though quite academic for a self-help book.

★★★★ *I Can't Get Over It: A Handbook for Trauma Survivors* (1996) by Aphrodite Matsakis. Oakland, CA: New Harbinger.

The author presents a full range of assessment and treatment options for PTSD. Her initial focus is to explain the diagnostic criteria, biochemical variables, feelings and thoughts of the trauma, concepts of victimization, and chart the triggers that evoke memory of the trauma. The healing process is framed as a growth rather than deficit model. Two special features of the book are customizing the growth model to specific types of trauma (e.g., crime, suicide, combat, domestic violence) and using the exercises and questionnaires sprinkled throughout. The author effectively explains the model through stages and then offers practical suggestions. Even though *I Can't Get Over It* was not written as a workbook, the exercises and questionnaires give it an action-oriented, problem-solving perspective.

Recommended

★★★ *Reclaiming Your Life after Rape* (1999) by Barbara Olasov Rothbaum and Edna B. Foa. Albany, NY: Graywind. (Also distributed by the Psychological Corporation.)

PTSD specifically manifested in rape assaults is the focus of this cognitive-behavioral workbook that lends itself both to self-help and therapy use. The book begins with a diagnostic explanation of PTSD, followed by an individualized assessment. Although the treatment options later in the workbook are solely cognitive-behavioral, a section is devoted to describing various therapeutic models. The second half of the workbook describes, in understandable detail, cognitive-behavioral treatments, including systematic desensitization, anxiety management, imaginal and *in vivo* exposure, and cognitive restructuring. A chapter on "other techniques" describes role playing, thought stopping, assertiveness, and self-talk. Complex principles of cognitive-behavioral treatment are effectively presented and accompanied by worksheets, assessment forms, and other application tools. This book is based on years of outcome research conducted by psychologist Foa and colleagues and is one of the highest rated self-help resources in our national studies. Only the comparatively low number of ratings kept it from achieving five-star status. Rothbaum and Foa have also coauthored a book for practitioners treating PTSD entitled *Treating the Trauma of Rape: Cognitive-Behavioral Therapy for PTSD.*

★★★   *The PTSD Workbook* (2002) by Mary Beth Williams and Soili Poijula. Oakland, CA: New Harbinger.

This is one of the few books written after September 11, 2001. Although it does not focus on that tragedy, the trauma and the aftermath are exemplified in the authors' approach to trauma. The book begins by helping readers understand the impact of PTSD on their lives, followed by descriptions of many creative exercises (e.g., drawing, journaling, identifying strengths), questions to be answered, and healing activities. Williams and Poijula explore reexperiencing trauma (e.g., dealing with flashbacks, nightmares, triggers of trauma), physical aspects, and associated symptoms (e.g., survivor guilt, shame, loss), with resulting recommendations for healing. A final section is devoted to complex PTSD and different means of coping with this chronic variation of trauma impact. The message of this book comes across powerfully in its workbook format and valuable content.

★★★   *Life after Trauma: A Workbook for Healing* (1999) by Dena Rosenbloom and Mary Beth Williams with Barbara E. Watkins. New York: Guilford Press.

The need for safety, trust, control, value, and connectedness are the basic human needs called into question as a result of a trauma. The book is designed to help individuals live their lives since the trauma (not relive the trauma) by assessing the status of each of their basic needs and working through ways to reevaluate and change those needs that have suffered as a result of the trauma. Each basic need is evaluated, and individualized means for change are designed. Specific attention is paid to the importance of self-care and coping with triggers of the past trauma. Strengths of the book are its workbook format and its flexibility as either a self-help or adjunct to therapy (with a letter to the therapist in an appendix).

Diamonds in the Rough

♦   *Rebuilding Shattered Lives* (1998) by James A. Chu. New York: Wiley.

The focus of this book is on severely traumatized individuals and the importance of implementing a balanced treatment plan. The first section describes the rediscovery of abuse after years of societal denial and the effect on survivors' psychological functioning. Chu presents a stage model of treatment and recovery: Early stage treatment is centered on relational aspects, symptom control, coping skills, and self care; the second stage of treatment emphasizes abreaction and catharsis; and the late stage concerns consolidation of gains and increased skills. The treatment model for complex PTSD is clearly articulated. Setting boundaries, managing countertransference, and confronting empathically are presented as key elements in the treatment plan. Case vignettes are presented in an informative way for mental health professionals, but the average layperson will find the book difficult as a self-help resource.

♦   *Survivor Guilt: A Self-Help Guide* (1999) by Aphrodite Matsakis. Oakland, CA: New Harbinger.

Guilt, in this book, is defined as a negative feeling created by the belief that one should have thought, felt, or acted differently. Survivor guilt is explained in terms of common causes, types of guilt, and its devastating effects. Existential survivor guilt (guilt for continuing to live) is differentiated from content survivor guilt (guilt for acts committed to stay alive). Matsakis reviews the psychological consequences for the survivor, including eating disorders, depression, anger, suicidal feelings, and substance abuse. Part Two of the book focuses on healing and the critical aspects of the process. Each chapter includes self-assessment guides that facilitate evaluation of the chapter topic. This book is intended for survivors and mental health professionals who work with them. It was favorably but infrequently rated in our national studies, leading to the Diamond in the Rough status.

AUTOBIOGRAPHIES

Diamonds in the Rough

♦ *Telling: A Memoir of Rape and Recovery* (1999) by Patricia Weaver Francisco. New York: HarperCollins.

In 1981, while her husband was away, an intruder broke into Francisco's home and raped her. She went into counseling but was unable to relieve her pain. Eventually, her marriage broke up, which she attributes to the rape. She carried the story inside her for more than 15 years before writing this frank memoir. She describes the horror of the assault and its aftermath. Francisco attended rape and domestic violence trials to collect additional material for the book. This well-researched and moving account was brand new at the time of one of our studies and thus not yet widely known, leading to a Diamond in the Rough designation.

♦ *The Bear's Embrace: A True Story of Survival* (2001) by Patricia Van Tighem. New York: Pantheon.

An unusual and devastating event leaves deep scars. It took the author many years to confront her demons and provide this frank portrayal of being attacked by a bear while hiking in the Canadian Rockies. The author, who had been a nurse, describes her pain, disfigurement, multiple surgeries, marital difficulties, and depression. Writing the book became a survival strategy and a step along the road to healing. A scary book in the sense that this type of random assault can happen to anyone, but uplifting in its description of life slowly returning after trauma, with new insights and wisdom. Recently published and not yet included in our national studies.

♦ *Miles to Go Before I Sleep: A Survivor's Story of a Terrorist Hijacking* (2001) by Jackie Nink Pflug. Center City, MN: Hazelden Foundation.

Accompanying her students to a basketball tournament, special education teacher Jackie Pflug's flight was hijacked. While negotiations proceeded on the ground, she was chosen for execution by the hijackers, shot in the head, and thrown out of the plane onto the tarmac. Fifty-eight passengers died as a result of the hijacking and the harrowing rescue attempt. Jackie Pflug suffered substantial brain injury but survived, and she provides this inspiring account of her continuing struggle to retrieve the skills she lost. The book provides valuable insights about courage, PTSD, and the slow, painful process of recovering lost abilities. The author became the special education client she was originally trained to teach. This autobiography was released the year before our latest study was conducted and was not yet widely known.

FILMS

Strongly Recommended

★★★★   *The Accused* (1988) directed by Jonathan Kaplan. R rating. 110 minutes.

Rape victims are often seen as complicit in their rape, particularly by the traditional, male-dominated judicial system, and especially when they act provocatively and are intoxicated. Jodie Foster is brutally, repeatedly raped in a bar in front of cheering men. She escapes and seeks legal help. Kelly McGillis, her public prosecutor, is unsympathetic to a woman so different and, at first, betrays Foster by accepting a reduced charge. Through their continuing relationship, the movie makes the point that no matter how a woman acts, she still has the right to say "no" and be heard. The film also convincingly shows the torment of trauma and the potential retraumatization associated with an insensitive judicial system.

Recommended

★★★   *Born on the Fourth of July* (1990) directed by Oliver Stone. R rating. 145 minutes.

This is the true story of a patriotic and excitement-seeking, small-town boy who volunteers to fight in Vietnam only to return wheelchair bound. Abandoned and condemned by his fellow citizens, he falls into drug use and PTSD but eventually finds himself by understanding the larger political picture and participating in antiwar activism. The movie might be used to show the possibility of redemption and making the best of a terrible situation by facing reality and seeing the truth beyond the culturally supported images.

★★★   *The Fisher King* (1991) directed by Terry Gilliam. R rating. 137 minutes.

Jeff Bridges portrays a radio talk-show host whose listener goes on a shooting spree. He quits his job and descends into a drinking binge, where he is rescued by a homeless man (Robin Williams) searching for the Holy Grail. Williams's character was traumatized by witnessing the death of his wife. Although an interesting and occasionally funny film, *The Fisher King* is not quite convincing or accurate about PTSD. (Also reviewed in Chapter 28, Schizophrenia.)

★★★   *Fearless* (1994) directed by Peter Weir. R rating. 122 minutes.

An ordinary man survives a plane crash that kills many people. He realizes that his assumptions about how life works and should be lived can be questioned. He begins to feel invulnerable but is laid low by a tiny accident. His wife offers loving support for his withdrawal and confusions, but only a fellow survivor can offer understanding. Their relationship avoids the sexual, and the movie shows how each grows. His PTSD and anxiety symptoms are shown and treated in group therapy. The film richly illustrates the psychic consequences of traumatic experiences and the ways we can overcome them with the help of our friends.

★★★ *The Client* (1994) directed by Joel Schumacher. PG-13 rating. 117 minutes.

Street-smart, 11-year-old Brad Renfro watches a suicide and gains information that puts his life in danger from the gangsters and politicians of a Southern Gothic town. He seeks out a lawyer, Susan Sarandon, and they bond and grow with each other. The film not only presents the boy's traumatization but also shows the healing power of relationships.

★★★ *The Deer Hunter* (1978) directed by Michael Cimino. R rating. 182 minutes.

Three working-class guys from a small town go to war and are greatly and differently affected by the experience. We witness the most graphic atrocities as they change. One is scarred but matures and can no longer kill even the deer he used to hunt. The other two are damaged, one physically and the other mentally. The film illustrates the way a person can endure PTSD and develop, even in the most hostile of environments, into a better human being. Winner of five Academy Awards.

★★★ *Full Metal Jacket* (1988) directed by Stanley Kubrick. R rating. 118 minutes.

The film moves from the induction into the military of naive recruits, though hellish training to toughen them, and into the war in Vietnam—the battles, killing, prostitution, drugs, and alcohol. It is a haunting film that demonstrates the genesis of PTSD, but not much else of clinical utility. Vivid scenes of the horrors of war and warriors mark a realistic, apolitical, and complex film.

Not Recommended

★★ *Beloved* (1998) directed by Jonathan Demme. R rating. 175 minutes.

★★ *The Legend of Bagger Vance* (2000) directed by Robert Redford. PG-13 rating. 127 minutes.

★ *Angel Eyes* (2001) directed by Luis Mandoki. R rating. 104 minutes.

INTERNET RESOURCES

Metasites

★★★★★ *David Baldwin's Trauma Information Pages*
         http://www.trauma-pages.com

This is the premier trauma resource on the Internet, with articles, resources, support, and books. Not specific for PTSD, it covers all kinds of traumatic experiences and reactions, so you may have to do some digging.

Psychoeducational Materials for Clients and Families

★★★★★ *Sexual Abuse: Guide Picks*
    http://incestabuse.miningco.com

A rich and edited resource for information and support about sexual abuse and its survivors. Especially of value are the less common resources on mother–daughter incest and male–male abuse.

★★★★★ *Caregiver Series* http://207.235.43.156/ctamaterials/caregivers.asp

Dozens of sophisticated articles on traumatized children for parents and caregivers.

★★★★ *Articles on Trauma and PTSD* http://www.sidran.org/trauma.html

This site provides numerous online resources for survivors, families, and helping professionals. A highly recommended resource.

★★★★ *National Center for PTSD* http://www.ncptsd.org/index.html

A great site, with everything from handouts to bibliographies, FAQs, and research. It covers disasters, terrorism, dissociation, and the like.

★★★★ *ISTSS Public Education Pamphlets*
    http://www.istss.org/publications/pamphlets.htm

Downloadable pamphlets on trauma-related issues. In addition, under the menu "Publications" (on the left), select "Childhood Trauma" to view Remembering *Childhood Trauma: Fact and Fiction–for Consumers.*

★★★★ *Psychology in Daily Life: Traumatic Stress*
    http://helping.apa.org/daily/traumaticstress.html

This APA site offers seven brief but packed pamphlets: *Managing Traumatic Stress; Coping with Terrorism; Handling Anxiety in the Face of the Anthrax Scare; Reactions and Guidelines for Children Following Trauma/Disaster; Resources on Coping with Traumatic Events;* and *Coping with the Aftermath of a Disaster.* They are ideal for public educational presentations.

★★★★ *PTSD Alliance* http://www.ptsdalliance.org/home2.html

A collaboration of four organizations concerned with trauma's effects, this site offers a dozens of short, informative materials for family, therapists, and the media.

★★★★ *Terrorism Fear: What You Can Do to Alleviate It* by Stephen Cox, MD
    http://www.lexington-on-line.com/naf.html

About 10 pages on specific irrational fears and their counters, when to seek professional help, many tips on coping better, and so on.

★★★ *Institute of Rural Health* http://www.isu.edu./irh/crisis.htm

This is a set of links to resources for coping with the consequences of September 11, 2001. The first nine are for citizens and clients; the latter nine for helpers.

★★★ *Common Responses to Trauma* http://www.trauma-pages.com/t-facts.htm

Dr. Patti Levin's two-page listing of symptoms and ways to cope. A friendly presentation.

★★★ *The National Center for PTSD: Research and Education on PTSD*
   http://www.ncptsd.org/index.html

Although oriented to military veterans, this site contains many readings of value for families and survivors. There are also assessment instruments, fact sheets, and the world's largest index of trauma literature.

★★★ *The Sidran Institute* http://www.sidran.org

The site focuses on traumatic memories and dissociation. Sidran is a publisher, and its annotated catalog is here. There are also about 20 valuable articles.

★★★ *Traumatic Stress and Secondary Traumatic Stress*
   http://www.isu.edu/~bhstamm/ts.htm

The site of Dr. Beth Hudnall Stamm, a major worker in this area. Her materials on traumatic stress and secondary or vicarious traumatization of helpers (family and professionals) are thorough, and the links are invaluable.

NATIONAL SUPPORT GROUPS

We have been unable to identify any national support groups specifically for PTSD. Similarly, the authors of the impressive *Self-Help Sourcebook* (White & Madara, 1995, p. 167) write, "Regrettably, we are unaware of any model or national self-help support groups that have yet been formed" for PTSD and accident victims. As a result, the following list is largely composed of educational and professional groups as opposed to self-help groups per se.

Anxiety Disorders Association of America (ADAA)
8730 Georgia Avenue, Suite 100
Silver Spring, MD 20910
Phone: 240-485-1001
http://www.adaa.org

   Dedicated to promoting the prevention and cure of anxiety disorders; their bookstore is excellent for its prices and the wide range of books.

International Society for Traumatic Stress Studies (ISTSS)
60 Revere Drive, Suite 500
Northbrook, IL 60062
Phone: 847-480-9028
http://www.istss.org

   More of a professional organization than a self-help association, but a valuable source of reliable information.

Emotions Anonymous
PO Box 4245
St. Paul, MN 55104-0245
Phone: 651-647-9712
E-mail: eaisc@mtn.org
http://www.emotionsanonymous.org

National Organization for Victim Assistance (NOVA)
1730 Park Road NW
Washington, DC 20010
Phone: 202-232-6682
E-mail: nova@trynova.org
http://www.trynova.org

Support for victims of violent crimes and disaster.

PTSD Support Services
PO Box 5574
Woodland Park, CO 80866
Phone: 719-687-4582
http://ptsdsupport.net

See also Abuse (Chapter 2) and Anxiety Disorders (Chapter 7).

CHAPTER 27

Pregnancy

Although Sara and Jim did not plan to have a baby right away, they did not take any precautions to prevent it, and it was not long before Sara was pregnant. They found a nurse–midwife they liked and invented a pet name—Bibinello—for the fetus. They signed up for birth preparation classes, and each Friday night for eight weeks faithfully practiced for contractions. They moved into a larger apartment so that the baby could have its own room and spent weekends browsing through garage sales and secondhand stores to find good prices on baby furniture—a crib, a high chair, a stroller, a changing table, a crib mobile, a swing, a car seat.

Jim and Sara also spent a lot of time talking about what kind of parents they wanted to be, what their child might be like, and what changes the baby would make in their lives. One of their concerns was that Sara's maternity leave would last only six weeks. If she wanted to stay home longer, she would have to quit her job, something she and Jim were not sure they could afford.

These are among the many scripts and questions expectant couples have about pregnancy. And there have been many resources created to help expectant parents like Sara and Jim better understand pregnancy and make more informed decisions about their offspring's health and well-being, as well as their own. We review, in this chapter, the most useful self-help books, films, and Internet resources for doing so.

SELF-HELP BOOKS

Strongly Recommended

★★★★★ *What to Expect When You're Expecting* (3rd ed., 2002) by Arlene Eisenberg, Heidi Eisenberg Murkoff, and Sandee E. Hathaway. New York: Workman.

This third edition of the best-selling "pregnancy bible" reflects advances in obstetrical practice but just as importantly incorporates new or expanded areas suggested by the

RECOMMENDATION HIGHLIGHTS

Self-Help Books

- On a month-by-month, step-by-step map of pregnancy:

  ★★★★★ *What to Expect When You're Expecting* by Arlene Eisenberg et al.

- On pregnancy in general:

  ★★★★★ *The Complete Book of Pregnancy and Childbirth* by Sheila Kitzinger

  ◆ *The Girlfriends' Guide to Pregnancy* by Vicki Iovine

- On becoming a father:

  ◆ *The Expectant Father* by Armin A. Brott and Jennifer Ash

Films

- On enduring pregnancy with the support of friends:

  ★★★ *Where the Heart Is*

- On making a life-threatening decision to maintain pregnancy:

  ★★★ *Steel Magnolias*

Internet Resources

- On pregnancy:

  ★★★★★ *Sabrina's Pregnancy Page*
  http://www.fensende.com/Users/swnymph/

  ★★★★★ *Childbirth.org* http://www.childbirth.org

- On infertility:

  ★★★★★ *Infertility FAQ* http://www.fertilityplus.org/faq/infertility.htm

  ★★★★ *Infertility* http://infertility.miningco.com

- On adoption:

  ★★★★ *Adoption.com* http://www.adoption.com

readers: alternative birthing, second pregnancies, postpartum depression, more on common pregnancy symptoms, and advice on traveling while pregnant. This is a month-by-month, step-by-step guide to pregnancy and childbirth. The authors are a mother–daughters team, and their book was the result of the unnecessarily worry-filled pregnancy of the second author (Heidi Murkoff). The book tries to put expectant parents' normal fears into perspective by giving them comprehensive information and helping them enjoy this transition in their lives. *What to Expect When You're Expecting* is an excellent self-help book for expectant parents. It is reassuring and thorough. The authors do an outstanding job of walking expectant parents through the nine months of pregnancy and childbirth.

★★★★★   *The Complete Book of Pregnancy and Childbirth* (1996) by Sheila Kitzinger. New York: Knopf.

This comprehensive guide to pregnancy and childbirth emphasizes an active and informed stance to giving birth. The expectant mother prepares for an active role in childbirth by learning about the changes that are occurring in her body, pregnancy and childbirth options, and who does what to her and why. Expectant parents learn about the early weeks of pregnancy, and the emotional and physical changes they are likely to experience at this time. Kitzinger educates expectant mothers about prenatal care and medical charts. She describes common worries of expectant mothers, lovemaking during pregnancy, and the father's role. The author recommends relaxation and breathing exercises, and provides advice about medical checkups. She covers what happens during the stages of labor, support during labor, coping with pain, the option of gentle birth, and what to expect in the first few hours and days after birth. The book has numerous charts, drawings, and photographs. Its enthusiasts especially liked Kitzinger's holistic approach to pregnancy and her emphasis on women's choices.

Recommended

★★★   *What to Eat When You're Expecting* (1986) by Arlene Eisenberg, Heidi Murkoff, and Sandee Hathaway. New York: Workman.

The book, written by the authors of *What to Expect When You're Expecting* (reviewed above), is based on 20 years of practical application in the Eisenberg family. They present the "best odds" diet, which they believe increases the probability of having a healthy baby by controlling the factors that can be influenced and minimizing the risk factors that cannot be controlled. The book describes the mother's nutritional needs during pregnancy and how they affect the baby. Daily recommended portions are given. The expectant mother learns how to assess her current eating habits and how to alter them if they are not good. Almost 100 pages of recipes and a lengthy appendix of nutritional charts are also included. The book is well-written, easy to read, and the nutritional plan for expectant mothers is sound, albeit perhaps slightly dated.

★★★   *Pregnancy after 35* (1976, reissued 1984) by Carole McCauley. New York: Pocket Books.

The older mother faces unique medical and emotional problems during pregnancy. This book is based on medical journal articles and interviews with physicians, psychologists, midwives, and older couples to address the special concerns of pregnancy in older women. Women over 35 learn about genetic counseling, risk factors, and psychological issues that arise throughout pregnancy. The book, published in 1976, is dated, especially in terms of nutritional advice. And, of course, it does not cover a number of tests that have been developed in recent years to assess the likelihood of having a healthy baby.

★★★   *The Well Pregnancy Book* (revised ed., 1996) by Mike Samuels and Nancy Samuels. New York: Summit.

This guide to pregnancy and childbirth emphasizes a holistic approach. It provides an overview of childbirth practices in different cultures and serves as an expectant parents' guide to pregnancy, childbirth, and the postpartum period. It covers nutrition and fitness, physical changes in the expectant mother and the offspring, and the medical aspects of hormonal and bodily changes in pregnant women. This book is better used in cases of uncomplicated pregnancies rather than high-risk ones. Critics also said that the book is too simplistic and poorly organized.

★★★   *From Here to Maternity* (1986) by Connie Marshall. Citrus Heights, CA: Conmar.

This self-help book is a general guide to pregnancy that emphasizes childbirth preparation and selection of a health care team. Its purpose is to improve the expectant couple's ability to communicate knowledgeably with their health care team. The book's three parts deal with (1) emotions during pregnancy, the expectant mother's body and prenatal growth, drug use, and choosing breast or bottle feeding; (2) selecting a doctor; and (3) labor and delivery. *From Here to Maternity* received a three-star rating, but some critics complained that the book is superficial and poorly illustrated.

Diamonds in the Rough

◆   *The Girlfriends' Guide to Pregnancy* (1995) by Vicki Iovine. New York: Pocket Books.

Pregnancy books are so "detached, calm, neat, and moderate" that the author would never ask a physician about the indelicate matters that her girlfriends discuss freely. Ninety percent of the good information she received came from girlfriends, not the experts. This is the backdrop for the hilarious *Girlfriends' Guide* that does, in fact, discuss every phase of pregnancy. Some topics are circumspect responses to serious concerns, such as being scared, fearing miscarriage, or worrying that something might be wrong with the baby. Other topics are funny responses to lighthearted thoughts, such as the likelihood of stretch marks, fear of turning into the husband's mother, and baby arrival anxiety (e.g., "What if the baby doesn't like me?"). The conversational style of the book is like lunch with a candid best friend. Much factual information is offered here, myths are dispelled, rumors are confirmed or denied, and lies about pregnancy are revealed. This book takes a funny, bold, and also knowledgeable view of pregnancy. In our earlier edition, this book was a Diamond in the Rough and for the same reasons it remains one: It was not rated frequently enough in our studies, but those who did read it rated it very highly.

◆   *The New Father's Panic Book* (1997) by Gene B. Williams. New York: Avon.

This self-help book is intended to eliminate panic and give expectant fathers a sense of belonging and an essential role in the birth and parenting process. The author points out that even today, in childbirth classes, specific instructions are still avoided and fathers are told, "Just be available and supportive." This book provides fathers with information important to decision making and to the father's sense of participation; topics include tests for pregnancy and for ruling out problems, group versus solo medical doctors, choosing a hospital or an alternative, stages of fetal development, the expectant mother's physical and emotional changes, and baby's first weeks. *The New Father's Panic Book* merits being a Diamond in the Rough for its recent publication date and its approach to the role of the expectant father.

♦ *This Isn't What I Expected: Recognizing and Recovering from Depression and Anxiety after Childbirth* (1994) by Karen R. Kleiman and Valerie D. Raskin. New York: Bantam.

The two authors/psychotherapists became aware of the symptoms of depression following childbirth from their patients. Although there was individuality in every case, common themes and precipitating patterns became evident, motivating the authors to help women understand postpartum depression and to engage them in recovery. The useful topics of coping, self-care, psychotherapy, fantasies, expectations, and recovery are presented sensitively and factually. A thorough postpartum assessment offered at the end is intended to assist those in doubt to focus their concerns. The recent publication of this book and its unique perspective make it a Diamond in the Rough selection.

♦ *1000 Questions about Your Pregnancy* (1997) by Jeffrey M. Thurston. Arlington, TX: Summit.

The author is an associate professor of obstetrics/gynecology at a major medical school. As a function of practice and teaching, he has developed answers to the 1,000 questions presented in this book. This easy-to-read reference gives the facts about pregnancy and childbirth and adds a little humor on the side. Questions are sequential by developmental stage of pregnancy, yet are subgrouped by subject areas (e.g., morning sickness, tests of fetal functioning, drugs, childbirth classes). The information carefully differentiates between fact and opinion, and coincides with the recommendations of the American College of Obstetrics/Gynecology. Because this question and answer book is up to date, factually accurate, and relatively recently published, it qualifies as a Diamond in the Rough.

FILMS

Recommended

★★★ *Where the Heart Is* (2000) directed by Matt Williams. PG-13 rating. 120 minutes.

Natalie Portman, a very pregnant 17-year-old, escapes to California hoping for a new life with her selfish and unreliable musician boyfriend. He dumps her in Oklahoma. With the assistance of an assortment of odd women, she lives in the Wal-Mart and delivers there, and eventually becomes part of a makeshift family of support. The plot is both too busy and full of holes, but the characters shine through. The folksy warmth about pregnancy and the message of nonstandard family love are the lasting lessons.

★★★ *Steel Magnolias* (1990) directed by Herbert Ross. PG rating. 118 minutes.

This movie spans several years in the lives of a group of women whose central meeting place is a beauty salon. One of the central characters, a diabetic woman, gives birth to a child her physician warned her not to have and subsequently lapses into a terminal coma. More generally, the film is about the support of good friends, accepting loss, and learning to grow beyond differences. Through troubling times, there is a rebirth of relationships and newfound support.

Not Recommended

★ *Father of the Bride II* (1995) directed by Charles Shyer. PG rating. 106 minutes.

★ *Nine Months* (1995) directed by Chris Columbus. PG-13 rating. 102 minutes.

★ *Baby M* (1988, made for TV) directed by James Stephen Sadwith. PG rating. 128 minutes.

INTERNET RESOURCES

Metasites

★★★★★ *Pregnancy/Birth* http://pregnancy.about.com

Under headings like Cesarean Section, Prenatal Tests, and Episiotomy are perhaps a thousand sites with comments, but no ratings.

★★★★ *Infertility* http://infertility.miningco.com

Under headings such as Infertility 101, Ovulation Software, Lifestyle Causes, Endometriosis, and others are hundreds of links with brief comments. It is very unlikely that you will fail to find what you seek or need in this massive collection.

Psychoeducational Materials for Clients and Families

General Sites

★★★★★ *Childbirth.org* http://www.childbirth.org

A very large and comprehensive site, with lots to read and do on every aspect. About 25 *FAQ*s are well done and cover some unusual areas, like Low Tech Fertility Methods and Amniotomy.

★★★★ *The Dad Zone* http://www.babycenter.com/dads

This commercial site offers about 25 fine articles from preconception to baby's first year, under headings of preconception, pregnancy, baby, toddler, and the like.

★★★★ *ParenthoodWeb*
        http://www.parenthood.com/parent_cfmfiles/pregnancy_labor.cfm
This site has dozens of short articles on every topic imaginable.

★★★★ *OBGYN.net: The Universe of Women's Health* http://www.obgyn.net

"This site, with original content by obstetrics and gynecology practitioners, is also an annotated subject directory of Web resources. Some of the topics covered in the For Women and Patients section are: contraceptives, medications, infertility, grief, pregnancy and birth, raising children, sexuality and reproductive health, and fitness. There's also an acronym glossary and it's searchable." The layout is complex, so the search engine is appreciated. Patients who still have medical questions after looking elsewhere can probably find the answer here.

Medical Aspects

★★★★★ *Sabrina's Pregnancy Page* http://www.fensende.com/Users/swnymph/

The gift of a knowledgeable midwife, this site has personal items, as well as dozens of well-considered links on pregnancy, parenting, breastfeeding, references, and good FAQs. The FAQ page also offers WebRings that change often and are more focused, so they should not be pursued until the stronger sites have been read.

★★★★★ *BabyZone* http://babyzone.com

An enormous site for any kind of question related to medication, diseases, symptoms, procedures, and so on.

★★★★ *Pregnancy Calendar* http://www.parentsplace.com

This site "will build a day-by-day customized calendar detailing the development of a baby from before conception to birth." The larger site (ParentsPlace.com) also offers interactive ways to create a plan for birth and has much material on nutrition, newborn care, and breastfeeding, as well as chat and bulletin boards.

★★★ *StorkNet's Week-by-Week Guide to Your Pregnancy!*
      http://www.pregnancyguideonline.com

Similar to the *Pregnancy Calendar* (above) but also includes Fetal Development, Maternal Changes, Checkups, Readings, and Ideas for Dad.

Getting Pregnant and Infertility

★★★★★ *Plus-Size Pregnancy Website*
      http://www.plus-size-preganancy.org/firstindex.html

Here are 20 very informative articles on preparing for and being pregnant, complications, clothing, and breastfeeding. Superb links and support for the large woman. A wonderful gift from Kmom. See also *FertilityPlus* at http://www.pinelandpress.com, which has a unique Infertility FAQ for Women of Size and 29 other solid articles.

★★★★★ *Infertility FAQ* http://www.fertilityplus.org/faq/infertility.html

Totaling about 40 pages, this is a well-organized and superb overview of the medical aspects that should be understood before exploring the psychological ones. It also covers online news groups, books and readings, and how to join online groups. The FAQs in section 12 are extremely informative about the more complex medical issues.

★★★★ *Preconception* http://www.babycenter.com/preconception

Although a commercial site, this offers about 100 short pieces on the issues, with specific information and some reporting of myths and errors.

★★★ *Infertility Resources* http://www.ihr.com/infertility/index.html

Under Infertility Educational Articles are hundreds of articles. The most relevant articles are under Male Factor and four of the articles under Psychological and Social Issues.

Pregnancy Loss

★★★★★ *Hygeia Foundation* http://hygeia.org

The gift of Michael R. Berman, MD, this site offers information and support for "families who have endured the loss of a pregnancy, newborn, or infant child." Hundreds of pages are available, after registration, under lists for those who have experienced a loss, for those parenting an ill newborn or older child, and for children with long-standing illnesses.

★★★★ *A Heartbreaking Choice* http://www.aheartbreakingchoice.com/

There are many short but useful articles here. It Happended Once—Will It Happen Again? by Helga V. Toriello, PhD, is for those in need of the three-page introduction to genetic risks.

★★★ *Waiting with Love* http://www.erichad.com/wwl/

"For parents who choose to continue a pregnancy knowing their unborn baby will die before or shortly after birth and for families who learn their newborn will die."

Untoward Pregnancies

★★★★★ *Planned Parenthood* http://www.plannedparenthood.org

Under the Health Info button on the left are about 10 headings leading to fact sheets, brochures, and readings. Parenting has eight superb guides on dealing with one's children's sexuality. Pregnancy has six informative readings. Abortion has about two dozen fact sheets and five very informative booklets.

★★★★ *Adoption.com* http://www.adoption.com

This site seeks to connect children (and pregnant women) with people seeking to adopt, and it offers commercial products. However, their Adoption Library is a searchable collection of thousands of articles on the literature, poetry, law, statistics, foster parenting, special needs kids, birthparents, and more. Probably the best starting site for those considering adoption.

★★★ *Pregnancy Centers Online* http://www.pregnancycenters.org

Offering addresses of local groups, this site is for women who have a crisis (unwanted) pregnancy, do not want to abort, and want support. It is vigorously antiabortion.

Birth Defects

★★★★★ *March of Dimes Fact Sheets*
      http://www.marchofdimes.com/professionals/681_1116.asp

This health library has about 30 well-written and supported fact sheets available on substances' effects on pregnancy, genetics, infections, pregnancy loss, and screenings.

Many deal with the psychological aspects, such as stress, drugs and alcohol, stillbirth, and pregnancy after 30. All are available in Spanish. See also their Resource Center (with online and phone answers to questions, local referrals, FAQs, and links) and Birth Defects Information sections, accessible from the left column, for additional information.

Childbirth Educators and Doulas

Doulas are trained to provide emotional, physical, and educational support to women and their families during and after childbirth.

★★★ *National Association of Postpartum Care Services* http://www.napcs.org
Some information and a doula finder. A similar site is *Doulas of North America* at http://www.dona.org.

★★★ *Association for Pre- and Perinatal Psychology and Health*
        http://www.birthpsychology.com
Many readings and directories, links, and media listings.

Other Resources

★★★★★ *Breastfeeding Resources on the Internet*
        http://www.prairienet.org/laleche/other.html
An organized and annotated listing of hundreds of sites. Comprehensive and authoritative. Thank you, Sue Ann Kendall.

★★★★ *ProMoM* http://www.promom.org
If a woman needs information or support, this site is enthusiastically in favor of breastfeeding.

★★★★ *Postpartum Support International* http://www.postpartum.net
A unique site with a good overview essay and a guide to prevention of depression.

NATIONAL SUPPORT GROUPS

Bethany Christian Services Pregnancy Crisis Hotline
Phone: 800-238-4269
http://www.bethany.org

   Information and counseling for pregnant women. Referrals to free pregnancy test facilities, foster care, and adoption centers.

Pregnancy Hotline
Phone: 800-848-5683
Fax: 609-848-2380

   Free, confidential information for pregnant women, shelters for women, baby clothes, adoption referrals.

Planned Parenthood
810 Seventh Avenue
New York, NY 10019
Phone: 800-230-7526
E-mail: communications@ppfa.org
http://www.plannedparenthood.org

Referrals to neighborhood Planned Parenthood clinics nationwide.

National Abortion Federation
1755 Massachusetts Avenue NW, Suite 600
Washington, DC 20036
Phone: 800-772-9100
http://www.prochoice.org

Provides information and referrals regarding abortions; financial aid.

National Adoption Center
1500 Walnut Street, Suite 701
Philadelphia, PA 19102
Phone: 800-TO-ADOPT
Fax: 215-735-9410
E-mail: nac@nationaladoptioncenter.org
http://www.adopt.org

Information on adoption agencies and support groups. Network for matching parents and children with special needs.

Compassionate Friends
http://www.compassionatefriends.org

The mission of the Compassionate Friends is to assist families in their grieving following the death of a child and to provide information to help others be supportive.

Helping after Neonatal Death (HAND)
PO Box 341
Los Gatos, CA 95031
Phone: 888-908-HAND or 408-995-6102
http://www.handonline.org

"HAND . . . is a non-profit, volunteer group founded in the early 1980's to provide support and information to bereaved parents, their families and friends following a miscarriage, stillbirth, or newborn death."

Resolve
1310 Broadway
Somerville, MA 02144-1779
Phone: 888-623-0744
E-mail: info@resolve.org
http://www.resolve.org

For those coping with infertility, this is the oldest and largest organization.

See also Infant Development and Parenting (Chapter 21) and Sexuality (Chapter 30).

CHAPTER 28

Schizophrenia

Schizophrenia, a serious mental disorder afflicting 1% of the population, is character-ized by disorganized thinking, impairment in reality testing, hallucinations, and delu-sions. Many scientific and academic books are available describing this disorder; how-ever, the resources reviewed in this chapter were explicitly chosen for their usefulness to individuals who deal with schizophrenia in their daily lives.

In recent years, mental health professionals have come to realize what laypersons touched by schizophrenia have known all along, namely, that schizophrenia can have as devastating an effect on family and friends as on the mentally ill individuals them-selves. Because the onset is typically during the late teens and early 20s, family mem-bers experience a deterioration of a loved one for whom the early years were normal. The person they had come to know is experiencing a metamorphosis before their very eyes. Parents and caretakers of children with schizophrenia suffer emotional up-heaval while also being responsible for seeking medical and psychological assistance, dealing with trauma within the family, and attending to financial, social, educational, and employment changes. Siblings of the mentally ill find their worlds turned upside down because their needs have suddenly become low priority. Extended family and friends are at loss, not knowing what to do or what not to do. And the financial costs of the disorder are staggering: $65 billion for medical costs and lost productivity alone.

The self-help resources reviewed here are primarily directed to patients, family, and friends who seek direction. We consider the evaluative ratings and descriptions, in turn, of self-help books, autobiographies, films, and Internet resources, followed by an alphabetical listing of national support organizations.

RECOMMENDATION HIGHLIGHTS

Self-Help Books

- For the families:

  ★★★★★ *Surviving Schizophrenia* by E. Fuller Torrey

  ★★★ *Coping with Schizophrenia* by Kim T. Mueser and Susan Gingerich

  ★★★ *How to Cope with Mental Illness in Your Family* by Diane T. Marsh and Rex M. Dickens

- For understanding the disorder and patient advocacy:

  ◆ *Understanding Schizophrenia* by Richard S. E. Keefe and Philip D. Harvey

  ◆ *Schizophrenia Simplified* by John F. Thornton and Mary V. Seeman

Autobiographies

- For a classic story of a teen's fantasy world and treatment:

  ★★★★★ *I Never Promised You a Rose Garden* by Joanne Greenberg

- For a spiritual quest following a schizophrenic breakdown:

  ★★★★ *Out of the Depths* by Anton T. Boisen

- For a critical look at treatment:

  ★★★★ *Too Much Anger, Too Many Tears* by Janet Gotkin and Paul Gotkin

- For a classic memoir of a schizophrenic episode among 1960s turbulence:

  ★★★ *The Eden Express* by Mark Vonnegut

- For memoirs and diary notes of youngsters suffering from schizophrenia:

  ★★★ *When the Music's Over* edited by Richard Gates and Robin Hammond

  ★★★ *Autobiography of a Schizophrenic Girl* by Marguerite Sechehaye

Films

- For largely true and inspiring stories of brilliant schizophrenics:

  ★★★★★ *A Beautiful Mind*

  ★★★★ *Shine*

- For examples of friendship despite catatonic schizophrenia:

  ★★★★ *Birdy*

- For a healing search despite mental disarray:

  ★★★★ *The Fisher King*

Internet Resources

- For just about anything you want to know:

  ★★★★★ *Schizophrenia.com* http://www.schizophrenia.com

  ★★★★★ *Internet Mental Health* http://www.mentalhealth.com/fr20.html

  ★★★★★ *The Experience of Schizophrenia* http://www.mgl.ca/~chovil

- For families:

  ★★★★ *Schizophrenia: A Handbook For Families*
  http://www.mentalhealth.com/book/p40-sc01.html

  ★★★ *Articles for the Patient and Caregiver*
  http://www.mhsource.com/schizophrenia/info.html

SELF-HELP BOOKS

Strongly Recommended

★★★★★ *Surviving Schizophrenia: A Manual for Families, Consumers, and Providers* (4th ed., 2001) by E. Fuller Torrey. New York: HarperPerennial.

The author, a renowned expert on schizophrenia, is both a psychiatrist and the brother of a person diagnosed with schizophrenia. As a result, this book is written with both a personal perspective and accurate medical information. The important aspects of this disease are addressed factually and encouragingly. View from the inside, view from the outside, what the disease is not, and questions asked are examples of topics discussed in an understandable and respectful way. The decline in outpatient services, rehabilitation, housing, and other needed assistance led to a closing section on how to be an effective advocate. The five-star *Surviving Schizophrenia* is widely regarded as the best self-help book on the subject.

Recommended

★★★ *Coping with Schizophrenia* (1994) by Kim T. Mueser and Susan Gingerich. Oakland, CA: New Harbinger.

This book is a comprehensive guide for families and individuals living with chronic mental disorder and for whom retaining some independence for the individual remains crucial. Until recent years, the families of the mentally ill have been denied explanations and have been shut out of treatment planning. Movement toward family education has begun, and this book is a significant contribution to helping family members improve their quality of life. The authors thoroughly present the disease and offer recommendations for coping and making decisions. The text provides an overview of diagnosis, symptoms, medication, side effects, and early warning signs of relapse. Other sections focus on solving problems, managing stress, establishing household rules, and dealing with depression, anxiety, and alcohol and drugs. The practical format, replete with numerous checklists and exercises, allows family members to gauge their own progress and that of the mentally ill member. Final chapters focus on the family quality of life, the importance of siblings, and planning for the future. An excellent self-help resource that, had it been better known, would have obtained a four- or five-star rating.

★★★ *How to Cope with Mental Illness in Your Family: A Self Care Guide for Siblings, Off-spring, and Parents* (1998) by Diane T. Marsh and Rex M. Dickens. New York: Jeremy P. Tarcher/Putnam.

This book is written from the point of view of a family affected by mental disorder. One author is a psychologist who works with families of the mentally ill, and the other is an adult who grew up with a mentally ill sibling. The book is directed to family members, particularly the siblings and adult children of the mentally ill. It describes the effect of the illness on the childhood and adolescence of the siblings and the effect that living with this disease may have on a person's worldview. Experiences of siblings are cited as illustrative of how they learned to cope and how they managed losses and challenges. Chapters are devoted to topics such as how the illness disrupts the family, the emotional burden of daily problems, peer relationships, vulnerability, and adaptation across developmental stages. The concluding focus is on strengths, coping skills, and hopefulness for family members developed through support groups and other resources.

★★★ *Helping Someone with Mental Illness* (1998) by Rosalynn Carter with Susan K. Golant. New York: Random House.

This refreshing first-person narrative gives a sense of storytelling between two people. Former First Lady Rosalynn Carter tells her story of initial involvement in mental health in 1970 and the motivating factors that continue to sustain her work. Chapters cover the biological and psychological nature of mental illness, known triggers, symptoms, and warning signs. The major mental illnesses of schizophrenia, manic–depression, obsessive–compulsion, anxiety, and depression are addressed. The authors articulate the importance of understanding mental illness in the workplace, insurance and managed care, and advocacy through the media and the public. Important information is summarized relative to new medications and treatment potential, known risk factors, and protective factors. This is a sensitive and personally written book on helping someone with mental illness.

Diamonds in the Rough

♦ *Understanding Schizophrenia: A Guide to the New Research on Causes and Treatment* (1994) by Richard S. E. Keefe and Philip D. Harvey. New York: Free Press.

In this self-help resource, schizophrenia is presented as researchers currently understand it. A valuable feature of the text is that it serves as a handbook for ongoing reference during the course of the illness and selection of treatments. It provides a description of the nature of schizophrenia, the impact on self and families, state-of-the-art treatments, and clinical advances. This book is a useful tool to help families gauge the knowledge and ability of the professionals with whom they are working. Families are the intended audience of this book, and the authors' optimism on improved treatments will provide them with plenty of encouragement. *Understanding Schizophrenia* remains a

Diamond in the Rough because it continues to receive very high ratings by those who read it.

♦ *Schizophrenia Simplified: A Field Guide to Schizophrenia for Frontline Workers, Families, and Professionals* (1995) by John F. Thornton and Mary V. Seeman. Toronto: Hogrefe & Huber.

Even though everyone who deals directly with schizophrenia has had experiences with the systems described here, *Schizophrenia Simplified* is one of the few sources that clearly explains the relationship between symptoms, the family, the medical and rehabilitation systems, and the legal system. Well-organized flowcharts characterize each section (color coded for convenience), and each of four sections focuses on one of the four systems (symptoms, family, medical, legal). A number of tables summarize section topics. This book is a road map for decision making and action that allows the reader to cross-reference material and better understand where any given person would be in the system and what the next step should be. The underlying purpose is to integrate and simplify the systems involved in the journey of a person with schizophrenia. Although not included in our national studies, the unique organizational perspective of this text gives it Diamond in the Rough status.

AUTOBIOGRAPHIES

Strongly Recommended

★★★★★ *I Never Promised You a Rose Garden* (1976) by Joanne Greenberg. New York: New American Library.

Originally published under the pseudonym Hannah Green, this slightly fictionalized version of the author's three years as an adolescent treated for schizophrenia is a classic in the mental health field. It is a sensitive portrayal of the relationship between a young girl in the throes of paranoid delusions, creating a fantasy world called the Kingdom of Yr, and her wise, comforting therapist. The treatment section is dated in not covering the use of the newer psychotropic drugs. Following the book's success, the author came out publicly, revealed her true name, and became active in the mental health movement. She acknowledges that the book was written deliberately to counteract attempts to romanticize mental illness. The book succeeds in that respect and does much more. There are not many clients with schizophrenia who can find and afford a therapist as wise and patient as the one described in the book, but their relationship can serve as a useful model of what the relationship can be under the best conditions. An especially moving book for teens.

★★★★ *Out of the Depths: An Autobiographical Study of Mental Disorder and Religious Experience* (1960) by Anton T. Boisen. New York: Harper.

This older book briefly describes the author's breakdown when he was a young theology student. He found a cause in his illness and dedicated himself to the mental health movement. It is an interesting account of the relationship between mental illness and religious experience. Boisen believed that many religious leaders, including George Fox,

Swedenborg, and John Bunyan, went through a psychotic experience. In his research, he assessed religious factors in 173 schizophrenic patients at Worcester State Hospital. He published several books on religion and was active in the mental health movement. Most useful for those with low self-esteem, who feel they cannot meet their own standards. The book is out-of-print and difficult to obtain.

★★★★ *Too Much Anger, Too Many Tears: A Personal Triumph over Psychiatry* (1992) by Janet Gotkin and Paul Gotkin. New York: HarperPerennial.

Janet exhibits many symptoms of schizophrenia, tries suicide on several occasions, is hospitalized numerous times, and receives drug treatment, ECT, and individual psychotherapy. Janet's recollections of her hospitalizations and treatment are interesting and often insightful. However, she rejects the diagnosis of schizophrenia and maintains that the treatments were not helpful. Both authors are active in the Mental Patients Liberation Movement. Critiques such as these are more useful for social reform than for personal assistance. The book will confirm the negative stereotypes held by those disenchanted with the mental health system.

Recommended

★★★ *Welcome, Silence: My Triumph over Schizophrenia* (1987) by Carol S. North. New York: Simon & Schuster.

The author is a psychiatrist who was chronically psychotic for almost eight years. She experienced auditory hallucinations and was hospitalized, receiving drug and megavitamin therapies. This book is out of print and difficult to secure. There are also some credibility concerns, because factual details have been changed and few professionals see a connection between the dialysis to which North attributes her recovery and relief from schizophrenia.

★★★ *Nobody's Child* (1992) by Marie Balter and Richard Katz. New York: Perseus.

At age 17, Marie Balter was diagnosed with schizophrenia and spent the next 17 years of her life at Danvers State Hospital. With the help of friends, she was released. She subsequently found an apartment, got married, obtained a PhD from Harvard, and became a vocal advocate for mental health patients. Recently, she returned to Danvers State Hospital as an administrator. The book presents a very hopeful message in showing that there is potential for achievement and career enhancement among long-term mental health clients.

★★★ *The Eden Express* (1988) by Mark Vonnegut. New York: Dell.

Now a pediatrician, Mark Vonnegut, a child of the 1960s and the son of a famous novelist, eloquently describes his hippie life in a British Columbia commune, his breakdown and diagnosis of schizophrenia, and the precarious road to recovery. In a note for this reprinting, Vonnegut believes that using today's definitions, he would probably be diagnosed as having a mood disorder. Whatever his diagnosis, the author suffered an acute episode that abated and did not return. In this engaging story of madness and eventual recovery, Vonnegut's optimism will have particular resonance for young people and demonstrate that a crazy period in a young person's life will not necessarily result in lifelong disability. Although the book is out of print, many used and library copies can be found.

★★★ *When the Music's Over: My Journey into Schizophrenia* (1996) edited by Richard Gates and Robin Hammond. New York: Plume.

This disorganized, semifictional account documents the brief life of David Burke, a young Australian who, before he committed suicide, asked his former psychology instructor, Richard Gates, to edit his notes for publication. Much of the manuscript was written while Burke was in a variety of jails, mental hospitals, and halfway houses. Both the disjointed format and the text illustrate the bizarre thinking characteristic of paranoid schizophrenia.

★★★ *Father, Have I Kept My Promise? Madness as Seen from Within* (1988) by Edith Weisskopf-Joelson. West Lafayette, IN: Purdue University Press.

A psychology professor describes in diary form her episode of paranoid schizophrenia, admission to a state hospital for a year, and life afterward as a teacher at Purdue University. The author is an inspiring person who positively views her breakdown as leading to constructive changes in her life. This hopeful book describes how a person with problems starting in childhood can mature and go on to a successful career in mental health.

★★★ *Beyond All Reason* (1965) by Morag Coate. Philadelphia: Lippincott.

A well-educated woman with a career in writing and white-collar jobs describes a history of acute schizophrenia with numerous hospital admissions. She was treated with drugs and with individual, group, and insulin coma therapy. After her initial denial and apprehension subsided, Coate had positive experiences in hospitals. There are descriptions of her religious life and insights. This is a somewhat confusing account; there are better books available on this topic.

★★★ *An Angel at My Table: An Autobiography, Volume Two* (1984) by Janet Frame. New York: George Braziller.

An Angel at My Table is a sequel to *Faces in the Water*, a fictional account of life in a mental hospital, which was published almost 30 years after the author was discharged from the last of her five hospitalizations. Frame is an accomplished New Zealand writer with an international reputation for fiction. The first volume of her autobiography traces her difficult childhood; this second volume covers her life at college and her treatment for schizophrenia; and the third volume covers her subsequent literary career. Because the author and her present physician doubt the accuracy of the original diagnosis of schizophrenia, the book seems most suitable for those who experience loneliness and difficulty fitting it.

★★★ *Autobiography of a Schizophrenic Girl: An Astonishing Memoir of Reality Lost and Regained* (1994) by Marguerite Sechehaye. New York: NAL/Dutton.

A reprint of a classic account of a young girl's schizophrenia compiled from case materials by her therapist Marguerite Sechehaye, the book has been republished several times under different titles and with different author names. Told in the young patient's own words, Renee describes bizarre perceptual experiences and feelings of unreality that started at age five. Similar to the protagonist in *I Never Promised You a Rose Garden*, Renee is brought back to reality with the aid of a caring therapist, whom Renee called Mama. It is not as tight a narrative as *Rose Garden* but still a good description of the thought disorder characteristic of childhood schizophrenia and of a skilled therapist's treatment.

★★★   *The Quiet Room: A Journey out of the Torment of Madness* (1996) by Lori Schiller and Amanda Bennett. New York: Warner Books.

Expanded from an article in the *Wall Street Journal*, this gripping account of Schiller's descent into schizophrenia and recovery, based on diary notes, is accompanied by interviews with family members and mental health practitioners. The book is particularly strong in demonstrating the effects of Lori's disorder on her friends and family, whose views are presented in the book. A sensitive inside view of a young woman's struggle against hallucinations and delusions.

FILMS

Strongly Recommended

★★★★★   *A Beautiful Mind* (2001) directed by Ron Howard. PG-13 rating. 136 minutes.

Russell Crowe plays the mathematician John Nash, whose work eventually wins a Nobel Prize but whose life is savaged by schizophrenia. His hallucinations and paranoid delusions are remarkably well portrayed. The disorder never takes precedence over Nash as a lovable albeit limited human. Treatment is shown positively, although the methods were then primitive and only partly effective. This Academy Award winning best film is hopeful about recovery but does not shy away from showing the terrible pain of Nash and his loving wife. An honest and beautiful film based on the book of the same title.

★★★★   *Birdy* (1985) and directed by Alan Parker. R rating. 120 minutes.

A powerful story about friendship and helping others survive the effects of the Vietnam War. One of the veterans suffers from catatonic schizophrenia, probably arising from both life and war experiences. These friends are fighting not only to overcome the ravages of war but also to rise above their lower socioeconomic existence in South Philadelphia. They refuse to abandon each other, and they celebrate their male bonding. This self-help resource is enthusiastically recommended by psychologists in our national studies, as well as by movie critics.

★★★★   *Shine* (1996) directed by Scott Hicks. PG-13 rating. 105 minutes.

A true and inspiring story of David Helfgott, an Australian piano prodigy whose brilliant career is interrupted by an unspecified mental illness, probably schizophrenia or bipolar disorder. As a child and then as an adult, he struggles to separate and individuate from his domineering father. The movie is described as glorious, powerful, and extraordinary. It takes you from David's childhood to his adulthood and shows all the joys and sorrows of this brilliant man's complex disorder.

★★★★ *The Fisher King* (1991) directed by Terry Gilliam. R rating. 137 minutes.

A substance-abusing talk-show host finds himself on the outs. His life is dramatically turned around when he meets a man who has been traumatized by witnessing the death of his wife. In what appears to be a psychotic state (or severe posttraumatic stress disorder), this man attempts to rediscover the meaning in life by searching for the Holy Grail. Both men struggle with their own demons, but together they secure the Grail and find healing. The movie is funny and inspiring but at times quite confusing. (Also reviewed in Chapter 26, Posttraumatic Stress Disorder.)

Recommended

★★★ *Benny and Joon* (1994) directed by Jeremiah Chechik. PG rating. 100 minutes.

The predominant themes here are accepting people and their limitations, struggling with mental illness, and learning to let go in a relationship. *Benny and Joon* is a love story; it reminds us that there is someone in the world for everyone. It reinforces the myth that love will conquer all. The movie creators walk a thin line between comedy and tragedy in their efforts to demonstrate the plight of a woman with schizophrenia. Overall, it emerges as a likable and effective comedy/drama.

Not Recommended

★ *Mad Love* (1995) directed by Antonia Bird. PG-13 rating. 93 minutes.

INTERNET RESOURCES

Metasites

★★★★★ *Schizophrenia.com* http://www.schizophrenia.com

This site offers basic information, more in-depth information, and discussion areas as well as a search engine with an effort-saving Most Common Searches list. This labor of love is the most complete and rich site on schizophrenia. No matter what you seek, you will find it here. Thank you, Brian Chiko.

★★★★★ *Internet Mental Health* http://www.mentalhealth.com/fr20.html

Click on Disorders and then Schizophrenia on the left to find hundreds of links and articles on all aspects of schizophrenia. This is one part of Phillip W. Long's vast, high-quality site. He is a Canadian and so can see both the American and European perspectives.

★★★★ *Mentalhelp* http://www.mentalhelp.net/poc/center_index.php

Mentalhelp has a large collection of articles from many sources as well as links to other sites and book reviews.

Psychoeducational Materials for Clients and Families

★★★★★ *Schizophrenia* http://www.nimh.nih.gov/publicat/schizoph.htm#schiz1

These well-written 15 pages are from the National Institute of Mental Health.

★★★★★ *The Experience of Schizophrenia* http://www.mgl.ca/~chovil

Ian Chovil's home page contains a biography, resources, advice, and diagrams for teaching.

★★★★ *Basic Facts about Schizophrenia*
　　　 http://www.mentalhealth.com/book/p40-sc02.html#head_2

These 40 pages cover almost all aspects of schizophrenia. The site is from a Canadian source, but the information is universal. The material is very realistic and may be too intense or complex for introducing clients or families. The FAQ is very good, as is the material on stigma and the Glossary.

★★★★ *Schizophrenia: A Handbook for Families*
　　　 http://www.mentalhealth.com/book/p40-sc01.html

About 50 pages, similar in format to the site above, but with mostly unique information.

★★★★ *Neuroleptic Malignant Syndrome Information Service* http://www.nmsis.org

The site offers three brochures for sale, six reprints at no charge, and an online FAQ.

★★★★ *The Center of Reintegration* http://www.reintegration.com

A good resource for the social rehabilitation perspective, with material on clubhouses, independent living, and family issues.

★★★ *Articles for the Patient and Caregiver*
　　　 http://www.mhsource.com/schizophrenia/info.html

Thirteen solid brochures.

★★★ *Schizophrenia*
　　　 http://www.mentalhealth.com

From the main page, scroll down and click on Books, then Schizophrenia, and then scroll down to Booklets, where you will find about 20 publications offering psychiatric perspectives on schizophrenia. The whole site is of great value.

★★★ *Recovery, Inc.* http://www.recovery-inc.com

The site offers about 10 readings describing the approach of Recovery, Inc.

★★★ *Center for Psychiatric Rehabilitation at Boston University*
http://www.bu.edu/cpr/

Perhaps the most useful part is "Handling Your Psychiatric Disability at Work and School," which offers readings on the Americans with Disabilities Act, job accommodation, dealing with a difficult boss, disclosing your disability, and so on.

Other Resources

Schizophrenia.com Home Page http://www.schizophrenia.com

Besides the Main Message Board, there are areas for People Diagnosed with Schizophrenia, Parents, Spouses, Siblings, Children/Offspring of Parents with Schizophrenia, Childhood Schizophrenia, Financial/Resources, Dual Diagnosis, and so on.

Schizophrenia Support Organizations http://members.aol.com/leonardjk/support.htm

J. K. Leonard provides both the mail and linked online addresses of local branches of national organizations.

NATIONAL SUPPORT GROUPS

National Alliance for the Mentally Ill (NAMI)
Colonial Place Three
2107 Wilson Boulevard, Suite 300
Arlington, VA 22201
Phone: 800-950-NAMI or 703-524-7600
http://www.nami.org

Support, information, conferences, and referrals; NAMI construes schizophrenia as a brain disease.

National Alliance for Research on Schizophrenia and Depression (NARSAD)
60 Cutter Mill Road, Suite 404
Great Neck, NY 11021
Phone: 516-829-0091
E-mail: info@narsad.org
http://www.narsad.org

National Mental Health Association (NMHA)
2001 N. Beauregard Street, 12th Floor
Alexandria, VA 22311
Phone: 703-684-7722
http://www.nmha.org

National Mental Health Consumers' Self-Help Clearinghouse
1211 Chestnut Street, Suite 1207
Philadelphia, PA 19107
Phone: 800-553-4539 or 215-751-1810
E-mail: info@mhselfhelp.org
http://www.mhselfhelp.org

Recovery Inc.
802 North Dearborn Street
Chicago IL 60610
Phone: 312-337-5661
E-mail: inquiries@recovery-inc.org
http://www.recovery-inc.org

Schizophrenia Society of Canada
50 Acadia Avenue, Suite 205
Markham, Ontario, Canada L3R 0B3
Phone: 905-415-2007
http://www.schizophrenia.ca

CHAPTER 29

Self-Management
and Self-Enhancement

"Don't worry, be happy!" are the words of a popular tune by Bobby McFerrin, " 'Cause when you worry, your face will frown, and that will bring everybody down ..." Is McFerrin's cheerful optimism an effective self-management strategy?

Starting with the earliest human writings, self-help resources have advanced strategies to cope successfully and manage undesirable behaviors. Some self-help writers suggest avoiding negative people; some preach trust in God; others teach positive thinking; and still others advocate perceiving reality as accurately as possible. In the early 1990s, a number of psychologists began recommending "positive illusions"—that is, happy people often entertain falsely high opinions of themselves, give self-serving explanations for events, and have exaggerated beliefs about their ability to control the world around them. In the early 2000s, the pendulum had swung to encouraging acceptance of life's inevitable travails and returning to spirituality, a topic considered in Chapter 31.

In a way, all self-help resources are about self-improvement. But in this chapter, we critically consider a multitude of self-help books and Internet resources devoted to self-management and self-enhancement. This is admittedly a broad topic; indeed, so broad and inclusive that we purposefully excluded films and autobiographies because they number in the hundreds.

SELF-HELP BOOKS

Strongly Recommended

★★★★★ *The 7 Habits of Highly Effective People* (1989) by Steven Covey. New York: Simon & Schuster.

Covey's best-selling and influential book provides an in-depth examination of how people's perspectives and values determine how competently they perform in their busi-

RECOMMENDATION HIGHLIGHTS

Self-Help Books

- On the success—and limitations—of changing behaviors:

  ★★★★★ *What You Can Change and What You Can't* by Martin Seligman

- On improving life and self-esteem with optimistic thinking:

  ★★★★★ *Learned Optimism* by Martin Seligman

  ★★★★ *Ten Days to Self-Esteem* by David Burns.

- On self-improvement, especially in business:

  ★★★★★ *The 7 Habits of Highly Effective People* by Steven Covey

- On the stages of change and what to do when:

  ★★★★ *Changing for Good* by James O. Prochaska and Associates

- On a cognitive approach to self-management:

  ★★★★ *A New Guide to Rational Living* by Albert Ellis and Robert Harper

  ★★★★ *Feel the Fear and Do It Anyway* by Susan Jeffers

  ★★★★ *What to Say When You Talk to Yourself* by Shad Helmstetter

- On optimizing natural healing and bodily functioning:

  ★★★★ *Spontaneous Healing* by Andrew Weil

- On learning to respond to life with ease:

  ★★★★ *Don't Sweat the Small Stuff . . . and It's All Small Stuff* by Richard Carlson

  ★★★★ *The Art of Happiness* by the Dalai Lama and Howard C. Cutter

- On conquering procrastination:

  ★★★★ *Overcoming Procrastination* by Albert Ellis and William Knaus

- On women's self-enhancement and not blaming mothers:

  ★★★★ *Don't Blame Mother* by Paula Caplan

Internet Resources

- On emotional intelligence:

  ★★★★★ *Emotional Intelligence* http://eqi.org

  ★★★★★ *Emotional Intelligence Test* http://www.queendom.com/tests/access/emotional_iq.html

- On self-esteem:

  ★★★★★ *Self-Esteem—What Is It?* http://www.positive-way.com/self-esteem%20what%20is%20it.htm

ness and personal lives. Covey argues that in order to be quality leaders in an organization, people must first become quality-oriented, identifying the underlying principles that are important in their lives and evaluating whether they are living up to those standards. Covey lists seven basic habits that are fundamental to anyone's efforts to become quality-oriented:

- Be proactive instead of reactive.
- Begin with the end in mind.
- Put first things first.
- Think win/win.
- Seek first to understand, then to be understood.
- Synergize.
- Sharpen the saw (renewal).

This five-star resource is a breath of fresh air among the superficial quick-fix books that populate the checkout counters across the nation. Covey's choices of personal, family, educational, and professional examples to illustrate the habits of highly effective people are excellent. Critics have said that no research has been conducted to confirm that these are the seven core habits of competent individuals.

★★★★★ *Learned Optimism: How to Change your Mind and Your Life* (1992, reissued 1998) by Martin Seligman. New York: Pocket Books.

This psychological approach to positive thinking was authored by Martin Seligman, a professor of psychology at the University of Pennsylvania. *Learned Optimism* is based on psychological research rather than spiritual belief. Seligman argues that optimism and pessimism are not fixed, inborn psychological traits but rather are learned explanatory styles—habitual ways we explain things that happen to us. Pessimists, says Seligman, perceive a defeat as permanent, catastrophic, and evidence of personal inadequacy; optimists, by contrast, perceive the same mishap as a temporary setback, something that can be controlled, and rooted in circumstances or luck. Seligman's positive message is that because pessimism is learned, it can be unlearned. Included are self-tests to determine the reader's levels of optimism, pessimism, and depression. Seligman reviews a great deal of research on explanatory styles, concluding that optimists do better in school, in athletics, and at work, because they persist even in the face of setbacks, whereas equally talented pessimists are more likely not to stay the course. Seligman also reviews research to demonstrate that pessimists have weaker immune systems, more health problems, and are more likely to be depressed. This five-star resource is an excellent self-help book on positive thinking. This well-documented but not overly academic book is psychobabble-free.

★★★★★ *What You Can Change and What You Can't* (1993) by Martin Seligman. New York: Fawcett.

Seligman, a leading authority on depression and motivation, also authored this five-star self-help resource. This book provides a wealth of scientific thought and scholarly opinions about the effect of biology, genetics, heredity, environment, and self-motivation on how we think and change. What we can change has definite limitations, but Seligman repeatedly reminds us that there is much we can do within the boundaries to influence our quality of life. In several chapters, Seligman gives his own evaluation of treatments for various disorders (e.g., anxiety, anger, depression). This book is written at a higher level than most self-help manuals but will be very informative for the interested general public.

★★★★ *Feel the Fear and Do It Anyway* (1987, reprinted 1996) by Susan Jeffers. New York: Fawcett.

This book applies a cognitive approach, much of it based on Ellis's rational–emotive therapy, to coping with fear. Jeffers believes that most inaction, whether it involves changing jobs, breaking off a relationship, or starting a relationship, stems from the fear of not being able to handle whatever comes along. She says that fear never completely goes away. Fear should be a sign to us that we are being challenged, and we should confront the fear by taking reasonable risks. Jeffers does a good job of showing how faulty thinking is the source of most people's unreasonable fears, and she gives valuable advice about how to modify such irrational thinking.

★★★★ *Changing for Good* (1995) by James O. Prochaska, John C. Norcross, and Carlo C. DiClemente. New York: Avon.

Prochaska, Norcross, and DiClemente bring their 20 years of federally funded research and 50 years of collective knowledge to bear on behavior change. The book is organized around the stages of change: precontemplation, contemplation, preparation, action, and maintenance. This scientific approach to self-change helps identify the stage of change for a particular problem and then reviews the common obstacles, best change methods, and interpersonal support for that particular stage. One of the few self-change books to be based on and backed by scientific research, this four-star resource will be helpful to laypersons who wish to understand the stages of change and valuable to the professionals working with them. (In the interest of full disclosure, *Changing for Good* was authored by one of the coauthors of this *Authoritative Guide to Self-Help Resources in Mental Health*.)

★★★★ *Ten Days to Self-Esteem* (1999) by David D. Burns. New York: HarperCollins.

Psychiatrist Burns is the author of the best selling *Feeling Good: The New Mood Therapy*. In this book, he provides a valuable resource for developing self-esteem and discovering the secrets of joy in daily life. In a clear and practical fashion, Burns advances 10 steps to self-esteem: the pride of happiness; you feel the way you think and you can change the way you feel; how to break out of a bad mood; the acceptance paradox; getting down to the root causes; how to get self-esteem; the perfectionist's script for self-defeat; a prescription for procrastination; and practice, practice, and practice. This self-help book is filled with logs, charts, and step-by-step guides to enhance self-esteem.

★★★★ *A New Guide to Rational Living* (1975) by Albert Ellis and Robert Harper. Englewood Cliffs, NJ: Prentice-Hall.

This cognitive approach to self-enhancement is coauthored by Albert Ellis, a well-known psychologist and prolific author of self-help books. His rational–emotive ther-

apy states that people develop psychological problems because they use irrational beliefs to interpret what happens to them and their world. In this view, people disturb
themselves by thinking in self-defeating, illogical, and unrealistic ways. According to
Ellis and Harper, years of lengthy psychotherapy are not needed to attack the root of
emotional problems. They believe that rational–emotive therapy can quickly help people learn how to detect their irrational thinking, overcome the influence of the past,
erase dire fears of failure, conquer anxiety, and acquire self-discipline. The book is
filled with conversations between irrational thinkers and therapists, and the subsequent
interchanges that led to successful living. This valued four-star book is widely known
(evaluated by 238 psychologists) and came close to achieving a five-star rating. The
book's enthusiasts say that Ellis's approach is very effective in motivating people to re-
structure their thinking and rid themselves of harmful beliefs.

★★★★ *Spontaneous Healing: How to Discover and Enhance Your Body's Natural Ability to*
  Maintain and Heal Itself (1995) by Andrew Weil. New York: Knopf.

This author and physician describes the mechanisms of the body's healing system; simply
put, the body can heal itself because it has a healing system. Weil delineates the ways an individual can optimize the functioning of his or her own system and incorporate alternative medicines and treatments to enhance the healing system. Using clear and concise language, this best-seller explains how the healing system operates and provides information
on how foods, environments, and lifestyles can maintain well-being. Included is an eight-
week program that can help the body's natural healing powers. Weil cleverly combines
current Western medical practice with alternative treatments (e.g., acupuncture, biofeed-
back, guided imagery, and herbal medicine). For the general public interested in the study
of the internal healing system, this book provides a wealth of knowledge.

★★★★ *What to Say When You Talk to Yourself* (1986) by Shad Helmstetter. Scottsdale,
  AZ: Fine.

The author examines the literature on success and concludes that in the many recommendations there are some missing ingredients: permanent solutions, knowledge of
mind–body functions, and word-for-word directions for programming the unconscious
mind. Helmstetter concludes that the only solution that includes all three ingredients is
self-talk and goes on to outline five levels of self-talk, the highest being the level of universal affirmation. The author spells out the self-talk strategies of silent self-talk, self-
speak, self-conversation, self-write, tape-talk, and creating self-talk tapes. Favorably evaluated but not particularly well-known, this book presents some helpful strategies for
coping with stressful circumstances, especially for negative thinkers and people low in
motivation. Helmstetter spells out what to say to yourself to improve your life instead of
just being a cheerleader, like so many motivational self-help authors. Critics contend
that the material about the nonconscious mind is fuzzy.

★★★★ *Don't Sweat the Small Stuff . . . and It's All Small Stuff* (1997) by Richard Carlson.
  New York: Hyperion.

A small best-selling book about simple ways to keep the little things from taking over
your life. Carlson argues that when you learn the habit of responding to life with more

ease, problems that seem insurmountable will begin to seem more manageable, and even the biggies won't throw you off track as much as they once did. The book consists of 100 strategies, covered in a single page each, to replace old habits of reaction with new habits of perspective. Many of the strategies apply not only to isolated events but also to many of life's most difficult challenges. For teens and adults who wish to live life more reflectively and fully.

★★★★ *Overcoming Procrastination* (1977) by Albert Ellis and William Knaus. New York: Institute for Rational Living.

Subtitled *How to Think and Act Rationally in Spite of Life's Inevitable Hassles*, the book applies rational–emotive therapy to the task of combating procrastination. Ellis and Knaus begin by explaining what procrastination means and then turn to its main causes—self-downing, low frustration tolerance, and hostility. They recommend a cognitive approach to overcoming procrastination and outline the basic ideas of Ellis's rational–emotive therapy. The last chapter includes a psychotherapy transcript of a therapist and procrastinator, and shows how rational–emotive therapy helped the client. *Overcoming Procrastination* just barely received a four-star rating, but it presents a creative, practical approach to solving procrastination.

★★★★ *Don't Blame Mother: Mending the Mother–Daughter Relationship* (1989) by Paula Caplan. New York: Harper & Row.

The thesis here is that society and psychology have shortchanged mothers, blaming them far too often and too much for their children's problems. Caplan argues that daughters are taught to criticize the work of mothering and to make their mothers the scapegoats. Caplan believes that myths of idealization give rise to impossible expectations and set mothers up for failure. However, mothers and daughters can move beyond these troublesome stereotypes and negative perceptions and gain a new appreciation for each other and their relationship. She gives advice on identifying conflicting messages and myths that weaken the mother–daughter bond. Caplan also underscores the value of women sharing experiences with other women as a means of personal change and self-improvement. Just making the four-star rating, this book rejects the notion, especially popular among those with a codependency perspective, that blaming mother is a means of psychological growth. *Don't Blame Mother* is a much-needed antidote. This is an excellent self-help book on mother–daughter relationships, especially on how to improve them in the adult years.

Recommended

★★★ *Opening Up: The Healing Power of Expressing Emotions* (1997) by James W. Pennebaker. New York: Guilford Press.

Opening up one's emotions is not "just getting feelings off one's chest," but a research-based means of releasing pain and restoring health. Psychologist Pennebaker explains various strategies for opening up, including his own extensive research on expressive writing. Case studies demonstrate the hidden price of silence and the reciprocal interaction of mind and body. An excellent resource for professionals and a useful self-help book, *Opening Up* would have received a four- or five-star rating had it been read by more experts in our national studies.

★★★   *Positive Illusions: Creative Self-Discipline and the Healthy Mind* (1989) by Shelley Taylor. New York: Basic Books.

Taylor's main themes are similar to Seligman's (reviewed above): Facing the complete truth about ourselves is often not the best mental health strategy. The healthy human mind has a tendency to block out negative information; positive illusions help us cope. Taylor believes that creative deceptions are especially beneficial when we are threatened by adversity. Taylor describes research on cancer patients, disaster victims, and other people facing crises to portray how mental and physical well-being can be improved by having an unrealistically positive view of one's self and abilities. This book was positively rated but by too few respondents to make the four- or five-star categories. It is a good book on positive thinking, but one that becomes too formal and academic in places. However, the quality of Taylor's documentation is outstanding, and intellectual readers will enjoy the book.

★★★   *Self-Directed Behavior: Self-Modification for Personal Adjustment* (2002) by David L. Watson and Roland G. Tharp. Belmont, CA: Wadsworth.

This book is, at once, a popular textbook and a valuable self-help resource. The authors take the behavioral position that all behavior is learned, practiced, and rewarded. Many behaviors are learned without awareness in childhood, but as adults, we can still acquire the skills necessary to function positively. The book teaches new actions, coping methods, and problem-solving skills. It can be used by the general public but is probably optimally used under the guidance of a mental health professional or a college professor. *Self-Directed Behavior* was very favorably evaluated in our studies; in fact, it would have received a rating of four stars if it had been read by more professionals.

★★★   *Emotional Intelligence* (1994, reprinted 1997) by Daniel Goleman. New York: Bantam.

This best-selling book reviews the importance of social and emotional competencies (e.g., self-awareness, self-discipline, and empathy) that can determine the quality of life. A *New York Times* reporter and social psychologist, Goleman gives equal weight to one's emotional quotient (EQ) and intelligence quotient (IQ). Goleman discusses how to understand and bolster emotional intelligence, which can be nurtured throughout life. Heavy on science reporting at times, this book has a more scholarly flare than most but appeals widely to educated laypersons. The book is written about EQ and contains little how-to information. Frequently rated in our national studies, it almost made the four-star listing.

★★★   *The 60-Second Shrink* (1997) by Arnold A. Lazarus and Clifford N. Lazarus. San Luis Obispo, CA: Impact.

The internationally known psychologist Arnold Lazarus and son distill 100 complex mental health topics into a back-pocket reference book for those who desire to cope more effectively with life's stressors. Depending on need, this book lends itself to time-efficient, selective reading. It is a technically eclectic, scientifically based, problem-solving self-help book, usable by professionals and laypersons alike. Topics traverse the mental health landscape: healthy thinking, action steps, relationship building, effective communication, handling emotions, stress reduction, weight management, and choosing various psychotherapies, for example. This valuable three-star resource just missed making the four-star category.

★★★ *The Art of Happiness: A Handbook for Living* (1998) by Dalai Lama and Howard C. Cutler. New York: Riverside.

The authors avow, "The very purpose of our life is to seek happiness. . . . I think that the very motion of our life is toward happiness." A book of deep reflection and Buddhist insight written for those seeking more happiness, it is more philosophy than self-help, but the Dalai Lama assists in finding sources of internal peace, training the mind, and reclaiming one's inner state of happiness. The book closes with reflections on living a spiritual life.

★★★ *Staying Rational in an Irrational World* (1991) by Michael Bernard. New York: Carol.

This book applies cognitive therapy to a number of different life domains—love, dating, sex, work, children, parents, women's issues, homosexuality, and death and dying. The basic theme of rational–emotive therapy is that to cope effectively, we need to replace irrational thinking with rational thinking. The book includes many examples in which individuals learn to talk to themselves more effectively and think in more rational ways. Two final chapters include an interview with Ellis about rational–emotive therapy and a long list of Ellis's books, tapes, and talks. Now quite dated.

★★★ *Positive Addiction* (1985) by William Glasser. New York: HarperCollins.

William Glasser became famous in the 1960s and 1970s for founding a school of therapy known as reality therapy—a results-oriented treatment designed to help people cope with their immediate environment. In *Positive Addiction*, Glasser turns from therapy to the problems virtually all of us have in developing our potential. He argues that every person can overcome self-imposed weaknesses by engaging in positive addictions or activities, such as running and meditation, that help people to expand their consciousness. Glasser says that when people do this, they "spin free" and almost mystically arrive at new strategies for coping with life. By contrast, negative addictions are escapes from the pain of striving for things people want but doubt they can accomplish, such as career or athletic achievements. This three-star resource contains ideas much more popular in the 1970s than today. *Positive Addiction* was written in 1976, and frequent references to well-known people of that time—Jimmy the Greek and Tim Galloway (*Inner Tennis*), for example—seriously date the book. Critics also say that, in places, the book regresses into mystical explanations.

★★★ *Talking to Yourself: Learning the Language of Self-Affirmation* (revised ed., 1991) by Pamela Butler. New York: HarperCollins.

Butler says that each of us experiences an inner self as a distinct person speaking to us, and we each engage this inner person in a dialogue throughout our lives. Through this inner dialogue with ourselves, we make decisions, set goals, and feel satisfied or dejected. Butler believes that our self-esteem is strongly influenced by such inner speech.

In this book, Butler provides a number of specific strategies for changing our self-talk and making it work better. Topics include anger and self-talk, sex and self-talk, and gender and self-talk. A three-star resource, this book provides good advice about how to improve the way we talk to ourselves.

★★★ *Life's Little Instruction Book* (1991) by H. Jackson Brown. Nashville, TN: Rutledge Hill.

This book of instruction was inspired by a father's love for his son and his desire to guide his son along life's many paths. The instructions start with (1) compliment people every day and ends with (511) call your mother. The compact booklet is filled with 511 one-liners that can be helpful for an adolescent or adult looking for good advice or recalling consensual wisdom of the ages.

★★★ *Life Strategies: Doing What Works, Doing What Matters* (1999) by Phillip C. McGraw. New York: Hyperion.

In this bestseller, Dr. Phil offers "Ten Laws of Life," starting with "Get Real" and continuing with "You Either Get It or Don't," "You Create Your Own Experience," "People Do What Works," "You Can't Change What You Don't Acknowledge," "Life Rewards Action," "There Is No Reality—Only Perception," "Life Is Managed—It's Not Cured," "We Teach People How to Treat Us," "There Is Power in Forgiveness," "You Have to Own It to Claim It," "A Guided Tour of Your Life," "The Seven Step Strategy," and "Finding Your Formula." Experts in our national studies found it to be a valuable but oversimplified recipe for self-enhancement.

★★★ *Self-Defeating Behaviors* (1991) by Milton Cudney and Robert Hardy. San Francisco: Harper.

This is a cognitive and behavioral approach to eliminating a wide range of self-defeating behaviors, such as procrastination, defensiveness, alcohol and drug abuse, shyness, and smoking. Cudney and Hardy argue that people can free themselves from these self-destructive patterns by doing the following:

- Identifying the problem-causing behavior.
- Specifying when, where, and with whom the behavior comes into play.
- Intercepting the behavior while it is being practiced.
- Developing replacement techniques.
- Facing fears.
- Overcoming setbacks.

The book received a three-star rating in one of our national studies. *Self-Defeating Behaviors* provides valuable steps for eliminating self-defeating behaviors, though it is difficult reading for a self-help book.

★★★ *A Short Guide to a Happy Life* (2000) by Anna Quindlen. New York: Random House.

The title fits the size of this self-help book: its 50 pages are composed of pictures and brief reflections. Anna Quindlen, author of best-selling novels and winner of a 1992 Pulitzer Prize, humbly offers her insights on what helps constitute a "happy life." She reveals her beliefs on what makes her life happy, emphasizing the twin imperatives of simplicity and clarity. Position and perspective are two other themes in her book; as a person shared with Anna one day at Coney Island, "Look at the view." A brief book for anyone interested in working toward happiness in his or her life.

★★★ *All I Really Need to Know I Learned in Kindergarten: Uncommon Thought on Common Things* (1998) by Robert Fulghum. New York: Ivy.

This best-selling author's approach to finding wonderment and meaning in the smallest of life's experiences is presented with wit and humor. Fulgum's book is one that you can read a little, put down, pick up later, and put it down again without worrying about the plot resolution or missing the overarching theme. His simple rules of life gleaned from early years in kindergarten—for example, share, play fair, clean up, say you're sorry, don't take things that aren't yours—are extrapolated into adult life. When you go out into the world, it is best to hold hands and stick together. The author concludes the book with "Peace is not something you wish for; it's something you make, something you do, something you are, and something you give away." A valued, insightful, perhaps overly simplistic book, it received a three-star evaluation in one of our national studies.

★★★ *Making Life Right When It Feels All Wrong* (1988) by Herbert Fensterheim. New York: Rawlins.

Psychologist Fensterheim recommends an eclectic mix of strategies for self-enhancement that combines changing actions with conquering long-standing, buried problems. This unusual approach to self-improvement actually combines behavioral and psychoanalytic strategies. Fensterheim says that you may not be able to control what happens to you, but you can control your reaction to it. The author applies his ideas to many different domains of life: love, assertiveness, work, friendships, and sports. The book includes many vignettes, anecdotes, and case studies. This three-star resource creatively integrates behavior therapy principles and psychoanalytic concepts of needs and blocks.

★★★ *Chicken Soup for the Soul* (1991) by Jack Canfield and Mark Victor Hansen. Deerfield Beach, FL: Health Communications.

These best-selling authors have selected a number of stories to illuminate life paths and motivate us to pursue a fulfilling lifestyle. Each of the 101 stories is designed to open our minds and hearts to our potential. The stories are divided into seven sections: love, learning to love yourself, parenting, learning, living your dream, overcoming obstacles, and eclectic wisdom. This three-star, entertaining book can be read at length or for 15 minutes and will leave one feeling inspired.

★★★ *Simple Abundance: A Day Book of Comfort and Job* (1995) by Sarah Ban Breathnach. New York: Warner Books.

Simple Abundance is a book of 366 evocative essays—one for every day of the year—written for women who wish to live by their own lights. The author describes the order of the essays as progressing from creating a manageable lifestyle to living in a state of grace. The essays are intended to help readers take stock in their life and find out what is working and what is not. A book written mainly for women, but a treasure of wisdom for all.

★★★ *Who Moved My Cheese?* (1998) by Spencer Johnson. New York: Putnam.

This brief and best-selling book offers a metaphor on the difficulties of change, organizational and individual. Four characters (Sniff, Scurry, Hem, and Haw) live in a maze and look for cheese to nourish them. The four characters are intended to represent the simple and the complex parts of ourselves. Cheese is the metaphor for what we want in life (job, money, relationship, etc.). The maze is where we go to find what we want. The characters are faced with unexpected changes and challenges. This small but valuable book provides indirect advice on effectively moving through the maze of life.

★★★ *Gentle Roads to Survival* (1991) by Andrew Auw. Boulder Creek, CO: Asian.

This book, in the humanistic tradition, is a guide to making self-healing choices in difficult circumstances. Auw believes that although some people may be born survivors, most of us have to learn survival skills. Auw addresses personal crises in religion, morality, parenting, marriage, cross-cultural adaptation, and many other stressful life circumstances. He especially advocates that each person has to discover his or her own unique path of adaptation and coping. This three-star book is an effective self-help resource for people facing highly stressful circumstances in their lives. Auw's tone is warm and compassionate throughout.

★★★ *I'm OK, You're OK* (1967, reissued 1996) by Thomas Harris. New York: Avon.

This 1960s best-seller presents a transactional analysis approach to self-management. Transactional analysis maintains that people are responsible for their behavior in the present and future, regardless of what has happened to them in the past. It distinguishes three main components in each person's makeup: the Parent, the Adult, and the Child. The Parent involves the many dont's and a few do's of our early years. The Child represents spontaneous emotion. Both Parent and Child have to be kept in proper relation to the Adult, whose function is maintaining reality through decision making. The goal of transactional analysis is strengthening and emancipating the Adult from the Parent and the Child. Harris identifies four life positions that underlie people's behavior: (1) I'm not OK—You're OK, the anxious dependency of an insecure person; (2) I'm not OK—You're not OK, a position of despair or giving up; (3) I'm OK—You're not OK, the criminal position; and (4) I'm OK—You're OK, the response of mature adults who are at peace with themselves and others. Harris believes that most people unconsciously operate from the I'm not OK—You're OK position. The three-star book is extremely well-known and was immensely successful when it was published. Despite its popularity, it receives a tepid evaluation from mental health professionals. Some experts still praise the book, and others are glad that it has lost much of its luster due to its superficiality, but all agree that its popularity has waned dramatically.

★★★ *How to Live 365 Days a Year* (1975, reissued 2002) by John Schindler. Englewood Cliffs, NJ: Prentice-Hall.

This book takes the stance that illnesses and problems in life arise out of emotions. The book is divided into two main parts. In Part I, How Your Emotions Make You Ill, readers learn that emotions produce most physical diseases and also about the good emotions and the bad emotions. Part II, How to Cure Your Emotionally Induced Illness, describes how to attain emotional maturity in many different areas of life—family, sexually, and at work, for example. *How to Live 365 Days a Year* received a three-star rating. On the positive side, it presents some important ideas about how emotional difficulties cause illness and how to take control of emotional life, but on the negative side, it is dated and inferior to more modern books.

★★★ *Unlimited Power* (1986) by Anthony Robbins. New York: Fawcett Columbine.

This book is based on the theory of neurolinguistic programming that claims that people can be programmed in ways that will make them highly successful. Robbins advocates a host of mental, emotional, and physiological programming strategies, especially developing confidence in the mind's power. To convince people of their mental powers, Robbins recommends firewalking, a barefoot jaunt over hot coals. A basic step in becoming successful, he says, is selecting a successful person as a model and learning about how the person became successful and conducts his or her life. Essential to Robbins's "ultimate success formula" are clarity of desired goals, energy, passion, persistence of action, effective communication skills, and altruistic motives. *Unlimited Power* barely received a mixed three-star rating: Mental health professionals said that this book has some good points mixed with some bad points. A good point is that Robbins's enthusiastic approach can motivate people to develop their talents and to select a competent model to emulate. The bad points are that research has generally not supported the postulates of neurolinguistic programming, that the mind-over-matter firewalking demonstrations are misleading (scientists have demonstrated that people can walk across hot coals without getting burned if they move quickly enough), and that Robbins's claims that just about anyone can develop "unlimited power" are unsubstantiated and outlandish.

Diamond in the Rough

◆ *Success Is a Choice: Ten Steps to Overachieving in Business and Life* (1997) by Rick Pitino with Bill Reynolds. New York: Broadway.

Pitino, a highly respected basketball coach, believes that success is not about shortcuts. He maintains the need to aim higher and work harder than ever before in order to succeed. His 10-step program teaches people to build self-esteem, identify goals, and use a positive attitude to accomplish what they want. Being better comes in many forms. Pitino speaks to the importance of communication, role models, and turning adversity into advantage. Before working on this 10-step program, a plan of attack needs to be formalized. Pitino ends his book: "Your real journey begins now." This book, a Diamond in the Rough because of its favorable but infrequent ratings, is for adolescents and adults who are willing to study and work hard to achieve their goals.

Not Recommended

★★ *Your Maximum Mind* (1987) by Herbert Benson. New York: Random House.

★★ *Self-Matters: Creating Your Life from the Inside Out* (2001) by Phillip C. McGraw. New York: Simon & Schuster.

★★ *Tough Times Never Last, but Tough People Do!* (1983) by Robert Schuller. New York: Bantam.

★★ *Your Erroneous Zones* (1976) by Wayne Dyer. New York: Funk & Wagnalls.

★★ *The Power of Optimism* (1990) by Alan McGinnis. San Francisco: Harper & Row.

★ *The Power of Positive Thinking* (1952) by Norman Vincent Peale. New York: Ballantine.

★ *How to Stop Worrying and Start Living* (1944) by Dale Carnegie. New York: Simon & Schuster.

★ *Steps to the Top* (1985) by Zig Zigler. Gretna, LA: Pelican.

★ *Awaken the Giant Within* (1991) by Anthony Robbins. New York: Fireside.

INTERNET RESOURCES

On this broad topic, the Internet is full of absolute junk. For example, self-growth.com (http://www.selfgrowth.com) offers, among others, Aging and Longevity, Aromatherapy, Body Language, Brain Enhancement, Feng Shui, Gurus, Happiness and Self-Improvement, Herbal Remedies, Memory Training, New Age, Spiritual Development, Subliminal Learning, Success Coaching, and Television Programming. In reviewing some of these sites, Dr. Ed Zuckerman, our computer whiz, could find nothing with empirical basis or noncommercial content. Therefore, reported here are only the sites with materials that he considered to have some research support or widespread agreement.

Metasites

★★★★★ *Emotional Intelligence* http://eqi.org

An enormously rich site by Steven Hein, PhD, offers reviews of other emotional intelligence sites, signs of high and low EQ, an enormous list of feeling words, and the like. EQ and Romantic Relationships might be useful for couples in some conflicts.

★★★★ *Mayo Clinic*
          http://www.MayoClinic.com/findinformation/healthylivingcenter/index.cfm

Each of these Healthy Living centers has many articles suitable for education. You can select materials on sexually transmitted diseases (use the Diseases and Conditions A–Z list as well), sexual dysfunctions, infertility, or other topics. They are all well written and quite thorough.

Psychoeducational Materials for Clients and Families

★★★★★ *Emotional Intelligence Test*
          http://www.queendom.com/tests/access/emotional_iq.html

Long, with 70 items, but a well-designed interactive test with multiple choices that really teach about emotional intelligence.

★★★★★ *Self-Esteem—What Is It?*
http://www.positive-way.com/self-esteem%20what%20is%20it.htm

After a good introduction, this site offers three more sections: a self-esteem question-naire; Stopping Your Inner Critic from *Self-Esteem*, by Matthew McKay, PhD, and Patrick Fanning; and 25 ideas to develop self-esteem. This site is a minicourse and worth exploring.

★★★★ *Self-Esteem: What It Is, Where It Comes from, and Why We Need It* by Steven Hein, PhD http://eqi.org/sebook.htm

In just four pages, Hein covers the development and definition of self-esteem.

★★★ *Emotional Intelligence Quiz*
http://ei.haygroup.com/resources/default_ieitest.htm

A nice 10-item questionnaire.

CHAPTER 30

Sexuality

Sex has its magnificent moments throughout the animal kingdom. Insects mate in mid-air, peacocks display their plumage, and male elephant seals have prolific sex lives. These are all instinctive behaviors. Experience plays an important role in human sexual behavior. We can talk about sex with each other, read about it in books, and watch it on television and in the movies.

Although we can talk about sex with each other, we often don't. Sex in America still comes cloaked in mystery and, as a nation, we are neither knowledgeable about sex nor comfortable talking about it. Although many people manage to develop a mature sexuality, even those who do handle sex maturely have periods of vulnerability and confusion. Many people wonder and worry about their sexual attractiveness, their ability to satisfy their sexual partner, and whether they will be able to experience their sexual fantasies. Our worries are fueled by media stereotypes of sexual potency and superhuman sexual exploits. Sexual concerns also prevail because of our inability to communicate about sex directly with one another.

In this chapter, we critically examine self-help books, films, and websites devoted to sexuality in its many manifestations.

SELF-HELP BOOKS

Strongly Recommended

★★★★★ *Becoming Orgasmic: A Sexual Growth Program for Women* (revised ed., 1988) by Julia Heiman and Joseph LoPiccolo. New York: Prentice-Hall.

This excellent resource offers women permission, encouragement, and specific behavioral exercises to become more sexually fulfilled. The book leads women through a personal sex history to understand their own sexual feelings and experiences, includes self-touch exercises for learning how to relax and gain sexual pleasure, and presents advice for sharing pleasures with a partner. The topics include looking at oneself, vaginal exer-

RECOMMENDATION HIGHLIGHTS

Self-Help Books

- For improving sexual relationships and communication:
    - ★★★★ *For Each Other* by Lonnie Barbach
    - ★★★★ *Illustrated Manual of Sexual Therapy* by Helen Kaplan
    - ★★★ *Sexual Awareness* by Barry McCarthy and Emily McCarthy

- For men:
    - ★★★ *The New Male Sexuality* by Bernie Zilbergeld

- For women:
    - ★★★★★ *Becoming Orgasmic* by Julia Heiman and Joseph LoPiccolo
    - ★★★ *For Yourself* by Lonnie Barbach
    - ★★★ *For Women Only* by Jennifer Berman and Laura Berman

Films

- For a powerful story of accepting homosexuality and then loss:
    - ★★★★ *Torch Song Trilogy*

- For a popular film on bisexual experimentation:
    - ★★★★ *Kissing Jessica Stein*

- For an intriguing look at the underground lifestyle of gay men:
    - ★★★ *Paris Is Burning*

Internet Resources

- For premier sexuality information:
    - ★★★★★ *Society for Human Sexuality* http://www.sexuality.org/index.html
    - ★★★★ *Sexuality Information and Education Council of the United States* http://www.siecus.org
    - ★★★★ *iVillage: Sex* http://www.ivillage.com/topics/relation/0,,166914,00.html

- For sexually active or curious teens:
    - ★★★★★ *Coalition for Positive Sexuality* http://www.positive.org/Home
    - ★★★★★ *Teenwire* http://www.teenwire.com

- For sexuality through the lifespan:
    - ★★★★ *Sex and Aging* http://www.sexhealth.org/sexaging/index.shtml

- For self-pleasuring methods:
    - ★★★★★ *Bianca's Good Vibration Masturbation Guide* http://shack.bianca.com/shack/goodvibe/masturbate

---

- For information on STDs:
  - ★★★★★ *American Social Health Association*
    http://www.ashastd.org/stdfaqs/index.html

- For birth control:
  - ★★★★★ *Birth Control Methods* http://www.plannedparenthood.org/bc
  - ★★★★★ *Ann Rose's Ultimate Birth Control Links*
    http://www.ultimatebirthcontrol.com

---

cises, erotic literature, fantasizing, using a vibrator, and intercourse. Attention is also given to potentially related conditions such as menstrual cycles, pregnancy, and general gynecological health. *Becoming Orgasmic* is a popular and effective self-help resource for preorgasmic women.

★★★★ *For Each Other: Sharing Sexual Intimacy* (1982) by Lonnie Barbach. Garden City, NY: Anchor.

For Each Other, like its precursor, *For Yourself*, is written for and about women who wish to improve their sexual fulfillment. This book focuses on sexual concerns within the sexual relationship with a partner. Basic aspects of sexuality and the cultural context in which women learn about sexuality are reviewed; orgasmic problems and recommendations are described; and general level of sexual interest is discussed. Various exercises that the author has found effective in her practice are suggested for each problem area. The subject of female sexuality is approached candidly and in support of the women for whom this book is written.

★★★★ *Illustrated Manual of Sexual Therapy* (1987) by Helen Kaplan. New York: Brunner/Mazel.

Kaplan espouses an integrated approach to improved sexual functioning through couples therapy and use of specific sexual exercises, which are outlined in this book. She does not incorporate psychotherapeutic strategies with the sexual exercises; however, an important context for the sexual aspects is an understanding of how the activities promote the relationship. Strategies are offered to counteract the difficulty some couples may have actually trying out these therapeutic exercises. Specific techniques are targeted for specific dysfunctions, for example, orgasmic problems and premature ejaculation. The narrative is accompanied by numerous drawings that show couples or therapists using this manual and how to carry out the exercises. A favorite of sex therapists for training, it is too academic and graphic for some couples.

Recommended

★★★ *The New Male Sexuality: A Guide to Sexual Fulfillment* (revised ed., 1999) by Bernie Zilbergeld. New York: Bantam.

The New Male Sexuality presents a number of specific methods to improve male sexuality and effectively disposes of a number of myths that have victimized men. One common myth Zilbergeld attacks is that all that men really want is sexual intercourse. When men want something else, such as love and sensitivity, they are inhibited by the stereotype. Zilbergeld believes that men have gotten themselves into a losing situation by adopting superhuman standards by which to measure their genitals, sexual performance, and satisfaction. Zilbergeld's book is not a sex guide full of gimmicks or gymnastics; it does not try to impose a lifestyle on anyone; and it does not accept the premise that all men are the same. Instead, Zilbergeld explains the most common sex problems, the importance of touching, how to relax in sexual situations, how to be sensitive to one's sexual partner, and sex for older adults and disabled individuals. The new edition also covers Viagra and recent medical discoveries. A series of exercises—verbal and physical—encourages men to understand their sexual feelings and preferences. Although rated by only 18 of our experts, its rating was one of the highest ever obtained in our national studies. Far above the crowd of how-to sex books, it is a literate, thoughtful analysis of male sexuality that can enhance the sexual lives of many men.

★★★ *For Women Only* (2001) by Jennifer Berman and Laura Berman. New York: Henry Holt.

Two sisters, one a urologist and one a psychologist, joined forces to write this book and to forge a new direction in medical and psychological practice for women with sexual dysfunction. Their view is that women have been treated in masculine terms for sexual concerns that have been typically been labeled emotional, relational, or due to fatigue from child rearing. They consider women's sexual concerns to have both medical and emotional roots. Berman and Berman hope to arm women with information they need about their bodies to provide them with a full spectrum of treatment options. They propose to demasculinize sexual concerns with different categorization: hypoactive sexual desire, sexual arousal disorder, orgasmic disorder, and sexual pain. They further suggest that many of the same health problems that apply to men's sexual concerns are applicable to women, including high blood pressure, diabetes, and high cholesterol. This book is comfortable to read; it establishes a holistic and positive viewpoint on women's sexual concerns.

★★★ *The New Joy of Sex* (1991) by Alex Comfort. New York: Crown.

This book is the revision and expansion of *The Joy of Sex,* published in 1973, which sold more than 8 million copies. It was a manual of uninhibited sexual techniques with boldly explicit illustrations. *The New Joy of Sex* continues the uninhibited approach to sexual expression and explicit illustrations that characterized its predecessor, along with new material on AIDS and other sexually transmitted diseases (including a stern lecture on the importance of using condoms). It contains six main sections, including several with unlikely titles. The first, Ingredients, covers topics such as love, fidelity, breasts, buttocks, lubrication, and penis. Appetizers examines exercises, kisses, and bites, among other topics. Main Courses includes mouth music, rear entry, standing positions, and the like. Sauces covers such topics as playtime, Chinese style, G-string, leather, vibrators, and bondage. Venues describes locations, such as beds, bathtubs, rocking chairs, railways, and motorcycles. Health and Other Issues explores topics such as AIDS, frigidity, age, bisexuality, fetishes, and transvestitism. This well-known book (rated by 173 psychologists) is educational and can be beneficial in helping people rid themselves of sexual anxieties and achieve greater sexual satisfaction. However, it's definitely more for liberal thinkers than for conservative ones.

★★★ *Making Love: A Man's Guide* (1984) by Barry White. New York: Signet.

As its title implies, this book is designed to help men improve their lovemaking and sexual skills. *Making Love* advises men about what they can give women, the role of appearance in sex, women's sexual hang-ups, how to make women feel like making love, foreplay, intercourse, women's sexual anatomy, what to do after having sex, how to keep sex exciting, and what to do about sexual problems. This is mainly a how-to book with specific recommendations to help men become better lovers. Although the book provides some good suggestions in places, too often it regresses to pop-psychology descriptions of sexuality. The consensus of the mental health professionals is that Zilbergeld's *New Male Sexuality* is a much better choice.

★★★ *Making Love: A Woman's Guide* (1983) by Judith Davis. New York: Signet.

Davis points out that at one time the woman was supposed to be the passive partner in making love, always waiting for the man to make the move and following his lead after that. She says that the rules have changed in today's world—that women can now take a more active, assertive role and can enjoy sex. This sexual how-to guide for women provides explicit instructions on how to become better lovers and attract men sexually. The book includes a number of recommendations, such as 20 sure-fire turn-ons, 7 come-love-me hints, and 9 "please-touch" erogenous zone tips. Some mental health professionals consider this to be a helpful guide for women who are too inhibited sexually, but others complain that the book contains too many sensationalist comments. In either case, it has become quite dated.

★★★ *Sexual Awareness: Enhancing Sexual Pleasure* (1993, revised 2002) by Barry McCarthy and Emily McCarthy. New York: Carroll & Graf.

This book is written for couples who want to improve their sexual communication, feelings, and functioning. Basic skills are presented within major book sections about comfort and pleasure, enhancing sexual satisfaction, and overcoming sexual problems. The approach utilizes both the research findings of Masters and Johnson and strategies consistent with social-learning theory. A variety of exercises are proposed for each presenting concern. The exercises are meant to provide choices and alternatives to couples, as well as ways they can explore, learn, and improve their sexual relationships. *Sexual Awareness* received very favorable ratings but relatively few evaluations, resulting in a three-star designation.

★★★ *The Soul of Sex* (1998) by Thomas Moore. New York: HarperCollins.

The author describes *The Soul of Sex* as a book about sexuality that contains no information on biology, anatomy, or health, and little about techniques and relationships. He says that the human soul is a composite of meanings: emotions, dreams, wishes, fears, a past, culture, thought, and fantasy. Therefore, he directs the reader to the soul of sex, meaning not the physical only, but a more spiritual and complex integration of all aspects of self. This book is written in a poetic, narrative form that draws on Greek mythology, English literature, and other sources, allowing symbolic representation in expression of meaning and interpretation. The author, a psychotherapist, intends this book to be read by psychotherapists, clients, and others who are drawn to his broader perspective of sex.

★★★ *What Really Happens in Bed* (1989) by Steven Carter and Julia Sokol Coopersmith. New York: M. Evans.

This self-help book presents a broad-based approach to improving sexual competence and relationships for both women and men. It represents an effort to cut through sexual expectations that too often are based on myths and romantic fantasies. The authors interviewed several hundred women and men to provide a profile of what people are really doing and saying in their sexual lives. Section 1, Talking about Sex, explodes a number of sexual myths and unrealistic expectations, and explores why people are reluctant to talk about what really happens in bed. Section II, Sexual Life Patterns and Stages, examines the single life and temporary sexual solutions, sexual fantasies and experimentation, marriage and sex, extramarital affairs, and what people can learn to improve their sex lives. The book includes a number of excerpts from the interviews the authors conducted. On the positive side, it cuts through many sexual myths and includes extensive material about communication and relationships. On the negative side, critics faulted the authors for the unscientific nature of their interviews.

★★★ *For Yourself: The Fulfillment of Female Sexuality* (1975) by Lonnie Barbach. New York: Doubleday.

Barbach addresses the worries that often distress nonorgasmic women and tells them how they can achieve orgasm. She attacks the negative cultural belief that women should not enjoy sex. A number of exercises that will enable women to achieve orgasm are presented, and each exercise is accompanied by an explanation of why it can be effective as well as pitfalls to avoid. The book also includes many examples from the sexual lives of women the author has counseled in her sex therapy groups. How to achieve an orgasm through masturbation and the eventual transfer to orgasms with a partner are covered. This book was very positively rated, but by relatively few experts in our studies. Its enthusiasts said that Barbach sensitively and clearly explains to women how they can achieve a more satisfactory sex life. The book is a bit dated, however.

Diamonds in the Rough

◆ *The Family Book about Sexuality* (1989) by Mary S. Calderone and Eric W. Johnson. New York: Harper & Row.

The authors cite the proliferation of misinformation and myth about sexuality as an important reason to write this book. They want people to understand the sexual part of their lives, the role sex plays in all lives, and the new information learned from research about sexuality. The topic is comprehensively discussed—from the human sexual response, reproduction, and family planning, to the family and its role, people with special problems, and sexually transmitted diseases. The second half of the book is what the authors call the Concise A–Z Encyclopedia, which defines and describes approximately 100 words related to sexuality. This combination of encyclopedia and information guide makes this book unique and useful for those who want to understand the subject more accurately. It is included as a Diamond in the Rough because of its strong rating, albeit by a small number of respondents.

♦ *Male Sexual Awareness* (1998) by Barry McCarthy and Emily McCarthy. New York: Carroll & Graf.

In this comprehensive approach to male sexuality, sexual functioning is addressed in topics such as performance expectations, sexual capacity, loss of sexual desire, masturbation, sexual trauma, contraception, and sexual fantasies. Medical and health issues are described in the sections on vasectomy, ejaculatory problems, sexually transmitted diseases (STDs), HIV, and other difficult subjects. Relational aspects of sexuality span divorce and widow status, marriage, extramarital experience, sexual orientation, and working through new roles in the "gender wars." *Male Sexual Awareness* was given a Diamond in the Rough classification because it was not read by the requisite number of mental health professionals, but it was highly rated by those who did read it.

Strongly Not Recommended

† *Dr. Ruth's Guide to Good Sex* (1983, reissued 1994) by Ruth Westheimer. New York: Warner Books.

† *Dr. Ruth's Guide to Erotic and Sensuous Pleasures* (1991) by Ruth Westheimer and Louis Lieberman. New York: Warner Books.

FILMS

Strongly Recommended

★★★★ *Torch Song Trilogy* (1989) directed by Paul Bogart. R rating. 117 minutes.

A story of gay men struggling to tell their families and friends about their mutual love. Tragedy strikes when one of them is murdered in a senseless killing. The theme is more about love and relationship struggles than about homosexuality. The movie shows the importance of being loved for who we are versus being loved conditionally. A highly regarded and rated film, it is a celebration of the tenacity of the human spirit with its often-thwarted search for love and acceptance.

★★★★ *Kissing Jessica Stein* (2002) directed by Charles Herman-Wurmfeld. R rating. 94 minutes.

Jessica Stein is a fastidious perfectionist who, after a series of hapless dates with hopeless men, decides to "choose" to be lesbian. She dates a bisexual, Heather Juergensen, whose personality is the opposite, experienced and cool. Jessica works enthusiastically with the novelty of lesbian sexuality but in her flightiness she never actually seems to become sexual. Although a comedy, the film does feature a few serious issues about "coming out" to family members. It serves as a light introduction to bisexual experimentation, the matrix of relational and sexual choices, and the discovery that one is not as straight as she (or he) thought.

Recommended

★★★ *Paris Is Burning* (1992) directed by Jennie Livingston. No rating. 78 minutes.

This film depicts an underground lifestyle in Manhattan where gay men work in fashion and dance shows to earn money. During the day, they prepare for the shows, and in the evening they perform. There are multiple story lines with different endings. More of a documentary than a commercial film, but it is effective in reminding clients of the centrality of accepting people for who they are.

★★★ *The Boys in the Band* (1970) directed by William Friedkin. R rating. 120 minutes.

A gathering of gay men at a birthday party turns into a sharing of intimate feelings and needs. At the end of the party, two of the men struggle with their personal relationships. This movie can be comforting for those who struggle with their sexual identity. Discovering oneself in any relationship is never easy, but it is worth the journey.

★★★ *Carnal Knowledge* (1971) directed by Mike Nichols. R rating. 97 minutes.

A story about a pair of college friends whose main mission in life is to meet women and have sex. As time passes, they both struggle to fill the emotional void in an intimate relationship. *Carnal Knowledge* has become a cult classic; whether teen or adult, you will get the messages woven throughout.

Strongly Not Recommended

† *9½ Weeks* (1987) and directed by Adrian Lyne. R rating. 113 minutes.

† *Eyes Wide Shut* (1999) directed by Stanley Kubrick. R rating. 159 minutes.

INTERNET RESOURCES

Metasites

★★★★★ *Society for Human Sexuality* http://www.sexuality.org/index.html

This is likely the premier sexuality information site on the Internet. Clients may benefit from readings under Learning More, such as Erotic Massage, Erotic Talk, Sex Toys, and G-Spot Play. Other topics and areas may too intense for some, such as BDSM (Bondage, Discipline, Slave, Master), Hosting Erotic Events, and Polyamory.

★★★★ *SIECUS: Sexuality Information and Education Council of the United States*
        http://www.siecus.org

"SIECUS is a 35 year old nonprofit organization, dedicated to affirming that sexuality is a natural and healthy part of life. SIECUS develops, collects, and disseminates information, promotes comprehensive education, and advocates the right of individuals to make responsible sexual choices." The Library and Informational Services button leads to the following publications that may be of use: How to Talk to Your Children about AIDS (six pages); fact sheets (typically two to three pages), including Sexually Transmitted Diseases in the United States; Sexual Orientation and Identity; Gay, Lesbian, and Bisexual Adolescents; and Adolescence and Abstinence.

★★★★ *iVillage: Sex*
   http://www.ivillage.com/topics/relation/0,,166914,00.html

For anyone with almost any question on sexuality, there are brief but well-written responses here. The site is well organized and comprehensive. Probably best as a good place to start exploring the vast landscape of human sexuality in an inviting format.

Psychoeducational Materials for Clients and Families

General Sites

★★★★★ *The Society for the Scientific Study of Sexuality*
   http://www.sexscience.org/publications/index.php?category_id=440

Here are three brochures of about three pages each: What Sexual Scientists Know about Compulsive Sexual Behavior, Rape, and Pornography. The contents are empirically based and may be used to counteract clients' hysterical reactions to these hot topics.

★★★★★ *Coalition for Positive Sexuality* http://www.positive.org/Home

This site offers an online tour (called Just Say Yes), with about 12 topics of special concern to sexually active teens (safe sex, birth control, homosexuality, pregnancy, STDs, and should I have sex?), presented without preaching or moralizing. The site is prochoice and in favor of needle exchange. The FAQ has about 10 questions and answers about HIV and other heavy topics such as abortion, sin, and abstinence.

★★★★★ *Guide to Sex for Large Couples* http://www.sexuality.org/l/sex/fatsex.html

The site examines negative attitudes toward the sexuality of fat people and offers clear advice on suitable positions. See also *Guide to Sexual Positions for Large People* at http://www.sexuality.org/l/sex/fatposit.html.

★★★★ *Sexual Disorders* by B. Green, MB http://www.priory.com/sex.htm

A seven-page overview of diagnoses and treatments, suitable as an introduction.

Self-Pleasuring

★★★★★ *Bianca's Good Vibration Masturbation Guide*
   http://www2.bianca.com/shack/goodvibe/masturbate

The site offers advice; directions; encouragement on clitoral, vaginal, G-spot, and anal masturbation for women; and penile, anal, and prostate masturbation for men. Toys, hang-ups, and positive values of masturbation are addressed briefly. A good site for the ambivalent or those with little experience.

Sexually Transmitted Diseases (STDs)

★★★★★ *American Sexual Health Association*
    http://www.ashastd.org/

The best site for STD information. Under the section Facts and Answers about STDS are 14 fact sheets with solid information. Under Programs and Resource Centers are links to several research centers. Under ASHA and CDC Hotlines are five ways to get almost instant answers to all kinds of questions on AIDS, herpes, and cervical cancer.

★★★★ *AVERT: AIDS Education and Research Trust*
    http://www.avert.org/yngindx.htm

This Young People's Section is a set of linked pages with good-quality information for teenagers on puberty, AIDS, homosexuality, relationships, and so on. Quite liberal and very complete.

Gay and Lesbian Issues

★★★★ *Queer Resources Directory* http://www.qrd.org/qrd

The Internet offers thousands of pages on homosexuality, and this is the best site for finding information on families, religion, the workplace, youth, and more.

★★★★ *Valuing a Gay or Lesbian Self-Identity* http://www.ksu.edu/ucs/gay.html

This set of seven linked pages from a university counseling center might be the best place to start for someone who has recently recognized a homosexual identity.

★★★★ *Coming Out* http://www.couns.uiuc.edu/brochures/comout.htm

A two-page brochure from a college counseling center on the process of coming out. Similar are *The Self-Discovery of Being Queer* at http://www.unhcc. unh.edu/resources/ glbt/queer.html, *Sexual Identity* at http://www.psc.uc.edu/sh/sh_ sexual_identity.htm, and *What Are Your Beliefs about Gays and Lesbians?* at http://ub-counseling.buffalo.edu/ orient.html.

Birth Control

★★★★★ *Birth Control*
    http://womenshealth.about.com/cs/birthcontrol/

Links to about 20 sites with complete, independent, and accurate information on birth control.

★★★★★ *Ann Rose's Ultimate Birth Control Links*
    http://www.ultimatebirthcontrol.com

Everything is here—all methods, decisions, and resources.

★★★★★ *Birth Control Methods* http://www.plannedparenthood.org/bc

As you might expect from Planned Parenthood, this site is comprehensive, accurate, detailed, timely, and well-organized. If a client needs any information to assist with making decisions about birth control methods, it is here.

★★★★★ *Emergency Contraception* http://ec.princeton.edu

For those who need to prevent pregnancy after unprotected sexual intercourse, all the methods and information are here.

★★★★★ *Ask NOAH: Family Planning and Contraception*
         http://www.noah-health.org/english/pregnancy/contraception.html

All the methods available are presented and considered in perhaps 100 articles with reliable and complete information.

★★★★ *Hoboken Family Planning: Sex Ed 101* http://www.sex-ed101.com

Some clients are ignorant about sexual health issues. Here they can find current but brief coverage of the facts of contraception, STDs, breast self-examination, mammography, testicular self-examination, and common vaginal infections.

Aging and Sexuality

★★★★ *Sexual Issues for Aging Adults* by Charette A. Dersch, Steven M. Harris, Thomas
         Kimball, James P. Marshall, and Michael A. Negretti
         http://www.hs.ttu.edu/sexuality&aging

This site offers only introductory information, so it may be suitable as introductory reading to orient or disinhibit a client.

★★★★ *Sex and Aging* http://www.sexhealth.org/sexaging/index.shtml

After a short introduction much valuable material is available under the links to Changes in Men, Changes in Women, and Tips for Better Sex Life. There are videos of panel discussions, in RealVideo, and transcripts of them as well.

For Teens

★★★★★ *Teenwire* http://www.teenwire.com

Addressing teen sexuality in an attractive and inviting format, this site from Planned Parenthood can be an source of solid social and medical information for the curious teen.

★★★★★ *All about Sex* http://www.AllAboutSex.org/aas_master_frameset.cfm

The For Teens and For Pre-Teens buttons lead to areas with about 20 articles. One example is First Sexual Intercourse, which offers about 12 pages of information and assistance in deciding and preparing. The Sex for One button goes to a very informative set of pages. The site is progressive and sex-positive and has several articles criticizing statements by members of the religious far right.

★★★★★ *Puberty 101* http://www.puberty101.com

Using a question-and-answer format, this site offers clear and complete information on difficult and important questions. The information on stages of development is unavailable elsewhere on the Internet. Thank you, J. Geoff Malta, MA.

★★★★ *Sex, Etc.* http://www.sxetc.org

Described as "a website by teens for teens," it offers a lot of information and answers. There are back issues of a newsletter here, and the site is searchable. It is sponsored by the Network for Family Life Education at Rutgers University. This could be the first place to refer curious teens for accurate information on gender, harassment, relationships, and other topics.

Hotlines

CDC National STD Hotline
Phone: 800-227-8922

National AIDS Hotline
Phone: 800-342-AIDS; 1-800-344-7432
     Español; 800-243-7889 Deaf Access
     (TTY)

National Gay and Lesbian Hotline
Phone: 888-843-4564

National Herpes Hotline
Phone: 919-361-8488

Teens and AIDS Hotline
Phone: 800-440-TEEN

NATIONAL SUPPORT GROUPS

This is a heterogeneous listing of groups. Some are support groups, others are consciousness-raising groups, and still others are political activism groups.

ACT UP (AIDS Coalition to Unleash Power)
332 Bleecker Street, Suite G5
New York, NY 10014
Phone: 212-966-4873
E-mail: actupny@panix.com
http://www.actupny.org

American Social Health Association
PO Box 13827
Research Triangle Park, NC 27709
Phone: 919-361-8400
E-mail: std-hivnet@ashastd.org
http://www.ashastd.org

Augustine Fellowship, Sex and Love Addicts Anonymous
PO Box 338
Norwood, MA 02062-0338
Phone: 781-255-8825
E-mail: slaaoffice@slaafws.org
http://www.slaafws.org

   A 12-step fellowship based on AA for those who desire to stop living a pattern of sex addiction or obsessive–compulsive sexual behavior.

Codependents of Sex Addicts (COSA)
PO Box 14537
Minneapolis, MN 55414
Phone: 763-537-6904
E-mail: cosa@shore.net

A 12-step program for those in relationships with people who have compulsive sexual behavior.

Dignity/USA
1500 Massachusetts Avenue NW, Suite 11
Washington, DC 20005-1894
Phone: 800-877-8797 or 202-861-0017
E-mail: diginity@aol.com
http://www.dignityusa.org

Organization of lesbian, bisexual, and gay Catholics and their families and friends.

Gay Men's Health Crisis
119 West 24th Street
New York, NY 10011
Phone: 212-807-6655
E-mail: hotline@gmhc.org
http://www.gmhc.org

Information is available in Spanish and Creole.

Family Pride Coalition
PO Box 65327
Washington, DC 20035-5327
Phone: 202-331-5015
E-mail: info@familypride.org
http://www.familypride.org

LLEGO (National Latino/a Lesbian and Gay Organization)
1420 K Street NW, Suite 200
Washington, DC 20005
Phone: 202-408-5380
http://www.llego.org

NARAL (National Abortion and Reproductive Rights Action League)
1156 15th Street, Suite 700
Washington, DC 20005
Phone: 202-973-3000
http://www.naral.org

National Advocacy Coalition on Youth and Sexual Orientation
1711 Connecticut Avenue NW, Suite 206
Washington, DC 20009
Phone: 202-319-7596

National Association of People with AIDS
1413 K Street NW
Washington, DC 20005-3405
Phone: 202-898-0414
E-mail: napwa@napwa.org
http://www.napwa.org

!OUTPROUD! (The National Coalition for Gay, Lesbian and Bisexual Youth)
369 Third Street, Suite B-362
San Rafael, CA 94901
Phone: 415-460-5452
E-mail: info@outproud.org
http://www.outproud.org

PFLAG (Parents and Friends of Lesbians and Gays)
1726 M Street, Suite 400
Washington, DC 20036
Phone: 202-467-8180
http://www.pflag.org

Planned Parenthood
810 Seventh Avenue
New York, NY 10019
Phone: 212-541-7800
E-mail: communications@ppfa.org
http://www.plannedparenthood.org

Sex Addicts Anonymous
PO Box 70949
Houston, TX 77270
Phone: 713-869-4902
E-mail: info@saa-recovery.org
http://www.sexaa.org

A 12-step program of recovery from compulsive sexual behavior.

Sexual Compulsives Anonymous
PO Box 1585
Old Chelsea Station
New York, NY 10011
Phone: 800-977-4325
E-mail: info@sca-recovery.org
http://www.sca-recovery.org

The Society for the Scientific Study of Sexuality
PO Box 416
Allentown, PA 18105
Phone: 610-530-2483
E-mail: thesociety@inetmail.att.net
http://www.sexscience.org

See also Love and Intimacy (Chapter 22), Marriage (Chapter 23), and Teenagers and Parenting (Chapter 34).

CHAPTER 31

Spiritual and Existential Concerns

Spirituality is far more than formalized religion. It's not simply a prayer we say on the Sabbath, but a prayerful life we live. Spirituality resides within our intellect, our emotions, our physical existence, and our daily lives.

The mental health professions and self-help authors have recently rediscovered the centrality of spirituality. But understanding spirituality is not new. More than 400 years ago, St. Ignatius compiled his notes into the *Spiritual Exercises,* a practical guide on discernment and living a life of spirituality.

Spirituality is inevitably concerned with the elusive search for the purpose and meaning of life. These existential concerns focus on life's ultimate questions—freedom, existence, meaning, authenticity, and death. Life, existence itself, is in a constant state of becoming; to live in the moment is a dynamic process of person and environment experiencing life.

In this chapter, we critically consider self-help books and Internet resources devoted to an assortment of spiritual and existential concerns.

SELF-HELP BOOKS

Strongly Recommended

★★★★★ *Man's Search for Meaning* (revised ed., 1998) by Viktor Frankl. New York: Pocket Books.

Viktor Frankl, a professor of psychiatry at the University of Vienna, takes an existential approach to the pursuit of self-fulfillment. After Frankl survived the German concen-

RECOMMENDATION HIGHLIGHTS

Self-Help Books

- For an existential approach to life and self-fulfillment:

  ★★★★★ *Man's Search for Meaning* by Viktor Frankl

- For rediscovering the joy of everyday life:

  ★★★★ *Finding Flow* by Mihaly Csikszentmihalyi

- For a spiritual approach to meaning and self-fulfillment:

  ★★★★ *The Road Less Traveled* by M. Scott Peck

  ★★★★ *When All You Ever Wanted Isn't Enough* by Harold Kushner

- For an inner-healing, mind–body approach to self-improvement:

  ★★★★ *Peace, Love, and Healing* by Bernie Siegel

- For finding one's way out of psychological pain:

  ★★★ *The Power of Now* by Eckhart Tolle

- For prayer and a religious approach to self-fulfillment:

  ★★★ *Illuminata* by Marianne Williamson

  ◆ *Sacred Contracts* by Caroline Myss

Internet Resources

- For the effect of depression on spiritual life:

  ★★★★★ *Depression and Spiritual Growth*
  http://chandra.astro.indiana.edu/bipolar/spirit.html

tration camp at Auschwitz, he founded a school of psychotherapy he called logotherapy, which maintains that the desire to find a meaning in life is the primary human motive. His mother, father, brother, and wife died in the concentration camps. Frankl emphasizes each person's uniqueness and the finiteness of life. He thinks that examining the finiteness of existence and the certainty of death adds meaning to life. Frankl believes that the three most distinct human qualities are spirituality, freedom, and responsibility. Spirituality, in his system, does not have a religious underpinning. Rather, it refers to a human being's uniqueness—to spirit, philosophy, and mind. Freedom is the freedom to make decisions. With the freedom to make decisions is responsibility for those decisions. Logotherapists often ask clients such questions as why they exist, what they want from life, and what the meaning of their life is. Originally published in 1946, *Man's Search for Meaning* is a five-star classic that still commands a great deal of respect among mental health professionals. This book challenges readers to think about the meaning of their lives. The reading is rough going at times, but for those who persist and probe Frankl's remarkable insights, the rewards are well worth the effort.

★★★★ *Finding Flow: The Psychology of Engagement with Everyday Life* (1997) by Mihaly Csikszentmihalyi. New York: Basic Books.

Csikszentmihalyi (pronounced "chik-sent-mee-high-yee") has been investigating the concept he calls "flow" for more than two decades. Flow is the state of deep enjoyment that people feel when they have a sense of mastering something. Supported by a number of research studies, this self-help resource addresses how people can better structure their everyday lives in joyful ways. What we do in our day can largely determine what kind of life we live, and how we emotionally experience what we do is even more important. When in flow, what we feel, what we wish, and what we think are in harmony. This excellent, four-star book offers engaging, research-supported information on creating and discovering flow in everyday life. The quality of life depends on what we do with what we have.

★★★★ *When All You Ever Wanted Isn't Enough* (1986) by Harold Kushner. New York: Summit.

Harold Kushner, rabbi and author of *When Bad Things Happen to Good People* (evaluated in Chapter 15), here offers a spiritual message of self-fulfillment. Subtitled *The Search for a Life That Matters*, the book maintains that material rewards create almost as many problems as they solve. Kushner believes that sooner or later we come face to face with a big question: What am I supposed to do with my life? We want to be more than just brief biological flashes in the universe that disappear forever. Kushner argues that there is no single, big answer to the meaning of life, but that there are answers. And the answers are found in filling day-to-day existence with meaning, with the love of friends and family, and with striving for integrity, instead of just reaching for the pot of gold. Kushner spends considerable time analyzing the biblical book of Ecclesiastes, because it asks us to think about life. Kushner believes, like the message in Ecclesiastes, that life is its own reward.

★★★★ *Peace, Love, and Healing* (1989) by Bernie Siegel. New York: Harper & Row.

Bernie Siegel, a surgeon and the best-selling author of *Love, Medicine and Miracles,* offers an inner resource to self-healing. Siegel believes that the medical field has ignored the power of self-healing for too long and argues that modern medicine and self-healing are not mutually exclusive. Among the self-healing techniques he recommends are meditation, visualization, relaxation, and developing peace of mind. Siegel describes a number of exceptional patients who used self-healing to improve physical and mental well-being. Although *Peace, Love, and Healing* received a four-star rating, it is controversial in the medical field. Some physicians feel that Siegel exaggerates the power of self-healing and that his ideas may keep some people from seeking medical treatment. Siegel's supporters among the mental health professionals say that he has inspired many patients, nurses, medical students, and even some doctors to look at healing in a larger context and to look at illnesses in new ways.

★★★★ *The Road Less Traveled* (1978) by M. Scott Peck. New York: Simon & Schuster.

This spiritual and psychological approach to life has been on best-seller lists for more than 10 years. M. Scott Peck, a psychiatrist, begins the book by stating that life is difficult and that we all suffer pain and disappointment. He counsels us to face up to life's difficulties and not be lazy. Indeed, Peck equates laziness with original sin, going on to say that people's tendency to avoid problems and emotional suffering is the root of mental disorders. Peck also believes that people are thirsting for integrity in their lives. They are not happy with a country that has "In God We Trust" as a motto and at the same time leads the world in the arms race. To achieve integrity, says Peck, people need to move spirituality into all aspects of their daily lives. Peck speaks of four important tools to use in life's journey: delayed gratification, acceptance of responsibility, dedication to the truth, and balance. After a thorough analysis of each, Peck explores the will to use them, which he calls love. Then he analyzes the relationship of growth and religion, which leads him to examine the final step of the road less traveled: grace. By grace, Peck means the whole range of human activities that support the human spirit. This immensely popular, four-star resource has developed a cultlike following, especially among young people. Peck has obviously recognized important voids in many people's lives, especially the need for an integrated, spiritually oriented existence. While many of Peck's ideas are not new, he has succeeded in packaging them in contemporary American language that has enormous appeal.

Recommended

★★★ *The Power of Now: A Guide to Spiritual Enlightenment* (1999) by Eckhart Tolle. Novata, CA: New World Library.

Though written in simple language and in a question-and-answer format, the book takes the reader on a spiritual and religious journey. We are not our mind; we can find our way out of psychological pain when we surrender to the now. Tolle helps us see that our relationships are yet another doorway into spiritual enlightenment if we use them wisely, if we use them to become more conscious and, therefore, more loving human beings. The result is real communication between self and others looking to be truly present. Drawing on the teachings of religious masters such as Jesus and Buddha, the book is designed to help on the spiritual journey through life.

★★★ *Further Along the Road Less Traveled* (2nd ed., 1998) by M. Scott Peck. New York: Touchstone.

Peck, the best-selling author of *The Road Less Traveled* (reviewed above), starts this book with the phrase "Life is complex." He describes the road each person has to travel as a rocky wilderness through which we must carve out our own individual paths. Searching for individual meaning and the center of spirituality is woven throughout this book. The author encourages us to glory in the mystery of life and not to be dismayed. Peck's book is interesting for the self-motivated layperson and the mental health professional. The author applauds the scientific advances of medicine but cautions of the danger of losing the centrality of psychological wisdom and of neglecting our spirituality.

★★★ *Care of the Soul* (1992) by Thomas Moore. New York: HarperCollins.

Moore, a former Catholic monk and presently a psychotherapist, makes a case for the loss of soul as the great malady of the 20th century. The soul is embodied in genuineness and depth, and is revealed in attachment, love, and community. This best-selling book is about living a soulful life. Moore repeatedly distinguishes between spirituality and soul. Those interested in the influence of philosophy and religion coupled with a modern view of spirituality and soulfulness will find this book both challenging and enlightening.

★★★ *The Seven Spiritual Laws of Success: A Practical Guide to the Fulfillment of Your Dreams* (1994) by Deepak Chopra. San Rafael, CA: Amber-Allen.

This book shatters the myth that success is the result of hard work, planning, and driving ambition. Chopra, a best-selling author, distills the way to create a successful and fulfilling personal life into seven principles. Essentially, personal understanding and harmony help promote fulfilling relationships. The overriding message is that once we understand our true nature and live in harmony with natural law, a sense of well-being, health, fulfilling relationships, enthusiasm, and mental satisfaction will flow effortlessly. This is a book you can reference time and again. It is for anyone looking for a spiritual and human perspective on living a successful life.

★★★ *Your Sacred Self* (2001) by Wayne W. Dyer. New York: Quill.

Popular self-help author Dyer concerns himself here with the sacred self, in which the spirit triumphs over the ego. Dyer advances a three-step plan: preparing for the sacred journey; implementing the keys to higher awareness; and transcending our ego identities toward the pursuit of an ego-less world. A book for the person desiring to become closer to his or her spiritual self.

★★★ *Flow: The Psychology of Optimal Experience* (1990) by Mihaly Csikszentmihalyi. New York: HarperCollins.

Flow is a state of enjoyable concentration in which a person becomes absorbed while engaging in an activity. We can develop flow by setting challenges for ourselves, by stretching ourselves to the limit, by developing competent coping skills, and by combining life's many experiences into a meaningful pattern. Flow can be found in many different experiences and walks of life. Rock climbers can become so absorbed that they feel at one with the cliff face. Chess masters play in a trancelike state. Artists dab paint on a canvas hour after hour in a state of immersed concentration. The famous humanistic psychologist Abraham Maslow described a similar sense of euphoria in the early 1960s. What distinguishes Csikszentmihalyi's concept of flow from Maslow's peak experiences is the frequency of flow experiences. Maslow thought people were fortunate if they caught a peak experience several times in their entire lives; Csikszentmihalyi, by contrast, says that if people cultivate flow experiences, they can have them several times a day. This three-star resource documents that the path to happiness does not lie in mindless hedonism but rather in mindful challenges. It is a serious, thoroughly documented, and well-researched book, but our mental health experts preferred Csikszentmihalyi's newer book, *Finding Flow,* reviewed earlier in this chapter.

★★★ *Illuminata: Thoughts, Prayers, Rites of Passage* (1994) by Marianne Williamson. New York: Random House.

A number-one best-seller, this book attempts to bring prayer into our daily life. Williamson provides prayers designed to heal our souls, hearts, body, and country. The prayers are designed for people of all ages and traverse the human experience—prayers to release anger, find forgiveness, discover great love, and achieve intimacy. Another section includes rites of passage, ceremonies for the signal events in our lives, blessing of the newborn, coming of age, marriage, and death. The author concludes that through prayer, we find what we cannot find elsewhere: a peace that is not of this world. A book for the young and old who find prayer an important part of their lives.

Diamonds in the Rough

♦ *Sacred Contracts: Awakening Your Divine Potential* (2001) by Caroline Myss. New York: Harmony.

This book addresses the question, "Why are we here?" The author guides readers in finding their divine potential by various approaches, one being to "pray for guidance," and another being to identify the underlying patterns of thought that color memories. The author writes that, after many thousands of readings, "I came to the conclusion that an organizing principle even greater than the interplay of the chakras is shaping the energy within each of us—and shaping our lives as it does so." Highly but rarely rated in our national studies, this book that will probably appeal to the spiritually inclined.

♦ *The American Paradox: Spiritual Hunger in an Age of Plenty* (2000) by David G. Myers. New Haven, CT: Yale University Press.

Myers reflects on the paradox of the richest country in the world having so many of its citizens growing less content with their lives. He notes that, since the 1960s, divorce rates have doubled, teen suicide has tripled, violent crime has quadrupled, and prison populations have quintupled. He believes the explanations for the paradox are individualism, the commercial culture, and normalizing of the worst of human behavior. Myers argues for a return to moral education; he states, "Religion is good for us." Less a self-help book than a cultural critique, it is nonetheless rich in reflective observations and cogent criticisms of individual and societal responsibility. A book for all to read and ponder.

♦ *The Search for Significance* (1990) by Robert McGee. Houston, TX: Rapha.

The Christian spiritual approach taken by this book suggests that self-fulfillment comes not from the ability to please others, but from the love and forgiveness of Jesus Christ. In Part I, McGee discusses the search for significance, good and evil, the process of hope and healing, and how a Christ-based approach is the only path to self-fulfillment and happiness in life. Part II is an extensive workbook, with many religiously based exercises. In two of our studies, *The Search for Significance* was positively rated, but by only 11 and 9 psychologists, respectively, thus receiving the designation of Diamond in the

Rough. This is a much stronger religious approach to life's meaning than the other spiritually based books in this category—for example, M. Scott Peck's *The Road Less Traveled* and Harold Kushner's *When All You've Ever Wanted Isn't Enough*. It will appeal mainly to Christians who seek self-fulfillment through religious commitment.

Not Recommended

★★ *The Celestine Prophecy: An Adventure* (1993) by James Redfield. New York: Warner Books.

★ *The Be (Happy) Attitudes* (1985) by Robert Schuller. Waco, TX: Word.

Strongly Not Recommended

† *The Way of the Wizard: Twenty Spiritual Lessons in Creating the Life You Want* (1995) by Deepak Chopra. New York: Harmony.

† *Clear Body, Clear Mind* (1990) by L. Ron Hubbard. Los Angeles: Bridge.

† *Dianetics: The Modern Science of Mental Health* (1950, reissued 2002) by L. Ron Hubbard. Los Angeles: Church of Scientology of California.

† *Scientology: The Fundamentals of Thought* (1988) by L. Ron Hubbard. Los Angeles: Bridge.

INTERNET RESOURCES

The Internet has exploded of late with a burgeoning interest in the intersection of religion and psychology, especially in psychotherapy, healing, and growth. In truth, all the concerns in this book contain existential and spiritual components. Yet, of the hundreds of mental health sites we reviewed, only a few had entries under religion or spirituality.

Of course, there are enormous numbers of links to specific religious traditions, especially Asian, and to alternative medicine. Sites in this area range from flaky (e.g., channeling, lightwork) to part psychological (e.g., transcendental meditation), to actively hostile (e.g., Scientology). We have excluded the sites of specific religions, science versus religion, and forms of existential psychotherapy.

Psychoeducational Materials for Clients and Families

★★★ *Religion and Spirituality*
    http://www.pastoralcounseling.net/religionandspirituality.html

A short page from a book by Jean G. Fitzpatrick on the differences between religion and spirituality, suggesting the need to live a spiritual life beyond the religious one.

★★★ *Psychotherapy and Spirituality Institute* http://www.mindspirit.org

Although sponsored by an organization of therapists in New York, this site offers some essays that address various aspects of living and relating.

★★★ *Psychology of Religion Pages* http://psychwww.com/psyrelig/index.htm

"This is a general introduction to the psychology of religion, for example, as it is studied by scientists in Division 36 of the American Psychological Association. Here you will find a description of what psychologists have learned about how religion influences people's lives." This may be useful for people who are struggling with social and psychological (but not spiritual) aspects of their faith. There are two dozen very relevant readings.

Other Resources

★★★ *Religious Studies Internet Links*
http://www.wlu.ca/~wwwrandc/internet_links.html

An excellent starting point, with links to collections and guides on religion and philosophy.

★★★ *John Templeton Foundation* http://www.templeton.org

After having made millions in international investing, Templeton set up a foundation to fund research on forgiveness, optimism, spirituality, and health, and to award a large monetary prize annually for progress in religion.

CHAPTER 32

Stress Management and Relaxation

We live in a stress-filled world. According to the American Academy of Family Physicians, almost two-thirds of all office visits to family doctors are for stress-related symptoms. Stress is also thought to be a major contributor to coronary disease, accidental injuries, cirrhosis of the liver, and suicide—four of the leading causes of death in the United States. Several of the best-selling drugs in the United States are antianxiety (Xanax, Ativan, Klonopin) and ulcer (Tagamet, Zantac) medications.

There are many ways to cope effectively with stress, just as there are many ways to cope ineffectively with stress. Converging research suggests that the most effective approach is to employ a variety of strategies instead of relying on a single method. For example, people who have had heart attacks are usually advised to change more than one aspect of their lives. The advice might go something like this: Practice relaxation; lose weight; confide in good friends; quit smoking; begin to exercise several times a week; reduce your anger; and take vacations on a regular basis. One of these alone may not turn the tide against stress, but a combination will maximize success.

In this chapter, we evaluate self-help books and Internet resources that deal directly with relaxation and stress management. Many other self-help resources reviewed in this book also provide advice on coping with stress; consult in particular Chapters 6 (Anger), 7 (Anxiety Disorders), 8 (Assertiveness), 14 (Communication and People Skills), and 29 (Self-Management and Self-Enhancement). In addition, for stress stemming from a particular source, such as career problems, the death of a loved one, or divorce, the recommended resources in those chapters may be appropriate.

RECOMMENDATION HIGHLIGHTS

Self-Help Books

- For comprehensive strategies to reduce stress:

  ★★★★★　*The Relaxation and Stress Reduction Workbook* by Martha Davis et al.

  ★★★★★　*The Stress and Relaxation Handbook* by James Madders

- For learning meditation and mindfulness:

  ★★★★★　*Wherever You Go, There You Are* by Jon Kabat-Zinn

- For mind–body, behavioral medicine approach to combating stress:

  ★★★★★　*The Wellness Book* by Herbert Benson and Eileen M. Stuart

  ★★★★　*Why Zebras Don't Get Ulcers* by Robert M. Sapolsky

- For learning relaxation to cope with stress:

  ★★★★★　*The Relaxation Response* by Herbert Benson

  ★★★★　*Beyond the Relaxation Response* by Herbert Benson

  ★★★　*Learn to Relax* by C. Eugene Walker

- For a spiritually based approach to coping with stress:

  ★★★★　*Each Day a New Beginning* by the Hazelden Foundation

  ★★★　*Touchstones* by the Hazelden Foundation

Internet Resources

- For alleviating headaches:

  ★★★★　*The Excedrin Headache Resource Center* http://www.excedrin.com

- For learning relaxation:

  ★★★★　*Basic Guided Relaxation* http://www.dstress.com/guided.htm

SELF-HELP BOOKS

Strongly Recommended

★★★★★　*The Relaxation and Stress Reduction Workbook* (5th ed., 2000) by Martha Davis, Elizabeth Robbins Eshelman, and Matthew McKay. Oakland, CA: New Harbinger.

This five-star workbook can be used as a general reference and a valuable resource to learn how to relax and manage stress in a number of environments. Now in its fifth edition, the book provides straightforward instructions on a variety of stress management techniques. The first two chapters are designed to help examine personal reactions to stress and understand the dynamics of stress and stressors. The book is easy to read and is accompanied by pictures of proper body positioning for specific techniques. The highest rated book in this category and among the most favorably evaluated in all our national studies, it is useful for laypersons in reducing stress and for professionals as a reference when using homework assignments with their clients. A very popular and apparently effective resource.

★★★★★ *Wherever You Go, There You Are* (1994) by Jon Kabat-Zinn. New York: Hyperion.

This book is a practical guide to meditation—in essence, a book about mindfulness/wakefulness. Psychologist Kabat-Zinn repeatedly reminds us that the moment is all we really have. To allow ourselves to be in the moment, we have to pause in our experience long enough to let the present moment sink in. Meditation is simply about being oneself and knowing something about who that is. Mindfulness has to do, above all, with attention and awareness. This engaging five-star resource will be of value to both the beginning and the experienced practitioner of meditation.

★★★★★ *The Stress and Relaxation Handbook: A Practical Guide to Self-Help Techniques* (1997) by James Madders. London: Vermilion.

Fully illustrated throughout, this book contains relaxation exercises to apply throughout the day. There are techniques designed for children, adults, and older adults. Some exercises are designed to help manage the pain and tension found in such problems as migraine, insomnia, digestive disorders, and the menstrual cycle. The message here is that we all suffer emotionally and physically from the strain of life, but that our reactions can be modified and controlled by training. Chapters begin with factual information about stress, our reactions to stress, and how we can reduce the negative effect of stress with proper relaxation techniques. The book was rated very favorably in our national studies, earning a five-star rating.

★★★★★ *The Relaxation Response* (1975) by Herbert Benson. New York: Morrow.

This influential book presents a particular strategy for reducing stress—learning how to relax. Benson believes that the relaxation response can significantly improve a person's ability to cope with stressful circumstances and can reduce the likelihood of a number of diseases, especially heart attacks and strokes. He points out that the relaxation response has been used for centuries in the context of religious teachings, usually in Eastern cultures, where it often is practiced on a daily basis. Benson developed a simple method of attaining the relaxation response and explains how to incorporate it into daily life. The relaxation response consists of four essential elements: (1) locating a quiet context; (2) developing a mental device, such as a word or phrase (e.g., *om*) that is repeated in a precise way over and over again; (3) adopting a passive attitude, which involves letting go of thoughts and distractions; and (4) assuming a comfortable position. Practicing the relaxation response 15–20 minutes once or twice a day improves well-being, according to the research. This important, five-star book was published at a time when Americans were skeptical about the spiritual and psychological practices of Eastern cultures. Many mental health professionals recommend Benson's approach to their clients because they have found that it works. The relaxation response is a simple, effective, self-healing technique for reducing stress.

★★★★★ *The Wellness Book: A Comprehensive Guide to Maintaining Health and Treating Stress Related Illness* (1992) by Herbert Benson and Eileen M. Stuart. New York: Fireside.

This book, coauthored by Benson of *The Relaxation Response* fame (reviewed above), is a comprehensive guide to implementing behavioral medicine into life and to treating stress-related diseases. Behavioral medicine combines the talents of mind and body, and uses psychological approaches to prevent illness and improve health. This book covers numerous wellness topics, principally the relaxation response, nutrition, exercise, body awareness, cognitive restructuring, stress management, coping, problem solving, and humor. This five-star book was highly rated by the experts in our national studies as an excellent and practical guide to mind–body interaction, but many advised that people should undertake major lifestyle changes under the supervision of a health care professional. The book provides sound advice for preventing disease and improving health, presents up-to-date material on the role of stress in disease, and is especially good at describing the powerful role of relaxation in reducing chances of incurring life-threatening diseases.

★★★★ *Beyond the Relaxation Response* (1984) by Herbert Benson. New York: Times Books.

This is Herbert Benson's sequel to *The Relaxation Response* (reviewed above). A decade after Benson coined the term *relaxation response,* he concluded that combining it with another strategy is even more powerful in combating stress. The other strategy is faith in a healing power either inside or outside the self. Benson arrived at this conclusion because of his own clinical studies of Tibetan monks in the Himalayas, which are described in detail in this book. The healing power can be belief in a certain dogma or a traditional religious system, or it can be faith in oneself, in the state attained while exercising, or in the relaxation response itself. Benson explains how to harness the power of faith in a number of different situations—while jogging, walking, swimming, lying in bed, or praying. *Beyond the Relaxation Response* is a four-star book that clearly conveys the power of mental strategies in influencing health and the healing process.

★★★★ *Minding the Body, Mending the Mind* (1987) by Joan Borysenko. New York: Bantam.

This book is mainly about the positive effects of relaxation on the mind and body. The author discusses how deep relaxation and meditation can shift disease-promoting physiological mechanisms into a healing mode. The focus of the book is on reducing anxiety and developing control over one's life. It also serves as a guide for conditioning the mind to function as a healer and health enhancer. The general public can use this book as a guide to coping with stress and disease more effectively. For those interested in the mind–body relationship to healing, this will be an informative resource. A solid book and a solid message.

★★★★ *Why Zebras Don't Get Ulcers: A Guide to Stress, Stress-Related Diseases and Coping* (revised ed., 1998) by Robert M. Sapolsky. New York: Freeman.

Drawing on current scientific research, this provocative and often amusing book looks at the interconnections between emotion and physical well-being. Sapolsky discusses the interactions between the body and the mind, and the ways in which emotions can affect the health of virtually every cell in the body. Stress and our vulnerability to disease are best understood in the context of the person who is suffering from that disease. Links are made between stress and increased risk for certain diseases, with specific chapters on the circulatory system, energy storage, growth, reproduction, the immune system, depression, and the aging process. The last chapter describes how to manage stress. For the interested reader or professional working with stressed clients, this is a very informative, four-star book. It is a scientific book for the nonscientist.

★★★★ *Don't Sweat the Small Stuff . . . and It's All Small Stuff* (1995) by Richard J.
       Carlson. New York: Hyperion.

Carlson offers meditations designed to help people keep their lives in perspective, giving priority to the important things. The book consists of 100 very brief, themed chapters that provide inspirational advice for individuals and help them understand why they shouldn't worry so much about life's minor irritations. A brief and focused bestseller. (Also reviewed in Chapter 29, Self-Management and Self-Enhancement.)

★★★★ *Each Day a New Beginning: Daily Meditations for Women* (1982, reissued 1996) by
       Karen Casey. Minneapolis: Hazelden Foundation.

This book of daily meditations for women follows the same format of *One Day at a Time in Al-Anon* and *A Day at a Time*, the daily meditative books described in Chapter 3. Each page of the book is devoted to one day—from January 1 through December 31—and contains three elements: a beginning quotation, a daily thought or meditation, and an ending self-affirmation. The book is a spiritually oriented approach for women coping with a wide array of stressors, not just addictions. Each day is perceived as a new opportunity for growth and successful coping. *Each Day a New Beginning* is well-conceived and presents thought-provoking ideas in a warm, personal tone. The book is especially appealing to women with a spiritual orientation.

Recommended

★★★ *Learn to Relax* (3rd ed., 1991) by C. Eugene Walker. New York: Berkley.

This book provides multiple methods for learning how to relax, including cognitive therapy, life structuring, realistic goal setting, relaxation exercises, assertion, nutrition, exercise, communication, friendships, self-hypnosis, and professional help. The book's subtitle—*Proven Techniques for Reducing Stress, Tension, Anxiety, and Promoting Peak Performance*—says it all. Psychologist Walker cleverly covers most of the relaxation territory with a minimum of jargon.

★★★ *Touchstones* (1986, reissued 1996) by the Hazelden Foundation. New York:
       HarperCollins.

This is the male counterpart of *Each Day a New Beginning* (reviewed above). It is a spiritually based approach to coping with stress for men, with each page devoted to a day of the year—from January 1 through December 31—and contains a quotation, a meditative commentary, and a self-affirming statement. The breadth of the quotations is extensive, ranging from comments by former New York Yankees baseball manager Billy Martin to passages from D. H. Lawrence and poems by Emily Dickinson. The meditative thoughts also are broad, from awareness of one's problems to letting go, to confession. The meditative commentary is warm and supportive, and the self-affirmations are motivating. This book will especially appeal to men with a spiritual orientation who are having difficulty coping with life's stress.

★★★   *The Male Stress Syndrome* (1986) by Georgia Witkin-Lanoil. New York: Berkley.

This self-help resource was written by a woman for men and presents strategies for helping men cope effectively with stress. Combining the results of a survey administered to more than 500 men and the women closest to them, with examples from her own clinical practice, Witkin-Lanoil isolates the key stressors common to most men. She also provides suggestions on how to recognize these factors and manage them. Relaxation exercises are among the suggested strategies for males. Some stress-reduction strategies are tailored to specific male problems, such as sex therapy for sex-related problems. This three-star book provides a good understanding of male-related stress factors and ways to reduce them.

Diamond in the Rough

♦ *Inner and Outer Peace through Meditation* (1996) by Rajinder Singh. Rockport, MA: Element.

The author has codified simple exercises, coupled with spiritual guidance and his own meditation experience, to help people achieve freedom from fear and achieve contentment. Singh explains how peace can be created by meditation and inner reflection. He connects the workings of inner (self) and outer (world) peace. The key to genuine world peace is inner peace founded on interpersonal respect and love. To create inner peace, it is necessary to calm the mind; hence, the importance of meditation. Highly but infrequently rated, thus earning Diamond in the Rough classification, this is a book for those who are already meditating or seeking to learn the art of meditation.

INTERNET RESOURCES

Psychoeducational Materials for Clients and Families

★★★★   *The Excedrin Headache Resource Center* http://www.excedrin.com

Although you cannot avoid the commercial aspects of this site, there are many educational materials on the types, causes, nonmedical treatment, and effects of headaches.

★★★★   *Basic Guided Relaxation: Advanced Technique* by L. John Mason, PhD
          http://www.dstress.com/guided.htm

A very good, four-page script.

★★★ *Progressive Muscle Relaxation* by R. Richmond, PhD
   http://members.aol.com/avpsyrich/pmr.htm
A five-page brochure on how to do progressive muscle relaxation.

★★★ *Stress Management* http://www.couns.uiuc.edu/brochures/stress.htm
A clear, two-page handout from a university counseling center.

★★ *Mastering Your Stress Demons* by Joseph Napora http://www.intelihealth.com
At the Intellihealth.com site, search for this title or for "stress." About 10 pages of a general talk Napora gave on what he calls "centering" to manage stress.

★★ *Meditation, Guided Fantasies, and Other Stress Reducers*
   http://www.shpm.com/articles/stress
At Self-Help and Psychology Magazine, there are some relaxing nature pictures, inspiring thoughts, and one- to two-page essays on stress topics.

See also Anxiety Disorders (Chapter 7), Communication and People Skills (Chapter 14), and Self-Management and Self-Enhancement (Chapter 29).

CHAPTER 33

Suicide

Suicide is a real and rising crisis. It is this country's 10th leading cause of death and the third leading cause of death among adolescents. Literally millions of people are struggling with thoughts of hurting themselves and battling the impulse to kill themselves. And it only takes one "successful" attempt to become a fatality.

Individuals contemplating or committing suicide are not the only people affected. Families, friends, and psychotherapists are continually worried about suicide contemplators. Those who commit suicide leave behind numerous friends and family members who will forever struggle to understand and accept the loss. The survivors may feel guilty and responsible, intensifying their grief.

In this chapter, we review mental health professionals' ratings on self-help resources that address (1) how to prevent suicide, (2) how to help people contemplating suicide, and (3) how to survive a loss due to suicide. We present self-help books, autobiographies, films, and Internet resources on this real and rising crisis.

SELF-HELP BOOKS

Recommended

★★★ *Choosing to Live* (1996) by Thomas Ellis and Cory F. Newman. Oakland, CA: New Harbinger.

A sensitive and persuasive case is made for choosing to live when confronted with suicidal impulses. This is one of the few cognitive therapy books that focuses specifically on suicidal risk. The message is written in the first person, directly to the reader, yet it is clear that the authors intend for the book to be used as an adjunct to psychotherapy. An appendix includes excellent guidelines for concerned family and friends on the warning signs, what to do, and what to do if the person refuses help. An early self-assessment asks readers to explore the hopeful versus the dark side of suicide. Ellis and Newman

---

RECOMMENDATION HIGHLIGHTS

Self-Help Books

- For individuals at high risk for suicide and their families:

    ★★★ *Choosing to Live* by Thomas Ellis and Cory F. Newman

- For partners of those who have committed suicide:

    ◆ *No Time to Say Goodbye* by Carla Fine

Autobiographies

- For a personal look at suicide by an authority and a survivor:

    ★★★★★ *Night Falls Fast* by Kay R. Jamison

Films

- On healing with psychotherapy after a suicide attempt:

    ★★★★★ *Ordinary People*

- On the trauma of a girl who announces and then commits suicide:

    ★★★★ *'Night, Mother*

- On the inexplicable suicide of teenage girls:

    ★★★★ *The Virgin Suicides*

- On stressors leading to a suicide attempt:

    ★★★★ *The Hospital*

Internet Resources

- On understanding suicide:

    ★★★★★ *American Society of Suicidology* http://www.suicidology.org

- On surviving a suicide crisis:

    ★★★★★ *A Comprehensive Approach to Suicide Prevention*
    http://www.lollie.com/suicide.html

    ★★★★★ *Suicide Prevention Help*
    http://members.tripod.com/~suicideprevention/index.html

    ★★★★ *Befrienders International*
    http://www.befrienders.org/mainindex.htm

---

present two profiles of suicide risk: the depressed and hopeless person, who needs restoration of hope and reduction of negative thinking; and the person with control concerns and communication problems, who needs reduction of conflict and problem-solving skills. The book offers a clear and well-developed series of steps on what one can do now: surviving the crisis, understanding one's own feelings and thoughts, implementing the cognitive treatment plan, looking forward to feeling better through coping, and solving one's problems without dying. *Choosing to Live* is an excellent choice for those at risk and their families. One of the most favorably rated self-help resources in our national studies, but not rated frequently enough to receive a five-star designation.

Diamond in the Rough

♦ *Living When a Young Friend Commits Suicide* (1999) by Earl A. Grollman and Max Malikow. Boston: Beacon.

The purpose of this book is to help those individuals who have lost friends or family members to suicide by answering questions often asked and some not so often asked. Adolescent and young adult suicide is implied in the title as the focus; however, the book can be equally helpful in other relationships. The chapters are clustered into themes of coming to grips with the reality of the suicide, the need to cope with the experience, and to continue with one's life. The needs to know why and to understand how people can feel boxed in, with no way out, are explained. The authors sensitively consider decisions about participation in the immediate grieving, such as attending the funeral, returning to school, and visiting the family. An informative section addresses the myths and misconceptions about suicide, such as "attempts are gestures of looking for attention," "it runs in the family," and "the friend had everything going for him(her)." A fine self-help resource not yet frequently known by the experts in our national studies.

AUTOBIOGRAPHIES

Strongly Recommended

★★★★★ *Night Falls Fast: Understanding Suicide* (2001) by Kay Redfield Jamison. New York: Vintage.

Not an easy topic to write about, but Kay Jamison brings to the task impressive credentials in this comprehensive yet personal book. Psychologist Jamison is one of the foremost authorities on mood disorders, in which suicide is a serious risk. She had a lifelong struggle with bipolar disorder, planned for her own suicide at 17, and made her first attempt at age 28. She considers suicide, especially in young people, to be a preventable public health problem. She identifies groups most at risk; the psychology of suicide notes; methods used to take one's life (including popular locations such as San Francisco's Golden Gate Bridge); effects of suicide on families; and the underlying genetic, biological, psychological, and cultural forces. This is a rational discussion of an action that appears irrational to others but the only rational solution to someone unable to cope. A well-researched, well-written book on a topic most people don't want to think about, it is essential reading.

Diamonds in the Rough

♦ *The Angel and the Dragon: A Father's Search for Answers to His Son's Suicide* (2002) by Jonathan Aurthur. Deerfield Beach, FL: Health Communications.

Using his 23-year-old son Charley's diary notes, letters, and poems, along with his own observations, an anguished father chronicles his son's short and troubled life. His son struggled with mental illness, underwent numerous hospitalizations, attempted suicide on multiple occasions, and finally completed suicide. There are warning signs that parents and others can look for and a discussion of the effects of psychotropic drugs. An excellent albeit ominous book for parents of a mentally ill child, especially in its description of the pressures that can bring about the suicide of a vulnerable young person. This book was recently published and too new for inclusion in our studies, and thus designated a Diamond in the Rough.

♦ *His Bright Light: The Story of Nick Traina* (2000) by Danielle Steele. New York: Dell.

Novelist Steele sensitively depicts her son's brief life, his struggle with bipolar disorder, and his tragic suicide at age 19. A brilliant and talented child, Nick was a good-looking, charming teenager who played in a rock band and experimented with drugs. His mother made repeated but unsuccessful attempts to find help for him. Nick's mental anguish comes through in his poems, songs, and diary notes. Although this is a sad book, it is also compassionate and respectful of Nick and his roller-coaster ride of a life. *His Bright Light* received the designation Diamond in the Rough because it was favorably but infrequently rated in our latest study.

FILMS

Strongly Recommended

★★★★★ *Ordinary People* (1980) directed by Robert Redford. R rating. 124 minutes.

Mary Tyler Moore and Donald Sutherland have an apparently happy family. Their older son dies suddenly in a boating accident. Their other son, Timothy Hutton, is so wracked by misplaced guilt and unshared grief that he attempts suicide and enters psychotherapy. The movie admirably demonstrates the emotional dynamics of the family, the denial and false coping, the feelings of shame and failure a suicide evokes in the survivors, and the fears of feeling deeply. One of the highest rated films in all of our national studies, this five-star resource was also an Academy Award winner. (Also reviewed in Chapter 15, Death and Grieving.)

★★★★ *Dead Poets Society* (1990) directed by Peter Weir. PG rating. 129 minutes.

The message of this coming-of-age movie is to "Seize the Day." Teacher Robin Williams demonstrates and inspires his teenage boys to live to the fullest. The evidence for this quest, at least in the movie, is rather simpleminded opposition to conventions. A student opposes his father's command and then, unable to maintain his defiance, kills himself. Williams is made the scapegoat for the suicide and is forced to leave the boarding school. The suicide is not directly explored, but the feelings of adolescent desperation and alienation are clearly expressed. This movie, probably better suited to examining the experiences of teenagers, is reviewed in Chapter 34, Teenagers and Parenting.

★★★★ *'Night, Mother* (1987) directed by Tom Moore. PG-13 rating. 96 minutes.

A traumatic story of a daughter who announces to her mother that she is going to commit suicide. The mother tries to dissuade her as they stay up late together laughing and reminiscing. Then, the daughter, in fact, takes her life. The daughter's painful struggle is revealed through the storytelling that night, and we see that the daughter is living with a lifetime accumulation of challenges with which she can no longer cope. The compelling message is to deal with life problems on a manageable scale rather than turning away and allowing the reserve of heartache to triumph. This four-star resource also reveals that suicide is the daughter's desperate way of taking charge after years of being dominated by others and being devalued as a person. The film is an adaptation of a Broadway play that received a Pulitzer Prize.

★★★★ *The Virgin Suicides* (2000) directed by Sofia Coppola. R rating. 97 minutes.

In their typical gawky and insecure ways, all the teenage boys in the suburb loved and lusted after the Lisbon sisters. Josh Harnett has an ideal sexual moment with Kirsten Dunst, abandons her, and goes on to a life of compromises and reality. This theme is worth more exploration, and perhaps sensitive adolescents and their parents might do so. A second theme is that the girl and her sisters kill themselves, and the movie explores why. Their mother is hysterical over the girls' blooming sexuality and the father is a nonentity, but these are not really explanations. We never really understand why, and that may be the best point of the suicide theme.

★★★★ *The Hospital* (1971) directed by Arthur Hiller. PG rating. 103 minutes.

Although a farce and "black comedy" from the 1970s, the scene of George C. Scott's suicide contemplation is superb. His wife and kids have left him, he is impotent, and someone is killing the patients in his hospital. He is rescued by a hippie chick, Diana Rigg, whose wisdom (and beauty) revive him through love. If you can ignore the trite Hollywood ending, the stresses leading to Scott's suicide contemplation are beautifully shown.

Recommended

★★★ *The Slender Thread* (1965) directed by Sydney Pollack. Not rated. 98 minutes.

This film is based on the true story of a college student working on a crisis hotline, who finds himself on the phone with a woman who has taken an overdose of sleeping pills and doesn't know where she is. She has reached despair because her husband has discovered that he is not the father of their son; she is deeply depressed and does not have the strength to go on. His frantic attempts to keep her on the phone while the police track her location is a story of caring about the life of a stranger and the desperate state that people come to before they reach out.

Not Recommended

★ *Last Tango in Paris* (1972) directed by Bernardo Bertolucci. X rating. 129 minutes.

INTERNET RESOURCES

Metasites

★★★★★ *American Society of Suicidology* http://www.suicidology.org

The button Suicide Warning Signs links to a good short list. In the left column, the button, About Suicide opens to Things You Should Know About Suicide links to some resources, the best of which is If You Are Feeling Suicidal. As you might expect, this site links to about everything available on the net.

Psychoeducational Materials for Clients and Families

★★★★★ *A Comprehensive Approach to Suicide Prevention*
            http://www.lollie.com/suicide.html

About eight intense pages of straight-from-the-shoulder information, perspectives, and metaphors. The best readings for someone contemplating suicide.

★★★★★ *If You Are Thinking about Suicide . . . Read This First* by Martha Ainsworth
            http://www.metanoia.org/suicide

Excellent suggestions, seven informational pages, three books, and links to resources for the actively suicidal.

★★★★★ *Suicide Prevention Help*
            http://members.tripod.com/~suicideprevention/index.html

This personal site of about 14 pages contains some of the best advice on coping with suicidal thoughts or friends. Realistic, practical, and sensitive, the site might be recommended to a client to bring to the surface hidden thoughts, or to family members to provoke discussions.

★★★★★ *Suicide and Suicide Prevention*
            http://www.psycom.net/depression.central.suicide.html

A comprehensive list of about 60 links to all kinds of materials on suicide. Many can be used for patient education and support, and many are for clinician improvement.

★★★★ *SA/VE—Suicide Awareness/Voices of Education* http://www.save.org

The site offers, besides support, a dozen well-written and helpful brochures on thoughts of suicide, telling children, misconceptions, and the like.

★★★★ *Befrienders International* http://www.befrienders.org/mainindex.htm

Readings for persons who feel suicidal and those worried about other's suicidality. Also, unique materials on homosexuality, bullying, and self-harm, and all, apparently, available in many languages.

★★★ *Now Is Not Forever* by J. Kent Griffiths, DSW
            http://members.aol.com/dswgriff/suicide.html

A six-page handout listing 69 things to tell yourself when feeling suicidal.

Self-Injury

★★★★   *Self-Injury: You Are NOT the Only One*
http://www.palace.net/~llama/psych/injury.html

An excellent site with presentations on What, Who, Why, and Causes, Self-Help (for stopping), and First Aid Living with Self-Injury. Absolutely comprehensive, sensitive, and organized.

NATIONAL SUPPORT GROUPS

American Foundation for Suicide Prevention
120 Wall Street, 22nd Floor
New York, NY 10005
Phone: 888-333-AFSP or 212-363-3500
E-mail: inquiry@afsp.org
http://www.afsp.org

American Suicide Foundation
1045 Park Avenue, Suite 3C
New York, NY 10028
Phone: 800-ASF-4042; 212-210-1111

Provides referrals to national support groups for suicide survivors.

Emotions Anonymous
PO Box 4245
St. Paul, MN 55104-0245
Phone: 651-647-9712
E-mail: eaisc@mtn.org
http://www.emotionsanonymous.org

A 12-step organization for people struggling with emotional difficulties.

Friends for Survival
PO Box 214463
Sacramento, CA 95821
Phone: 916-392-0664; 800-646-7322
http://www.friendsforsurvival.org

For family, friends, and professionals after a suicide death.

National Suicide Hotline
Phone: 800-SUICIDE or 800-784-2433

Suicide Awareness Voices of Education (SAVE)
7317 Cahill Road, Suite 207
Minneapolis, MN 55424-0507
Phone: 952-946-7998
E-mail: save@winternet.com
http://www.save.org

Ray of Hope
PO Box 2323
Iowa City, IA 52244
Phone: 319-337-9890
E-mail: eroff1@juno.com

Mutual support after suicide bereavement.

SOLOS—Survivors of Loved Ones' Suicides
PO Box 592
Dumfries, VA 22026-0592
E-mail: solos@1000deaths.com
http://www.1000deaths.org

"Those left behind die a thousand deaths." Support, testimony, and 10 trifold brochures.

Yellow Ribbon Suicide Prevention Program
PO Box 644
Westminster, CO 80036-0644
Phone: 303-429-3530
E-mail: ask4help@yellowribbon.org
http://www.yellowribbon.org

See also Bipolar Disorder (Chapter 10) and Depression (Chapter 17).

CHAPTER 34

Teenagers and Parenting

Growing up has never been easy. It wasn't easy for the parents of today's adolescents when they were teenagers. It isn't easy for today's youth. What will become of this younger generation? It will grow up and start worrying about the next generation.

In matters of taste and manners, the youth of every generation seem radical, unnerving, and different from adults—different in their behavior, music, hairstyles, clothing, and activities. Acting out and boundary testing are time-honored ways in which teenagers move toward accepting, rather than rejecting, parental values. Many parents have a difficult time coping with the acting out and boundary testing of their adolescents. They want to know why their adolescents talk back to them and challenge their rules and values. They want to know whether they should be authoritarian or permissive. They want to know why adolescents have such mercurial moods—happy one moment, sad the next. And they want to keep their adolescents from drinking alcohol, taking drugs, dropping out of school, becoming depressed, getting involved with the wrong peer group, and being sexually permissive.

As parents worry about these treacherous roads, adolescents have their own concerns. For them, the transition from childhood to adulthood is a time of evaluation, of commitment, and of carving out a place in the world. They try on one face after another, trying to find an identity of their own. They want to discover who they are, what they are all about, and where they are going in life. They move through a seemingly endless preparation for life. They want their parents to understand them but often feel that they don't. And in the end, there are two paradoxical gifts they hope parents will give them—one is roots, the other is wings.

Self-help resources on teenagers and parenting fall into three main categories: resources written to help adolescents navigate the muddle of the middle years; those that provide parenting recommendations; and those that focus exclusively on parent–adolescent relationships. Let us now consider self-help books, films, and Internet resources for adolescents and their parents.

RECOMMENDATION HIGHLIGHTS

Self-Help Books

- For adolescent girls and their parents:

  ★★★★★ *Reviving Ophelia* by Mary Pipher

- For improving parent–adolescent relationships:

  ★★★★★ *Between Parent and Teenager* by Haim Ginott

  ★★★ *Positive Parenting Your Teens* by Karen Joslin and Mary Decher

  ★★★ *You and Your Adolescent* by Laurence Steinberg and Ann Levine

- For teenagers:

  ★★★★ *All Grown Up and No Place to Go* by David Elkind

  ★★★ *When Living Hurts* by Sol Gordon

  ◆ *Bringing Up Parents* by Alex J. Packer

Films

- On friendship and the rites of adolescent passage:

  ★★★★★ *Stand by Me*

- On identity development and authority conflicts:

  ★★★★ *Dead Poets Society*

- On teenagers genuinely encountering each other and themselves:

  ★★★★ *The Breakfast Club*

- On coming of age:

  ★★★★ *Circle of Friends*

  ★★★★ *Little Women*

- On struggling with giftedness and buried child abuse:

  ★★★★ *Good Will Hunting*

- On grappling with identity, relationship, and peer conflicts:

  ★★★★ *A Bronx Tale*

Internet Resources

- On the social, emotional, and sexual development of adolescents:

  ★★★★★ *Adolescence Directory On-Line (ADOL)*
  http://education.indiana.edu/cas/adol/adol.html

  ★★★★★ *TeenWire* http://www.teenwire.com/index.asp

  ★★★★★ *TeensHealth* http://www.teenshealth.org/teen/index2.html

SELF-HELP BOOKS

Strongly Recommended

★★★★★ *Reviving Ophelia: Saving the Selves of Adolescent Girls* (1994) by Mary Pipher. New York: Grosset/Putnam.

This is a sensitive, insightful journey into the torn lives of adolescent girls who, as children, were eager, confident, and curious, and who, upon the arrival of adolescence, lose their way and their selves. Mary Pipher observes the dark turn of culture in which adolescent girls are pressured to conform, compete, and be superficially physically attractive. She tells moving stories of many adolescent clients and her experiences with them in psychotherapy. Chapters on families, mothers, fathers, divorce, depression, and other forces that touch adolescent girls present ways parents can support their daughters and also identify ways in which parents become agents of culture and unknowingly steer girls toward self-doubt. The author discusses healthy directions that she takes in therapy, including teaching skills on centering, separating thinking and feeling, making conscious choices, holding boundaries, managing pain, modulating emotions, and enjoying altruism. *Reviving Ophelia* is the highest rated selection in its category and a very popular book for adolescent girls.

★★★★★ *Between Parent and Teenager* (1969) by Haim Ginott. New York: Avon.

Despite the fact that this valuable book is well past adolescence itself (it was published more than 30 years ago), it continues to be one of the most widely read and recommended books for parents who want to communicate more effectively with their teenagers. It has sold several million copies. Ginott describes a number of commonsense solutions for parents who are having difficulty understanding and communicating with their teenagers. At the same time that parents are trying to shape up their teenagers, the teenagers are fighting to be the masters of their own destiny. For Ginott, parents' greatest challenge is to let go when they want to hold on; only by letting go can parents reach a peaceful and meaningful coexistence with teenagers. Throughout, Ginott connects with parents through catchy phrases such as "Don't collect thorns" and "Don't step on corns"; "Don't talk in chapters," that is, don't lecture, but rather be a good listener; "Accept teenagers' restlessness and discontent," which reminds parents that normal adolescents experience a great deal of uncertainty; and "Don't put down their wishes and fantasies," which underscores that normal adolescents are idealists. Ginott's nontechnical, easy-to-read writing style and many examples of interchanges between parents and adolescents give parents a sense of what to say (and how and when to say it). His strategies can make the life of parents and teenagers a kinder, gentler world.

★★★★ *All Grown Up and No Place to Go: Teenagers in Crisis* (revised ed., 1997) by David Elkind. Reading, MA: Addison-Wesley.

Elkind believes that raising teenagers is more difficult than ever. He argues that today's teens are expected to confront adult challenges too early in their development. By being pressured into adult roles too soon, they are all grown up with no place to go—hence the title of his book. The book is divided into three main parts. Part I, Needed: A Time to Grow, describes today's teenagers as in the midst of a crisis, informs parents about how adolescents think, outlines the perils of puberty, and provides details about peer shock. Part II, Given: A Premature Adulthood, analyzes American society and informs parents that adolescents don't have any rites of passage to guide them, how the hodge-podge of American family structures has made adolescence a difficult transition, and how bad secondary schools really are. Part III, Results: Stress and Its Aftermath, examines the effects of these family and societal problems on teenagers' identity and ability to cope with stress and other problems. A very helpful appendix provides a list of services for troubled teenagers. This four-star book provides important recommendations for how parents, teachers, and other adults can communicate and interact more effectively with teenagers. Elkind does an especially good job of showing how adolescents develop and how our society has neglected their needs. Parenting recommendations are scattered through the book, embedded in discussions of different areas of adolescents' lives.

Recommended

★★★ *You and Your Adolescent: A Parent's Guide for Ages 10–20* (2nd ed., 1997) by Laurence Steinberg and Ann Levine. New York: HarperCollins.

This book presents an excellent overview of adolescent development and mixes in wise parenting strategies along the way. Steinberg and Levine tackle the dual task of giving parents a solid understanding of adolescent development and prescribing parenting strategies. Part I, The Basics, paints a picture of what makes a good parent, the nature of family communication, and what today's families are like. Part II, The Preteens: From 10 to 13, discusses the nature of physical health and development (puberty, sexual awakening, and drugs), psychological health and development, and the social world of the young adolescent (peers, dating, middle schools and junior high, and achievement). Part III, The Teens: From 14 to 17, focuses on sex and the high school student; drug and alcohol use in high school; the search for identity; a number of problem behaviors, such as delinquency and running away; friends and social life, school, and work. Part IV, Toward Adulthood: From 18 to 20, explores the transition from adolescence to adulthood and how parents can ease this transition for themselves and their offspring.

Two aspects of Steinberg and Levine's book especially set it apart from other self-help books on teenagers and parenting. First, the authors accurately tell readers that some of the horror stories they have heard about adolescents are false. They believe that boundary testing and acting out are time-honored traditions that, if not taken to extremes, are a normal part of adolescent development. Second, Steinberg and Levine's book is organized developmentally. Adolescent experts increasingly recognize that the 12-year-old is different in many ways from the 17-year-old. Our mental health experts opined that *You and Your Adolescent* presents a good balance between educating parents about the nature of adolescence and parenting recommendations.

★★★ *Positive Parenting Your Teens* (1997) by Karen Renshaw Joslin and Mary Bunting Decher. New York: Fawcett Columbine.

The organizational style of this book is unique. The book is intended to be a sequel for parents of teens to the book *Positive Discipline A–Z* (reviewed in Chapter 13, Child Development chapter). Several short sections describe the goal of creating an atmosphere of cooperation and responsibility, and explain how to have discussions, engender trust, and accomplish follow-through. The major focus of the book is teaching how to solve the 100 common concerns of parents and teens. For each concern, the authors offer an example, explain how to understand the situation, tell what to say and do, suggest preventative measures, and indicate how to know when to seek help. The list is thorough (e.g., rebelliousness, friends, depression, clothes, swearing), and the authors effectively addresses each concern. Our mental health experts consistently rated this book very favorably, but not enough rated it to move it to the four- or five-star category.

★★★ *When Living Hurts: For Teenagers and Young Adults* (revised ed., 1994) by Sol Gordon. New York: Union of American Hebrew Congregations.

The table of contents of this book is labeled "A table of wisdom, worry, and what to do," which gives the reader a sense of the book's style, sincerity, and good old-fashioned advice. The topics are timely (e.g., suicide, depression, sex, religion, parents, purpose of life). More important, however, is the person-to-person approach and the format, which includes thoughts for the day, slogans, advice, short writings of teenagers, funny poems, photos, and short narratives, such as "What's a mensch?" This book reads as if the teenager is having a confidential conversation with a favorite uncle. It is written for teenagers, but it is applicable for parents of all faiths. Highly regarded but not particularly well-known by the psychologists in our national studies.

★★★ *Surviving Adolescence: Helping Your Child through the Struggle* (1991) by Larry Dumont. New York: Villard.

This book is especially geared toward educating parents about the early warning signs of adolescent disorders, ranging from substance abuse and eating disorders to learning disabilities, depression, and suicidal behavior. In addition, Dumont describes a number of treatments for troubled teens, including inpatient hospitalization, outpatient psychotherapy, group therapy, behavior therapy, and drug therapy. He spends considerable time explaining to parents how to make a decision about whether to hospitalize an adolescent. This three-star book is especially good for helping parents make a decision about hospitalizing a teenager and provides excellent coverage of a number of adolescent disorders. Critics argue that *Surviving Adolescence* may cause some parents to overreact to adolescent misbehaviors that are not serious but rather part of the normal course of adolescent development.

★★★ *Chicken Soup for the Teenage Soul on Tough Stuff: Stories of Tough Times and Lessons Learned* (1997) by Jack Canfield, Mark Hansen, and Kimberly Kirberger. Deerfield Beach, FL: Health Communications.

Adolescents from around the world express their opinions and share their stories about coping with adolescence. More inspiration than self-help per se.

★★★ *Queen Bees and Wannabes: A Parent's Guide to Helping Your Daughter Survive Cliques, Gossip, Boyfriends, and Other Realities of Adolescence* (2002) by Rosalind Wiseman. New York: Crown.

Wiseman describes the problems that teenage girls might experience in the gossip and clique-filled world of adolescence. The "Queen Bee" is the teenage girl who dictates rules, such as who wears what and who dates whom; the "Wannabe" is the teenage girl who strives to get in a clique or is the target of a clique's wrath. Wiseman offers parents of teenage daughters advice on how to help their daughters understand and cope with this world.

★★★ *Toughlove* (reissued ed., 1997) by Phyllis York, David York, and Ted Wachtel. New York: Bantam.

This book squarely places the blame for adolescents' problems on the adolescents, not the parents. The book communicates that many parents are victimized by the guilt caused by their teenagers' behavior. According to the authors, many parents are too hard on themselves instead of on the teenager and the peer group when their adolescent takes drugs, fails at school, engages in promiscuous sex, or commits delinquent acts. *Toughlove* teaches parents how to face crises, take stands, demand cooperation, and meet challenges by getting tough with teenagers. Although toughlove may in the short run cause the gulf between parents and teenagers to widen, in the long run, it is the only way the teenager will develop maturity, according to toughlove advocates. This book barely received a three-star rating in one of our national studies. Most of the mental health experts preferred the gentler, more balanced approach of Pipher, Ginott, and Elkind to the harsh approach of *Toughlove*. Its problems, in addition to its punitive approach, are that controlled research has not been conducted on the method; it may lead parents to exaggerate their teenagers' problems; and it may inadvertently blame individual adolescents for societal or family problems.

Diamonds in the Rough

♦ *Get Out of My Life, But First Could You Drive Me and Cheryl to the Mall? A Parent's Guide to the New Teenager* (revised ed., 2002) by Anthony E. Wolf. New York: Farrar Straus & Giroux.

A helpful and humorous self-help resource that was released in a revised edition just after our latest national study. The newer edition contains additional information on sex, drugs, and life after September 11, 2001. Psychologist Wolf is reassuring about the inherent difficulties in raising teenagers, while providing realistic survival tips. He beautifully captures the ambivalence of many teenagers and their loving, hostile, dependent relationship with their parents.

♦ *What Teenagers Want to Know about Sex: Questions and Answers* (1988) by Boston Children's Hospital, Robert P. Masland, and David Estridge. Boston: Little, Brown.

This book is written for teenagers to provide truthful information about sexuality and help them understand the physical and emotional changes that occur during adolescence. The Boston Children's Hospital staff visited many schools, asking students to share questions and educators to recount their most frequently asked questions. The results are the comprehensive questions that appear in this book (e.g., hygiene, human reproduction, thoughts and feelings, puberty, STD, alcohol and drugs). The authors respond objectively to the questions by answering factually and sensitively. The questions and answers are well-formed, accurately geared to teenagers, and are not judgmental or patronizing. Its scientific orientation and its positive ratings by the mental health experts give *What Teenagers Want to Know about Sex* a Diamond in the Rough designation.

♦ *Bringing Up Parents: The Teenager's Handbook* (1992) by Alex J. Packer. Minneapolis: Free Spirit.

The humorous slant of this book is unique in giving advice to teenagers. Packer's informal, matter-of-fact, and collaborative writing style are consistent with the principles of the text. The book targets 12- to 17-year-old readers and is not written from an "us against them" perspective, but rather as "how to take the first step in making the relationship better." Chapter titles include "Taking Charge of the Fight Brigade," "Tricks and Treats," and "Close Encounters of the Worst Kind." The book focuses on the perennial conflicts and developmental tensions between parents and teenagers. Parents will not feel ganged up on by this book, but might instead agree with the author on the identified problems and solutions. The strong albeit infrequent ratings and interesting slant of this text give it a Diamond in the Rough status.

Not Recommended

★★ *Preparing for Adolescence* (1978) by James Dobson. Santa Ana, CA: Vision House.

FILMS

Strongly Recommended

★★★★★ *Stand by Me* (1987) directed by Rob Reiner. R rating. 89 minutes.

An excellent film about the rites of passage of four adolescents who grow toward manhood through a series of events ignited by the accidental death of a young boy. The boys learn the importance of friendship and loyalty. During their two-day journey, they encounter a number of adventures that further clarify for each what kind of a person he is becoming. As their journey progresses, each boy is put to the test, and each responds with a mixture of childish fear or grief within his evolving person. One of the highest-rated movies in our national studies.

★★★★ *Dead Poets Society* (1990) directed by Peter Weir. PG rating. 129 minutes.

An English teacher struggles to fit in at a conservative prep school. His passion for poetry and charismatic personality help establish a strong bond with his male students. Several of the boys revive a secret society. Conflict ensues between the boys and adults, with tragedy befalling one of the boys as his father tries to pull him out of the theater society. The teacher's inspirational motto is "Seize the Day." This powerful and uneasy movie received four Academy Award nominations.

★★★★ *A Bronx Tale* (1993) directed by Robert De Niro. R rating. 121 minutes.

A boy is offered two models of manhood by two men who care about him. His hardworking father says that a hero works hard, providing for his family, and living honestly. A Mafio tells him to live a fancier life, be loyal, and live by his own values. In another relevant plot, at 17, the boy falls in love with a black girl and, because this is forbidden in 1968 among both the Italians and blacks in the Bronx, he seeks men's advice. He is told that he must do what he thinks is best and face the consequences. In a different subplot, he finds himself, because of peer pressure, about to do a terrible thing and affect his whole future. The themes are universal in teenagers, even if the circumstances are not. This film offers teenagers much to ponder and discuss.

★★★★ *The Breakfast Club* (1986) directed by John Hughes. R rating. 95 minutes.

Five high school students from different walks of life in suburban Chicago serve Saturday detention together. As the day progresses, they delve into each other's private worlds and struggle to be honest with themselves and one another. The realistic diversity and separation of roles among the students is likely to resonate with many adolescents. A valuable lesson on how misleading first impressions and preconceived ideas often get in the way of nurturing relationships.

★★★★ *Circle of Friends* (1995) directed by Pat O'Connor. PG-13 rating. 112 minutes.

This roommate comedy set in Ireland in 1957 is a good old-fashioned, coming-of-age story about three friends who confront their changing lives in unique ways. The combined and complex forces of church, economics, social class, and sex weigh heavily on their choices.

★★★★ *Little Women* (1933) directed by George Cukor. Not rated. 117 minutes.

A timepiece; a movie about transition to adulthood during the Civil War era, detailing the ups and downs of teenage sisters. It is a humorous story of how four sisters learn moral lessons and grow from childish pleasures to adult joys. The film, which received many Academy Award nominations, is based on the Louisa May Alcott novel of the same title.

★★★★ *Good Will Hunting* (1997) directed by Gus Van Sant. R rating. 126 minutes.

Will Hunting, a brilliant 20-year-old man, is acting out his conflicts through oppositional behavior, which lands him in a life-altering relationship with a psychologist portrayed by Robin Williams. Will, a college janitor, is discovered to be a mathematical genius and is mentored by a math professor who sees a great future for Will. There is no future, however, until Will is able to resolve several dilemmas in his turbulent psychotherapy. He must accept that his intellectual gift will lead him away from his blue-collar culture and the friends who have been his mainstay; he must heal his rage and shame from unacknowledged early childhood abuse; and he must recognize that his intellect and his secret have squelched his ability to feel. This powerful story illuminates class struggle, the responsibility of giftedness, and the centrality of human connection. This film won an Academy Award for Best Original Screenplay in 1997, and Robin Williams won the Best Supporting Actor award.

Recommended

★★★ *My Bodyguard* (1980) directed by Michael Hayes. PG rating. 96 minutes.

The son of a hotel manager finds himself the target of a school bully, then employs a school outcast, the biggest kid in class, to be his bodyguard. The adolescents struggle with communication and conflict resolution, friends and support systems, and parent–child relationships. Filmed in and around Chicago, this comedy/drama is entertainment with an enduring message.

★★★ *Splendor in the Grass* (1961) directed by Elia Kazan. Not rated. 124 minutes.

This is the story of a blue-collar girl and rich boy who fall in love in the 1920s. They are young, passionate, and very conflicted about where their relationship is leading. The girl, played by Natalie Wood, attempts suicide and is placed in a psychiatric institution. In the meantime, the devil-may-care boy, played by Warren Beatty, continues with his free-spirited, fast-paced lifestyle. The film presents the personal moral conflicts and gender differences characteristic of the 1920s. The moral of the story, however, is in the awakening and maturing of Natalie Wood's character to see the shallowness and limitations of her boyfriend as she develops herself.

★★★ *Powder* (1995) directed by Victor Salva. PG-13 rating. 111 minutes.

On her way to the delivery room, a mother is struck by lightening and dies. Her child is born an albino, and the distraught father calls him Powder because of his white skin. Left to be raised by his grandparents, Powder lives in a basement. He possesses a photographic memory, an exceptionally high IQ, and telepathic powers. All of these qualities provide Powder with his greatest ability: compassion. This well-meaning film goes to supernatural heights to demonstrate acceptance and rejection, love and hate, and identity development.

★★★ *Pretty in Pink* (1987) directed by Howard Deutch. PG-13 rating. 96 minutes.

A high-school girl lives with her loving father, who must budget their money wisely. Accompanied by her insecure best friend, she feels threatened when a wealthy and well-meaning boy asks her out on a date. An entertaining and sensitive movie about growing pains and the meaning of money.

★★★ *Sixteen Candles* (1985) directed by John Hughes. PG rating. 93 minutes.

A fresh comedy about a 16th birthday party that turns out to be anything but sweet. The parents forget the girl's birthday party, and she doesn't receive an invitation to the big dance. The story focuses on the feelings of a 16-year-old girl who dreams of finding Mr. Right, who already has his eye on her.

Not Recommended

★★ *St. Elmo's Fire* (1986) directed by Joel Schumacher. R rating. 110 minutes.

INTERNET RESOURCES

Metasites

★★★★★ *Adolescence Directory On-Line (ADOL)*
        http://education.indiana.edu/cas/adol/adol.html

This "is a collection of World-Wide-Web (WWW) documents that focus on the social and emotional growth and development needs of adolescents. . . . ADOL exists as a way to help educators, parents, health practitioners, researchers, and teens access the many resources available on the WWW." Although we have not visited all the linked sites, they are very impressive, and appear to be of high quality and well-chosen. The sections are Conflict and Violence, Mental Health Issues, Health and Health Risk Issues, Counselor Resources, and Teens Only.

Psychoeducational Materials for Clients and Families

★★★★★ *Teen Center* http://www.wholefamily.com/aboutteensnow/dramas

In scripts, 26 realistic conflicts are played out and commented on by a psychotherapist. The topics are Divorce, Anorexia, Teen Sex, Loneliness, Suicide, Slob City, Teen Pregnancy, Dad's Affairs, and Family Fights. These might be useful for teens and their parents to read so that they can see how typical their conflicts and relating styles are and how a therapist might view them. The therapy is not shown, but there are comments by the therapists—which is an advantage for a therapist referring clients to this site.

★★★★★ *TeensHealth* http://www.teenshealth.org/teen/index2.html

There are perhaps 150 readings of value here. For example, under Your Body is Compulsive Exercise, and under Sexual Health are Sexually Transmitted Diseases. Many of these readings can be of use to teens regarding depression, suicide, body image, and conflicts with parents. The site is like a text on teens.

★★★★★ *TeenWire* http://www.teenwire.com/index.asp

A large, high-quality, and rich site, as would be expected from Planned Parenthood. It offers information written for adolescents on relationships, sexuality, and pregnancy. The Warehouse has articles about dating, love, sex, birth control, infections, diseases, abortion, sexual orientation, parents and friends, feelings, and more. World Views presents teen issues from other parts of the world. Hothouse is a teen-written e-zine.

★★★★ *Adolescence: Change and Continuity*
        http://www.personal.psu.edu/faculty/n/x/nxd10/adolesce.htm

This site must have a thousand papers written by students at Penn State, all clearly organized and in accessible English. There are hundreds under these headings: Relationships; Parenting; Grandparents; Family Problems; and Intimate Violence. When you go to any of these, all the papers in that section will be on one page and indexed at the top, so finding relevant ones is easier. The papers generally summarize an area, and many offer links.

★★★★ *The Teenager's Guide to the Real World!*
http://www.bygpub.com/books/tg2rw/tg2rwtoc.htm

Sections from the book of the same name include essays on dating and relationships, sexuality, studying, volunteering, jobs, cars, college, and others.

★★★★ *Self-Help Brochures* http://www.couns.uiuc.edu/brochures/brochure.htm

The Counseling Center at the University of Illinois has posted online brochures for their students addressing issues with which many teens deal. Titles of those available that are not listed elsewhere in this book include Addictive Relationships; Coming Out; Committed Relationships and School; Understanding Dysfunctional Relationship Patterns in Your Family; and When Your Parent Has a Mental Illness.

★★★★ *10 Things You Oughta Know About . . .*   http://teenadvice.about.com/cs/teenfactsheets/index.htm?PM=ss13_teenadvice

Here are about 30 well-written fact sheets that could be useful for opening discussions of topics such as date rape, oral sex, marijuana, lying, and so on.

★★★ *The Family Resource File*
http://www.kidspeace.org/HealingMagazine/resource.asp

About 30 briefly described books and websites that you are unlikely to come across on your own, but of specialized use.

★★★ *Friends First* http://www.friendsfirst.org/about.html

This program "asks kids to begin to reason through the tough choices and consequences of being sexually involved before marriage and stresses monogamy as the safest and best choice in marriage." Abstinence means no genital contact here. The site emphasizes decision making and assertiveness and provides research findings showing less divorce among those who have not been sexually intimate before marriage. Only bibliographies are available online, and materials are for sale, but we include this site because it is almost the only one available from this perspective.

Hotlines

Girls and Boys Town National Hotline
Phone: 800-448-3000
http://www.girlsandboystown.org

   Provides crisis intervention, information, and referrals for the general public. It is free, confidential, short-term crisis intervention for children and families.

Kid Save
Phone: 800-543-7283
http://www.kidspeace.org

   They offer information and referrals to public and private services for children and adolescents in crisis.

NineLine
Phone: 800-999-9999

A nationwide crisis/suicide hotline. Referrals are made for youth or parents for drugs, domestic violence, homelessness, runaways, and so on.

National Youth Crisis Hotline
Phone: 800-HIT-HOME

A crisis hotline and referral service for runaways or youth (17 and younger) with other problems and their parents.

NATIONAL SUPPORT GROUPS

Families Anonymous
PO Box 3475
Culver City, CA 90231
Phone: 800-736-9805
E-mail: famanon@FamiliesAnonymous. org
http://www.FamiliesAnonymousorg

A 12-step fellowship for relatives and friends concerned about substance abuse and behavioral problems.

Parents Anonymous
675 West Foothill Boulevard, Suite 220
Claremont, CA 91711-3416
Phone: 909-621-6184
E-mail: parentsanonymous@ parentsanonymous.org
http://www.parentsanonymous.org

Professionally facilitated, peer-led group for parents who are having difficulty.

Parents Without Partners
1650 South Dixie Highway, Suite 510
Boca Raton, FL 33432
Phone: 800-637-7974 or 561-391-8833
E-mail: pwp@jti.net
http://www.parentswithoutpartners.org

Brings teens from single-parent homes together to share ideas and problems, develop leadership skills, and plan fun activities.

SADD (Students Against Destructive Decisions)
PO Box 800
Marlboro, MA 01752
Phone: 508-481-3568
http://www.saddonline.com

See also Child Development and Parenting (Chapter 13), Families and Stepfamilies (Chapter 20), and Violent Youth (Chapter 37).

CHAPTER 35

Weight Management

Even ancient Romans were known to starve themselves, but never before have so many people, especially women, spent so much time, energy, and money on their weight. Since its inception in 1963, Weight Watchers alone has enrolled more than 24 million members. And understandably so: More than half of the U.S. population is considered overweight. The Surgeon General reports that some 60% of American adults are overweight or obese, as are 13% of children. And the rates continue to rise.

The hundreds of self-help resources for losing weight reflect our national obsession with being thin, or at least thinner. Some materials that encourage dietary modifications combined with exercise are based on sound nutritional and health principles. However, many materials aimed directly at weight loss itself are based on a gimmick, some quick fix for obesity, that is either nutritionally unsound or impossible to follow for any length of time, or both. Research has repeatedly demonstrated that those who lose weight quickly are, in 90% of the cases, unable to keep it off.

The quick-fix books received neutral or downright negative evaluations in our national studies. In fact, there are more negative ratings—and thus daggers—for weight loss books than in any other category in this volume. Our experts' negative evaluations of many weight loss books is in keeping with the research evidence: A recent report released by the Federal Trade Commission found that at least 40% of advertisements for weight loss products made at least one representation that was patently false.

The weight management resources in this chapter revolve around three interrelated topics: weight loss programs; comprehensive weight management plans that involve changes in eating, exercise, and lifestyle; and weight acceptance messages. As you read about the ratings of weight management resources, keep in mind that they were made by mental health professionals who frequently treat individuals who want to lose weight, not by nutritionists or physicians who specialize in weight loss.

RECOMMENDATION HIGHLIGHTS

Self-Help Books

- On managing weight and enhancing your healing system:

  ★★★★ *Eight Weeks to Optimum Health* by Andrew Weil

  ★★★ *Eating Well for Optimum Health* by Andrew Weil

- On the cultural and psychological underpinnings of women's weight loss:

  ★★★★ *Fat Is a Feminist Issue* by Susie Orbach

- On losing weight and maintaining it by changing your lifestyle:

  ★★★ *The LEARN Program for Weight Control* by Kelly Brownell

Autobiographies

- On overeating, semistarvation, and inspiring recovery:

  ★★★★★ *Feeding the Hungry Heart* by Geneen Roth

- On overcoming compulsive overeating:

  ★★★★ *Breaking Free from Compulsive Eating* by Geneen Roth

- On overcoming stigma against fatness:

  ◆ *Wake Up, I'm Fat!* by Camryn Manheim

Internet Resources

- On the cultural influences on weight, health, and body image:

  ★★★★★ *Weight Loss* http://weightloss.about.com/mlibrary.htm

- On size acceptance:

  ★★★★★ *Size Wise* http://www.sizewise.com

  ★★★★★ *National Association to Advance Fat Acceptance*
  http://naafa.org/documents/brochures

  ★★★★ *Fat!So!* http://www.fatso.com/index.html

- On diet ratings and other reliable information:

  ★★★★★ *Nutrition Navigator* http://www.navigator.tufts.edu

SELF-HELP BOOKS

Strongly Recommended

★★★★ *Eight Weeks to Optimum Health* (1997) by Andrew Weil. New York: Knopf.

In this book, Weil translates the information contained in his best-seller *Spontaneous Healing* into a practical plan. The program takes full advantage of the body's natural healing power. Weil fine-tunes current eating habits, incorporates antioxidant supplements, and adds walking and stretching the weekly regimen. He provides basic breathing exercises that create greater relaxation and energy, explains the techniques of visualization, and shows how to avoid environmental hazards. Weil suggests making art, music, and the natural world a greater part of life. The book has a dozen additional customized plans for specific ages, genders, lifestyles, and medical needs. This informative, four-star book is roundly recommended to the layperson willing to commit to an eight-week program that works with the body's own healing system.

★★★★   *Fat Is a Feminist Issue: The Anti-Diet Guide for Women* (1997) by Susie Orbach. New York: Galahad.

This book, a compilation of two international best-sellers, *Fat Is a Feminist Issue* and *Fat Is a Feminist Issue II*, is a psychological exploration of why so many women are compulsive overeaters. It is not a diet book per se. Orbach states that because compulsive overeating is primarily a women's problem, it may have something to do with being a female in today's society. Examining compulsive overeating from feminist and psychoanalytic perspectives, Orbach believes that being fat serves a number of purposes for women: It prevents them from being perceived as sex objects, expresses anger they have been conditioned to deny, or reflects problems of separation from their mothers. Orbach presents a program to help women learn the difference between hunger and boredom or loneliness, and to show them how to use food to satisfy only their hunger, rather than more profound longings. These ideas are then presented in a workbook fashion to facilitate behavior change. The book deals with food, fatness, thinness, compulsive eating, bulimia, anorexia, and body image. *Fat Is a Feminist Issue* is favorably evaluated for its important insights into the nature of obesity and the psychological underpinnings of compulsive overeating. It is one of the few self-help books in this category that received a positive rating.

Recommended

★★★   *The LEARN Program for Weight Control* (7th ed., 1997) by Kelly Brownell. Dallas: American Health Publications/Brownell & Hager.

The LEARN Program for Weight Control advocates a change in lifestyle in order to lose weight. LEARN is an acronym for lifestyle, exercise, attitudes, relationships, and nutrition. The book includes 16 lessons that guide effective, medically sound weight loss. The LEARN program promises an average weight loss of 20 to 25 pounds, translating into a 1- to 2-pound weight loss each week for the 20 weeks the program usually lasts. Self-assessment questionnaires and homework assignments accompany each of the lessons. These exercises show which techniques are working and how much progress has been made. Yale University psychologist Brownell teaches when, how, and why habits occur, and how to change them. In two of our studies, the *LEARN Program for Weight Control* was rated very positively, but by relatively few mental health professionals. In both studies, its average rating would have placed it as a five-star book had more psychologists been aware of it. This book presents an excellent strategy for weight loss that has a much better chance of helping people lose weight and maintain the loss than quick-fix diet books. It contains no gimmicks and no false promises; rather, readers are encouraged to alter their exercises, lifestyles, and eating patterns in order to lose weight and keep it off. The book is clear, well-written, and nicely organized. Its only problem is that it is not widely available.

★★★ *Make the Connection: Ten Steps to a Better Body—and a Better Life* (1996) by Bob Greene and Oprah Winfrey. New York: Hyperion.

In this book, Green, a professional trainer, and Winfrey, a national television host, show what to do physically and mentally to lose weight and feel good about oneself. The book starts with Oprah's personal stories about her own work to get into shape. Oprah's inspiring journey and Green's professional knowledge combine for a realistic model of a healthy lifestyle. The authors cover reasons we eat, methods of enhancing self-awareness, the purpose of body fat, the physics of body weight, and their 10-step program on physical, emotional, and dieting changes. People looking for inspiration and usable information will find this three-star book helpful.

★★★ *Eating Well for Optimum Health* (2000) by Andrew Weil. New York: Knopf.

The primary principles of diet and nutrition are addressed in this text by Weil, who also authored *Eight Weeks to Optimum Health* (reviewed above). He views dietary habits in relationship to patterns of health and illness. The purpose of his book is to provide basic nutritional facts, address weight reduction, teach the reading of food labels, discuss popular diets, and provide customized dietary advice for common ailments. A very informative chapter on basics of human nutrition revisits carbohydrates, protein, and fat, and includes several tables and charts, including the glycemic index of popular foods. The worst diets in the world and the best diets in the world (e.g., raw foods, Japanese, Asian, vegetarian, the Mediterranean foods) are interestingly presented and contrasted. Each chapter includes "A Healing Story" of a patient or acquaintance who changed nutritional intake and demonstrated concrete health improvement as a result of diet. The last section of the book is devoted to health-conscious recipes.

★★★ *Eat More, Weigh Less* (1993) by Dean Ornish. New York: HarperCollins.

Cardiologist Ornish discusses what really motivates people to make and maintain lifestyle changes, based on three research studies conducted during the past 16 years. He believes that being overweight is not solely a physical problem; it needs to be addressed in a broader context. On his Life Choice program, meals are so low in fat that you get full before you consume too many calories. Your metabolism doesn't slow down, so you can eat more frequently, eat a greater quantity of food, and still lose weight. The author notes that the Life Choice program is an adjunct to, not a substitute for, conventional medical therapy. In the process of making this lifestyle change and losing weight, you may want to share this book with your physician. The latter section of the book presents 250 gourmet recipes containing less than 10% fat. This is an educational and helpful book for people looking for a lifestyle change and not just weight loss.

★★★ *The New Fit or Fat* (revised ed., 1991) by Covert Bailey. Boston: Houghton Mifflin.

This book describes ways to become healthy by developing better diet and exercise routines. Bailey argues that the basic problem for overweight people is not losing weight, which fat people do periodically, but gaining weight, which fat people do more easily than those with different body chemistry. He explores the way our body stores fat and analyzes why crash diets don't work. He explains the relation between fat metabolism and weight, concluding that the ultimate cure for obesity is aerobic exercise coupled with a sensible low-fat diet. Originally published in 1977, the 1991 edition is greatly expanded with new information on fitness lifestyles and recent scientific advances. A new chapter answers readers' most frequently asked questions about Bailey's views on diet and exercise. A new section suggests strategies for getting started. This three-star book offers solid, no-nonsense advice about how to lose weight and become more physically fit.

★★★ *Sugar Busters: Cut Sugar to Trim Fat* (1995, reprinted 1998) by H. Leighton Steward, Morrison C. Bethea, Samuel S. Andrews, and Luis A. Balart. New York: Ballantine.

This book takes the position that low-fat foods are full of sugar, which is related to the production of insulin, which in large amounts keeps you from losing weight, no matter how strictly you diet or how often you exercise. The authors show how to reduce the sugar in the daily menu. You develop a diet plan, determine the glycemic levels of foods, decide which foods to eat at what time of the day, avoid certain food combinations, and learn various myths about calories, fats, cholesterol, and weight gain. Also included is a 14-day meal plan. The book provides a history of refined sugar, and the biological and metabolic usage of sugars in our body. Included is a useful glossary to assist understanding some of the technical terms. In consultation with a physician, this best-seller could be a helpful book for individuals with sugar-related concerns or those willing to follow this diet plan.

Not Recommended

★★ *Diet for a Small Planet* (20th anniversary ed., 1991) by Frances Lappe. New York: Ballantine.

★★ *Body for Life* (2000) by Bill Philips and Michel D'Orso. New York: HarperCollins.

★★ *The Zone* (1995) by Barry Sears. New York: HarperCollins.

★ *The Pritikin Program for Diet and Exercise* (1979) by Nathan Pritikin. New York: Bantam.

★ *One Meal at a Time: Step-By-Step to a Low-Fat Diet for a Happier, Healthier, Longer Life* (1991) by Martin Katahn. New York: Norton.

★ *Dr. Atkins' New Diet Revolution* (1992) by Robert C. Atkins. New York: Evans.

Strongly Not Recommended

† *The T-Factor Diet* (1989, revised 2000) by Martin Katahn. New York: Norton.

† *The Rotation Diet* (1986) by Martin Katahn. New York: Norton.

† *The Diet Center Program: Lose Weight Fast and Keep It Off Forever* (revised ed., 1990) by Sybil Ferguson. Boston: Little, Brown.

† *The 35-Plus Diet for Women* (1987) by Jean Spodnik and Barbara Gibbons. New York: Harper & Row.

† *Dr. Atkins' Diet Revolution* (1972) by Robert Atkins. New York: Evans.

† *Dr. Abravanel's Anti-Craving Weight-Loss Diet* (1990) by Elliot Abravanel and Elizabeth King. New York: Bantam.

† *The Carbohydrate Addict's Diet* (1991) by Rachael Heller and Richard Heller. New York: Dutton.

† *The 5-Day Miracle Diet* (1997) by Adele Puhn. New York: Ballantine.

† *The Beverly Hills Diet* (1981) by Judy Mazel. New York: Macmillan.

AUTOBIOGRAPHIES

Strongly Recommended

★★★★★ *Feeding the Hungry Heart: The Experience of Compulsive Eating* (1993) by Geneen Roth. New York: NAL/Dutton.

The author discusses her personal history of overeating followed by semistarvation and her recovery as she learned to control her eating. She includes stories from other people in the weight management seminars that she conducts. It is not so much a diet book as the author's philosophy of weight management through self-understanding and self-love. More specific recommendations for weight loss follow in Roth's sequel, *Breaking Free from Compulsive Eating*, reviewed below. Many overeaters find this five-star autobiography to be an inspiring and realistic account that motivates them to change their destructive eating habits.

★★★★ *Breaking Free from Compulsive Eating* (1993) by Geneen Roth. New York: NAL/Dutton.

Speaking from personal experience, the author of numerous books about eating and dieting (*Why Weight?*; *When You Eat at the Refrigerator, Pull Up a Chair*; and *Feeding the Hungry Heart*) advises readers about how they can free themselves from compulsive eating. She outlines the techniques developed in her weight loss workshops. Roth shows women struggling with weight management that they are not alone and maintains that self-understanding can bring self-acceptance.

Recommended

★★★ *Diary of a Fat Housewife: A True Story of Humor, Heartbreak, and Hope* (1995) by Rosemary Green. New York: Warner Books.

Now married with six children, this one-time beauty queen describes a 10-year battle with obesity. She began keeping a brutally honest journal at age 30 and tried various self-treatments. It is a good portrayal of what it means to be an obese woman in American today. By destigmatizing the topic, the book will be useful to those who are obese and their families.

Diamond in the Rough

♦ *Wake Up, I'm Fat!* (2000) by Camryn Manheim. New York: Broadway.

This very funny book is based on the one-woman show of the same name. At the ceremony where she received an Emmy award, Manheim announced to the delighted audience, "This is for all the fat girls." She faced stigma about her weight throughout high school and experimented with pills and cigarettes for weight reduction. She recounts the cutting remarks, cruel jokes, relationship problems, and discrimination she faced. Manheim is a peppy, smart, colorful, and persuasive advocate for fat acceptance. This is not a health or diet book; there is no mention of research findings on weight issues, but the book goes far in debunking the stick figure quest so prevalent in the dominant culture. Not many of the mental health experts in our studies were acquainted with autobiographies on weight management, but those who had read this book, rated it highly.

INTERNET RESOURCES

Metasites

★★★★★ *Weight Loss* http://weightloss.about.com/mlibrary.htm

Jennifer R. Scott maintains this site and offers many high-quality subsites about the cultural aspects of weight, health, body image, and the facts of weight loss. There are several hundred pages here, covering anything one might want to know or explore.

★★★★★ *Size Wise* http://www.sizewise.com

This site serves as an on-line companion to the book *Size Wise—A Catalog of More Than 1000 Resources for Living with Confidence and Comfort at Any Size*. A searchable and well-organized guide to all aspects of size acceptance, including clothing, medical care, kids, fitness, and groups.

★★★★ *Calorie Control Council* http://www.caloriecontrol.org

Centered on minding calories, this site offers abundant information on exercise, eating differently, and other materials to support healthy eating.

Psychoeducational Materials for Clients and Families

★★★★★ *Nutrition Navigator* http://www.navigator.tufts.edu

Tufts University School of Nutrition Science offers ratings of various diets as well as the most reliable advice. Materials are for health professionals, journalists, and educators, so you can find any information. Highly recommended.

★★★★★ *NAAFA: National Association to Advance Fat Acceptance*
http://naafa.org/documents/brochures

A dozen brochures offer facts and guidelines about dieting, hypertension, eating disorders, and legal rights. Under Official Documents are policy statements based on research related to drugs, surgery, fitness, and those who admire fat people. Very enlightening.

★★★★★ *About-Face* http://www.about-face.org/index.html

Designed to combat negative and distorted images of women in the media, this site might be a good referral for women too concerned with appearance and too controlled by the consumer culture.

★★★★ *Fat!So?* http://www.fatso.com/index.html

A site with attitude. The readings at Greatest Hits offer facts and stories that are very helpful for acceptance. Click on the exclamation points on the pages to go on.

★★★★ *Largesse, the Network for Size Esteem* http://www.eskimo.com/~largesse

A comprehensive list of books, links, and organizations. The section on Size-Positive Support and Educational Materials offers affirmations and help with using them.

★★★ *Big Folks Health FAQ* http://www.faqs.org/faqs/fat-acceptance-faq/health

This document contains information about often-exaggerated health costs for fat people.

NATIONAL SUPPORT GROUPS

**Council on Size and Weight
Discrimination**
PO Box 305
Mt. Marion, NY 12456
Phone: 845-679-1209
E-mail: info@cswd.org
http://www.cswd.org

  Information, referrals, advocacy.

Food Addicts Anonymous
4623 Forest Hill Boulevard, Suite 109-4
West Palm Beach, FL 33415
Phone: 561-967-3871
E-mail: info@foodaddictsanonymous.org
http://www.foodaddictsanonymous.org

  A 12-step fellowship to recover from the disease of food addiction.

Healthy Weight Network
402 South 14th Street
Hettinger, ND 58639
Phone: 701-567-2646
E-mail: hwj@healthyweight.net
http://www.healthyweight.net

  Obesity watchdog organization, advocate for healthy eating and fitness.

**ISAA (International Size-Acceptance
Association)**
PO Box 82126
Austin, TX 78758
Phone: 512-371-4307
E-mail: Director@size-acceptance.org
http://www.size-acceptance.org

  Advocacy, activism, chapters, brochures, newsletter.

Largely Positive
PO Box 170223
Milwaukee, WI 53217
E-mail: contact@largelypositive.com
http://www.largelypositive.com

Promotes health and self-esteem for larger people through newsletters and local support groups.

NAAFA: National Association to Advance Fat Acceptance
PO Box 188620
Sacramento, CA 95818
Phone: 916-558-6880
E-mail: mabnaafa@aol.com
http://www.naafa.org

Their Book Service has excellent materials. Membership newsletter, educational materials, regional chapters, annual convention, pen-pal program.

National Center for Overcoming Overeating
PO Box 1257
Old Chelsea Station
New York, NY 10113-0920
Phone: 212-875-0442
http://www.OvercomingOvereating.com

Home of the Women's Campaign to End Body Hatred and Dieting.

Overeaters Anonymous
PO Box 44020
Rio Rancho, NM 87174-4020
Phone: 505-891-2664
E-mail: info@overeatersanonymous.org
http://www.overeatersanonymous.org

A 12-step program of recovery from compulsive eating disorders.

Shape Up America!
c/o Web Front Solutions Corporation
15757 Crabbs Branch Way
Rockville, MD 20855
Phone: 301-258-0540
E-mail: info@shapeup.org
http://www.shpaeup.org

A nonprofit organization started by former Surgeon General C. Everett Koop to advance the benefits of keeping active and maintaining a healthy weight.

Take Off Pounds Sensibly (TOPS)
PO Box 07360
4575 South Fifth Street
Milwaukee, WI 53207-0360
Phone: 800-932-8677
http://www.tops.org

For overweight people who wish to attain and maintain their goal weight.

Trevose Behavior Modification Program®
PO Box 11674
Philadelphia, PA 19116
http://www.tbmp.org

Self-help groups of 10 people meet for an hour a week to substitute good habits for bad habits and to learn to keep the lost weight off permanently. The organization, largely located in Pennsylvania and New Jersey, is advised by professionals, and the early research on its effectiveness is quite promising (Latner, Wilson, Stunkard, & Jackson, 2002).

See also Eating Disorders (Chapter 19).

CHAPTER 36

Women's Issues

The mental health professions have historically portrayed human behavior in male-dominant themes. While much progress has been made in recent decades, sexism is still evident in society, and women continue to be discriminated against in the workplace, in politics, at home, and perhaps in self-help resources.

Critics argue that self-help materials have perpetuated many stereotypes and myths harmful to women. What are some of these stereotypes? We can journey through the chapters of the *Authoritative Guide to Self-Help Resources in Mental Health* and find books that condemn women for dysfunctional personalities, that treat codependency as a woman's disease, that consider eating disorders as uniquely female problems, and that blame mothers for most of their children's problems. We find books that overdramatize sex differences and that favor the male "difference" (women are described as overly invested in romantic love, dependent on others, and incapable of controlling their emotions). Few authors, historically, have written about the positive features of being female, and fewer still give credence to many of the daily responsibilities women have traditionally performed and continue to manage.

The best self-help resources on women's issues address such concerns and help women become aware that what have been labeled as character defects in the past are actually strengths that should be nurtured, rewarded, and cherished. Of course, many resources in other categories address women's issues and provide self-help advice for women. In other chapters, we recommend a number of excellent self-help books on specific aspects of women's lives, such as assertion, communication, parenting, intimacy, pregnancy, and sexuality.

In this chapter, we describe and evaluate self-help resources—books, autobiographies, films, and websites—that address quintessentially women's issues. These include work and parental roles, gender stereotypes, sex differences, feminist concerns, and women's health.

RECOMMENDATION HIGHLIGHTS

Self-Help Books

- On women's health and well-being:

  ★★★★★ *The New Our Bodies, Ourselves* by the Boston Women's Collective

- On women's work and parenting roles:

  ★★★★ *The Second Shift* by Arlie Hochschild

- On women's life stages and transitions:

  ★★★★ *The Seasons of a Woman's Life* by Daniel J. Levinson and Judy D. Levinson

  ★★★ *Life Preservers* by Harriet Lerner

  ★★★ *The Wisdom of Menopause* by Christiane Northrup

- On inspiring and nurturing women:

  ★★★★ *Chicken Soup for the Woman's Soul* by Jack Canfield et al.

- On gender stereotypes, myths, and sex differences:

  ★★★★ *The Mismeasure of Woman* by Carol Tavris

- On women's bodies and their self-image traps:

  ★★★ *Body Traps* by Judith Rodin

Autobiographies

- On the remarkable lives of multitalented woman:

  ★★★★★ *Heart of a Woman* by Maya Angelou

  ★★★ *Reason for Hope* by Jane Goodall

- On an insider's and Jewish look at the women's movement:

  ★★★ *Deborah, Golda, and Me* by Letty Cottin Pogrebin

- On influential women and mothering experiences:

  ◆ *Mothers* by Alexandra Stoddard

Films

- On women bonding on the baseball field and thriving without men:

  ★★★★ *A League of Their Own*

- On the interdependence of women and the ability to change:

  ★★★★ *Fried Green Tomatoes*

- On quilting as a metaphor for women sharing experiences:

  ★★★★ *How to Make an American Quilt*

- On the balance between family and career and midlife reevaluations:

    ★★★★ *The Turning Point*

- On insightful conversations about food and life:

    ★★★★ *Eating*

Internet Resources

- On solid information on a broad topic:

    ★★★★★ *WWWomen* http://www.wwwomen.com

    ★★★★ *Femina: Web Search for Women* http://femina.cybergrrl.com

- On the medical aspects of women:

    ★★★★★ *North American Menopause Society* http://www.menopause.org

    ★★★★ *Health and Sexuality*
    http://feminist.com/resources/links/links_health.html

- On employment discrimination:

    ★★★★★ *Equal Employment Opportunity Commission* http://www.eeoc.gov

- On feminism:

    ★★★★★ *On the Issues* http://www.echonyc.com/~onissues/about.htm

SELF-HELP BOOKS

Strongly Recommended

★★★★★ *The New Our Bodies, Ourselves* (25th anniversary ed., 1996) by the Boston Women's Health Book Collective. New York: Touchstone.

This highly rated book updates an earlier edition with new information on AIDS, older women, birth control methods, and disorders that primarily affect women, to name a few topics. The new edition keeps women updated on physical and mental health, along with legal, political, and social organizational realities of women's identity and roles. A mission for the authors is to encourage women to get together—to meet, talk to, and listen to each other. Women interested in women's passions and potentialities will thoroughly enjoy this resource. This five-star book will probably leave women feeling, to use one of the most overused words of the decade, empowered. One of the most highly regarded self-help resources in any of our studies, and deservedly so.

★★★★ *The Second Shift* (1989) by Arlie Hochschild. New York: Viking.

This self-help resource focuses on the inequality of gender roles in two-career couples with children. Hochschild conducted extensive interviews and home observations of 50 two-career couples with children under the age of six to discover how they allotted their time and responsibility to careers, child rearing, and household chores. Not surprisingly, she found that women handled the bulk of child care and housework in addition to holding down full-time jobs outside the home. Hochschild labels married couples as traditional (the husband works and the wife stays at home), transitional (both work, and he does less than she thinks he should around the house), or egalitarian (both spend equal time on work and home responsibilities). In her study, all the families were in the last two categories, and the majority were transitional. Hochschild believes that men and women use gender strategies that are based on deep-seated emotional beliefs about manhood and womanhood as they try to define how to juggle jobs, child-rearing, and household responsibilities. One of Hochschild's main goals in *The Second Shift* is to bring these gender strategies into the open so that married couples can discuss and benefit from them. Multiple solutions—from the personal to the societal—are presented to rectify the inequalities. What separates *The Second Shift* from standard feminist fare is the texture of the reporting and the subtlety of the insights. A valuable, if disconcerting, book.

★★★★   *The Mismeasure of Woman* (1992) by Carol Tavris. New York: Simon & Schuster.

This book explores the stereotyping of women and comparative characteristics with men. Topics include the question of women's inferiority or superiority to men; premenstrual syndrome; postmenstrual syndrome; diagnostic bias that women get sick and men have problems; and fables of female sexuality. Tavris hypothesizes that no matter how hard women try, discrimination determines that they can't measure up. They are criticized for being too feminine or not feminine enough and are judged by how well they fit into a male world. The book contains a review of research that documents how women continue to be ignored, misrepresented, and even harmed by male-dominated health professions. Tavris believes that more evidence exists for similarities between the sexes that for differences between them. She explores how society pathologizes women through psychiatric diagnoses, sexist divorce rulings, and images of women as moody, self-defeating, and unstable. This is an excellent analysis of gender stereotyping and how women should be measured by their own standards. *The Mismeasure of Woman* is well documented and captivating, presenting a witty feminist portrayal of women's dilemmas and what can be done about them.

★★★★   *The Seasons of a Woman's Life* (1996) by Daniel J. Levinson and Judy D. Levinson. New York: Knopf.

This book, the counterpart to Levinson's *Seasons of a Man's Life* (reviewed in Chapter 4), traces the developmental themes and stages of women's adulthood. It is based on lengthy interviews conducted in the 1980s of 55 randomly selected women from various professions and at various stages in their lives. This study confirms that in every woman's life, there is a mixture of joy and sorrow, success and failure, and self-fulfillment and self-defeat. This four-star book is favorably regarded and compellingly addresses women's development throughout the life cycle.

★★★★ *Chicken Soup for the Woman's Soul* (1996) by Jack Canfield, Mark Victor Hansen, Jennifer Read Hawthorne, and Marci Shimoff. Deerfield Beach, FL: Health Communications.

These best-selling *Chicken Soup* authors have written another inspiring book, this time specifically for women. The book is designed to reinforce the bond between women using 101 stories describing the unique and the common life experiences that reflect lifestyles of girls and women. Some of the experiences shared in this book address goals, relationships, giving birth, job responsibilities, family, and friendships. This is a book you can pick up for two minutes or two hours that will make you feel moved and guided.

Recommended

★★★ *Too Good for Her Own Good: Breaking Free from the Burden of Female Responsibility* (1990) by Claudia Bepko and Jo-Ann Krestan. New York: Harper & Row.

The authors sensitively examine low self-esteem in women that results from feeling that they are not good enough. The Goodness Code requires women to be attractive, ladylike, unselfish, of service to others, the moving force in making relationships work, and competent—all without complaining. The authors argue that goodness comes to most women almost instinctively; they feel they must be competent in virtually everything they do while remaining responsible for the happiness of others around them. Yet no matter how hard women work to please others, they often feel inadequate, because part of being good is knowing that they are never good enough. The results: Far too many women have a low self-image, feel insecure, and are overworked. The authors then discuss how to break free by changing the balance of various factors. A number of case histories buttress the authors' points. The book's enthusiasts said that many women with low self-esteem who have lived their lives in the service of others' needs will find themselves described on almost every page of this book.

★★★ *Body Traps* (1992) by Judith Rodin. New York: Morrow.

This book addresses how society has constructed a negative and destructive perception of female bodies and how women can free themselves from this trap. Psychologist Rodin argues that good looks, appearance, and fitness have become the measures women use to evaluate their self-worth. A number of the traps discussed by Rodin are the variety trap, the shame trap, the competition trap, the food trap, the dieting rituals trap, the fitness trap, and the success trap. Mental health experts in our studies consistently rated the book favorably but not frequently. The book is a thoughtful, penetrating look at society's preoccupation with women's appearance and the unrealistic expectations and harmful effects the preoccupation has produced. *Body Traps* is informative, well-written, and very helpful guide to what women's bodies mean to them.

★★★ *The Wisdom of Menopause* (2001) by Christiane Northrup. New York: Bantam.

From her perspective as an obstetrician–gynecologist and from her own menopausal journey, Northrup movingly traces women's changes through the menopausal experience. Initial chapters chronicle her movement toward authenticity, self-fulfillment, and an excitement for life that is unleashed as a result of menopausal changes. The author argues that women's ease in showing anger, intolerance for disrespect, and rejection of diminished roles at perimenopause are not the negative result of raging hormones, but rather the beginning of clarity in self-perception and a confrontation with the cultural prescription of women as relational caretakers. Many topics will hit home with women of a wide age range, such as cultural ambivalence about the meaning of money, the decision about hormone replacement, and understanding the physiological effects of menopause including hot flashes, mental fuzziness, headaches, and mood swings. Valuable information is offered regarding brain functioning, skin changes, bone density and osteoporosis, cardiac protection, and breast cancer screening. A fine self-help resource grounded in both medical science and feminist analysis.

★★★ *Life Preservers: Good Advice When You Need It Most* (1996) by Harriet Lerner. New York: HarperCollins.

Life Preservers, a Diamond in the Rough in our earlier edition, is a compilation of questions and answers published in the author's monthly *New Woman* magazine column "Harriet Lerner's Good Advice." Questions came from women over many years, whose inquires are in some cases frequently asked and in others rarely voiced. The questions and answers are clustered into significant areas, including work and creativity, anger and intimacy, friendship and marriage, children and parents, loss and betrayal, and sexuality and health. The questions are diverse, poignant, and candid—questions many would want to ask but do not. Lerner's answers are thoughtful and straightforward, well-developed directions that walk the reader through a decision-making process; she identifies as she goes the potential consequences of taking action. Her writing style contains a colorful and humorous flare that is compatible with the seriousness of her work, yet facilitates a welcomed light side.

★★★ *The Silent Passage* (revised ed., 1998) by Gail Sheehy. New York: Random House.

As reviewed in Chapter 4, this best-seller addresses menopause. Sheehy's objectives are to erase the stigma of menopause, normalize the process, and direct women to medical and psychological resources. An engaging and easy read on a neglected topic.

★★★ *Women Who Run with the Wolves: Myths and Stories of the Wild Women Archetype* (1992) by Clarissa Pinkola Estes. New York: Ballantine.

Estes's work as a Jungian analyst influences her psychic-archeological portrait of the female archetype. She draws a parallel between healthy wolves and healthy women in two ways: (1) They share certain psychic characteristics, keen sensing, a playful spirit, and a heightened capacity for devotion; and (2) both have been hounded, harassed, and falsely imputed to be devouring, devious, and overly aggressive by their detractors. Estes maintains that once women reassert their relationship with their wild nature, they will be gifted with a permanent and internal watcher, a visionary, who will guide them. In this book, *wild* means to live a natural life, one in which a creature has innate integrity and healthy boundaries. On the positive side, this three-star (almost four-star) resource can be deeply inspiring and insightful. On the negative side, some mental health experts contend that it can be easily misinterpreted and misapplied, and complain that the Jungian orientation has little scientific support.

★★★ *Backlash: The Undeclared War against American Women* (1991) by Susan Faludi. New York: Crown.

This book concerns the way women and feminism are portrayed by the media. Faludi uncovers a growing backlash against women and feminism in the United States. This backlash has hurt women in two main ways: first, by convincing women that their feelings of dissatisfaction are the result of too much feminism and independence; and second, by simultaneously undermining the minimal progress that women have made at work, in politics, and in their own minds. She cites the (in)famous Harvard–Yale study, which in 1988 reported that a single, college-educated woman over the age of 30 has only a 20% chance of ever getting married, and that by the time she is 40, she will have only a 1.3% chance. Faludi says that the man shortage is only one of the myths propagated by the media (another is the infertility epidemic) and finds evidence of other antifeminist orientations in movies, television, and fashion advertising. The result is that feminism declined in the 1980s and early 1990s. *Backlash* received a three-star rating, and though a best-seller when published, it has received mixed reviews. Some of the book's supporters say that it makes a brilliantly argued case for feminist backlash in the media. However, several critics argue that it is another 1980s-type bashing book that, although scholarly, makes stick-figure stereotypes of relationships between women and men. Clearly, it is a controversial book about which people rarely feel neutral.

★★★ *We Are Our Mother's Daughters* (1998) by Cokie Roberts. New York: Morrow.

This chief congressional analyst for ABC News discusses significant concerns facing women today. She explores the diverse roles women have assumed as they have traveled the personal and political pathways of American history. Each essay is an introduction to several of the fascinating women the author has encountered during her career and to significant women in her life. This book celebrates the diversity of choice and perspective available to women today. Roberts's position is that women are connected throughout time and, in turn, are their mother's daughters. A three-star book that helps women experience the great conversation all women have shared throughout history.

★★★ *My Mother/My Self* (1977, reissued 1987) by Nancy Friday. New York: Delacorte.

Nancy Friday has authored a number of best-selling books on women's sexuality, including this one and *My Secret Garden*, about women's sexual fantasies. *My Mother/My Self* was based on more than 200 interviews with women (most were mothers and, of course, all were daughters), as well as consultations with a number of mental health experts. Its basic premise is psychoanalytic in nature: Daughters identify with their mothers while becoming their mothers' rivals, and the influence of this complex relationship is felt throughout a daughter's life. Friday also describes the conflicting messages daughters receive from their mothers about their bodies and sexuality, as well as unconscious introjection of the mothers' bad qualities. She describes the mother–daughter relationship in early childhood, then moves through a number of women's milestones, such as loss of virginity and menopause. One of her basic themes is that society's denial of women's sexuality often conflicts with their role as mothers. This book was easily the most widely rated book in the Women's Issues category, evaluated by 187 psychologists. The book's supporters said that it broke new ground when it was published in the late 1970s by providing a probing, insightful analysis of mother–daughter relationships and society's negative portrayal of women's sexuality. However, critics argued that Friday overdramatizes and stereotypes the body inferiority and sexual difficulties of women. All told, an interesting if dated resource on women's sexuality.

Strongly Not Recommended

† *Secrets about Men Every Woman Should Know* (1990) by Barbara DeAngelis. New York: Delacorte.

AUTOBIOGRAPHIES

Highly Recommended

★★★★★ *Heart of a Woman* (1982) by Maya Angelou. New York: Bantam.

Maya Angelou continues to chronicle the remarkable trajectory of her life in this fourth volume of her best-selling autobiography. She overcame many obstacles to become a premier poet, film writer, director, and activist. In this book, she has a young son and is working as a nightclub singer in Los Angeles when she decides to become part of the vibrant art scene in New York City. She joins the Harlem Writers Guild, becomes northern coordinator for the Southern Christian Leadership Conference, marries an African freedom fighter, travels to Africa as a journalist, where the marriage dissolves, and returns to the United States to resume her extraordinary life and career. Throughout all the excitement and turbulence, she remained close to her young son. A candid account of being a black single mom in New York City with an amazing life and talent, this is an inspiring story for anyone, especially young women.

Recommended

★★★ *Reason for Hope: A Spiritual Journey* (2000) by Jane Goodall. New York: Warner Books.

A National Geographic cover story and PBS special brought Jane Goodall's groundbreaking research with chimpanzees in the Gombe Reserve to public attention. In this spiritual autobiography, she recounts the inner life that sustained her. Goodall had been a young waitress in England when she went to Africa, became secretary to paleontologist Louis Leakey, and without formal training or academic degrees, undertook her pioneering studies of chimpanzees. She tells the joys and frustrations of building a research institute, arduous fundraising and public speaking to gain support, the opposition she had to overcome, and the personal tragedies in her life. Throughout it all, her faith in the sacredness of all life and belief in the moral evolution of humanity remained strong. This autobiography shows how determination and intelligence, without formal credentials, can lead to a successful career, and how the inner and outer worlds are connected. A very favorably rated autobiography in our national studies, but unfortunately not yet widely known.

★★★ *Deborah, Golda, and Me: Being Female and Jewish in America* (1992) by Letty Cottin Pogrebin. New York: Doubleday.

A founding member of *Ms.* magazine and a noted feminist thinker, Pogrebin uses this book to reconcile her Jewish faith, which she rejected for much of her life, with her feminism. The book touches on a variety of related issues, including anti-Semitism within the women's movement and the sometimes strained relations between blacks and Jews. A very helpful book for those who want to integrate their Judaism and feminism.

Diamond in the Rough

◆ *Mothers: A Celebration* (1997) by Alexandra Stoddard. New York: Avon.

In this color-illustrated book, the popular author Alexandra Stoddard (*Grace Notes, Living a Beautiful Life, Living in Love*) recounts her experiences as a mother and stepmother, and writes about the women who influenced her life. There are many poignant anecdotes and stirring personal recollections about what it means to be a mother. It was favorably evaluated by just a few respondents in our national studies, thus earning a Diamond in the Rough designation.

FILMS

Strongly Recommended

★★★★ *Fried Green Tomatoes* (1992) directed by Jon Avnet. PG-13 rating. 130 minutes.

Kathy Bates is dowdy, unhappily married, and generally trapped. On a visit to a nursing home she meets a spunky elderly lady, Jessica Tandy, who tells her an old story of rural life filled with memorable characters, racial bigotry, a mysterious murder, and, most importantly, how a varied group of women helped each other thrive. Through the story and the modeling, Bates gathers courage, stops overeating, confronts her slovenly husband, and recaptures her life. An inspiring tale for women on two levels: the interdependence of women in the past and the ability to change in the present.

★★★★ *A League of Their Own* (1993) directed by Penny Marshall. PG rating. 124 minutes.

An excellent film depicting the formation of the All American Girl's Professional Baseball League. The film starts in the 1990s at the Baseball Hall of Fame and then flashes backs to the 1943 season, a time the female players cherish forever. This feminist film shows team sports building character and binding women together. It also effectively demonstrates women's societal struggles during World War II and the attendant changes in gender roles. Widely known and favorably evaluated in our national studies.

★★★★ *The Turning Point* (1977) directed by Herbert Ross. PG rating. 119 minutes.

Two former friends and rivals meet years after following different paths, one to pursue a single life of a professional ballerina and the other to raise a family. Both envy the other's path, wondering about roads not taken. Their earlier rivalry is reignited when the ballerina mentors the other's daughter. A dated film, but one that poignantly illustrates women's life choices (and losses), midlife reevaluations, and the balance between career and family.

★★★★ *How to Make an American Quilt* (1995) directed by Jocelyn Moorhouse. PG-13 rating. 116 minutes.

A gathering of women to make a wedding quilt turns into a social support network. The quilt serves as a metaphor for their varied experiences with life and love. Although not an uplifting film, it refreshingly shows strong women alive and doing well. It deservedly received a bevy of awards.

★★★★ *Eating* (1990) directed by Henry Jaglom. R rating. 110 minutes.

A group of women attending a birthday party sit and talk about food and life. Their conversations are realistic, fascinating, and often hilarious. Not as well known as other movies in this category, but a valuable and entertaining flick. (Also reviewed in Chapter 19, Eating Disorders.)

Recommended

★★★ *The Piano* (1993) directed by Jane Campion. R rating. 121 minutes.

This complex film is, among other things, a gothic romance dressed in Victorian clothes. A mute mother with modern and unconventional sensibilities travels with her daughter to New Zealand, where the mother meets her new husband. The bond among mother, daughter, and music (the piano) provides them with a mutual security and vehicle for expression during some dark times, which include physical abuse. A beautiful and haunting picture nominated for multiple Academy Awards, *The Piano* effectively demonstrates women's struggles for emotional and physical survival.

★★★ *My Breast* (1994) directed by Betty Thomas. Not rated. 90 minutes.

A New York journalist has an unsatisfying relationship with her boyfriend. The diagnosis of breast cancer leads her to dramatically change her life. This television movie received modest and mixed reviews by our mental health experts, but it is one of the few that addresses breast cancer forthrightly.

★★★ *Working Girl* (1988) directed by Mike Nichols. R rating. 116 minutes.

Melanie Griffith has fabulous ideas but is a secretary and is too working class to move up to management. She gets a new female boss, who has the right voice, clothes, and hair for her managerial job. When Griffith finds that her boss plans to steal her great idea, she pretends to be an executive, finds a guy at another firm who can make this happen, and, unfortunately, sleeps with him. Both a comedy and a thriller, this film fully illustrates some of the difficulties women face in the workplace and in relation-ships. In the end, authenticity and initiative pay off.

★★★   *Thelma and Louise* (1992) directed by Ridley Scott. R rating. 129 minutes.

Two women find each other when all seems hopeless in their lives. This controversial movie follows their cross-country jaunt. Searching for freedom and fighting for sur-vival, the women ride into a tragic ending. The movie is unsettling, with easy justifica-tion of murder, rape, and escape. It is bound to precipitate heated discussions about women's power and choices.

INTERNET RESOURCES

What is a woman's issue, or better yet, what part of human behavior is not? Everything has a women's angle, so the number of topics and therefore Internet sites is enormous. As a result, this section offers a larger-than-usual number of metasites—places from which you can find many sites on just about any topic of relevance to women.

Metasites

★★★★★   *WWWomen* http://www.wwwomen.com

Links to thousands of sites, each with a brief and accurate description. The site is non-commercial, positive, and offers solid information; it is the best metasite we have lo-cated on this broad topic.

★★★★★   *Women's Issues—Home Page* http://home.about.com/index.htm

Because this site is always changing, enter "Women" in the search box and follow your interest. Thousands of links under about 25 headings such as Discrimination, Domestic Violence, Self-Defense, Self-Image, Sexual Assault, Sexual Harassment, and Workplace Rights.

★★★★   *WWWomen: Mothers*
         http://www.wwwomen.com/category/mother/general.html

Many interesting sections, each with dozens of sites for MOMs (makers of memories) and about motherhood. It contains support, chat, inspiration, tips, and kid-safe materi-als. Lots of state sites offering support and information for new mothers, stay-at-home moms, work-at-home mothers, employed moms, single parents, older parents, and so on.

★★★★   *Femina: Web Search for Women* http://femina.cybergrrl.com

This site offers thousands of links that are well-organized under the headings most use-ful to clients: Girls, Health, Computers, Family, and so on, and a good search engine. To start a woman exploring the Internet and to seek specific information, this is an excel-lent place to start.

★★★   *Black Stump Women Page: Girls Guide*
        http://home.mira.net/~lions/women.htm

They claim to list 16,128 sites under 22 headings, such as artists, history, childbirth, politics, sports, and travel.

Psychoeducational Materials for Clients and Families

Health

★★★★   *Health and Sexuality* http://feminist.com/resources/links/links_health.html

Here are about a hundred site links under the headings of General Health, Breast Cancer/Cancer, Reproductive Health, and Women and AIDS. The last two have unique and valuable links. It is a good place to start but does not have a search engine.

★★★★   *Alcohol and Women* http://www.niaaa.nih.gov/publications/aa10-text.htm

About four pages of still valuable research information, though written in 1990. "Drinking behavior differs with the age, life role, and marital status of women." A good introduction to the differences gender makes from the National Institute on Alcohol Abuse and Alcoholism.

★★★★   *How Stress Affects the Body* by Jeanne Spurlock, MD http://www.
        amwa-doc.org/publications/WCHealthbook/stressamwa-ch09.html

In eight pages, this site contains "information on why women are vulnerable to stress, how to cope, how to change behavior, and the psychological signs of stress" from the American Women's Medical Association.

★★★★   *Women's Health Issues* by American College of Obstetricians and Gynecologists http://www.acog.org/from_home/pubqry.cfm

They offer to mail up to 5 of their 150 pamphlets to anyone who asks for them. These appear to be well written, comprehensive, and authoritative. You can use either this fill-in to find pamphlets or the Search Public Website on the left to explore the 1,500 publications available. The pamphlets are for sale and not online at the ACOG site. However, a generous physician, Joe Heyman, MD, has placed about 50 of them online at his site. The site is also highly informative about political health care issues. Very highly recommended (http://www.heyman.yourmd.com/ypol/user/usermain.asp?siteid=216202).

Feminism

★★★★★   *On the Issues* http://www.echonyc.com/~onissues/about.htm

This is a progressive woman's magazine with articles (under Features) offering well-written, sometimes hard-hitting feminist perspectives on contemporary issues.

★★★★   *Feminist Utopia* http://www.amazoncastle.com/feminism/feminism.htm

A good starting place because of its breadth; everyone will find something of value from statistics on health and work to nonsexist language, from suffragettes and Herstory to definitions and wise quotations. Thank you, Colleen McEnearny.

★★★★ *Feminist.com* http://www.feminist.com
Offering a variety of resources about activism, nonviolence, and support for women in business. Under Resources, on the left, are stimulating and inspiring readings, quotes, and links.

Menopause

★★★★★ *North American Menopause Society* http://www.menopause.org
A complete presentation of all medical aspects of menopause in about 50 pages. The FAQs are quite informative but very medical.

★★★★ *Menopause* http://fbhc.org/patients/betterhealth/menopause/home.html
A seven-part primer on menopause, simply written, with good links for more information.

★★★★ *Menopause* http://www.docguide.com
Type "Menopause" into the Search field to find current medical information designed for physicians. You don't need to register to be connected.

Lesbian Issues

★★★★★ *Gay/Lesbian Issues* http://home.about.com
Enter "Lesbian" into the search box. A metasite with many subsites on mental health issues, such as Families/Parenting, Out and Outing, Hate Crimes, Religion and Bible Abuse, Work Issues, and Marriage.

★★★ *Lesbian Links* http://femina.cybergrrl.com
Enter "Lesbian" in the search box for a hundred good links.

Workplace Rights

★★★★★ *Equal Employment Opportunity Commission* http://www.eeoc.gov
If you have concerns about employment discrimination, this is the place to start. The Quick Start sections are excellent, and all the laws and policies are here.

★★★ *Employment Discrimination*
    http://www.law.cornell.edu/topics/employment_discrimination.html
The site is quite legal and offers links to all the important documents and decisions. It is likely to be of use to sophisticated readers needing legal support before contacting a lawyer.

★★★ *National Committee on Pay Equity* http://www.feminist.com/fairpay/index.htm

Lots of information on the wage gap between the sexes and what to do about it. See also *Working Women: Equal Pay* at http://www.aflcio.org/yourjobeconomy/women/equalpay/.

NATIONAL SUPPORT GROUPS

Business and Professional Women
1900 M Street, Suite 310
Washington, DC 20036
Phone: 202-293-1100
E-mail: memberservices@bpwusa.org
http://www.bpwusa.org

Organization comprised of working women to promote workplace equity and provide networking opportunities.

National Black Women's Health Project
600 Pennsylvania Avenue SE, Suite 310
Washington, DC 20003
Phone: 202-548-4000
E-mail: nbwhp@nbwhp.org
http://www.blackwomenshealth.org

Committed to the empowerment of all women through wellness.

National Organization for Women
733 15th Street NW
Washington, DC 20005
Phone: 202-628-8669
E-mail: now@now.org
http://www.now.org

Women Employed
111 North Wabash, 13th floor
Chicago, Illinois 60602
Phone: 312-782-3902
E-mail: info@womenemployed.org
http://www.womenemployed.org

See also Abuse (Chapter 2), Eating Disorders (Chapter 19), Pregnancy (Chapter 27), Sexuality (Chapter 30), and Weight Management (Chapter 35).

CHAPTER 37

Violent Youth

Violent acts committed by children and adolescents have become shockingly public in recent years. The Columbine High School shooting sensitized and confronted us with the increasing prevalence of violent youth. The number of offenders under age 18 admitted to state prisons more than doubled from 1985 to 1997; in fact, 61% of persons admitted to prisons under age 18 have been convicted of a violent offense (U.S. Department of Justice Bureau of Statistics, 2002). We are beginning to realize that violent youth are a reality that cannot be ignored. Families, clinicians, educators, and community members alike are searching for effective ways to predict, prevent, and treat violent children.

For our purposes, youth violence includes school violence, criminal behavior, and bullying, as well as the formal diagnoses of oppositional defiant disorder (ODD) and conduct disorder. These disorders are similarly defined as persistent patterns in which children behave aggressively, violate the basic rights of others, and repeatedly defy social rules. The major difference between the two is severity: ODD is less severe than conduct disorder. Both disorders are more common among boys than girls.

In this chapter, we showcase self-help books, films, autobiographies, and websites for violent youth. In each case, the resources are divided between those written for the troubled youths themselves and those written for the people with the task of caring for them.

SELF-HELP BOOKS

In our national studies, only 8 of 27 listed self-help books on violent children were rated by five of more mental health experts. Unfortunately, the self-help books in this area are not yet widely known among the mental health community.

Strongly Recommended

★★★★★ *Your Defiant Child* (1998) by Russell A. Barkley and Christine M. Benton. New York: Guilford Press.

This thorough self-help book offers an eight-step plan for families struggling with a combative child. The program emphasizes consistency and cooperation, promoting

RECOMMENDATION HIGHLIGHTS

Self-Help Books

- On reducing oppositional, defiant, and explosive behavior:

  ★★★★★ *Your Defiant Child* by Russell Barkley and Christine Benton

  ★★★★ *The Explosive Child* by Ross Greene

  ★★★ *The Defiant Child* by Douglas Riley

- On understanding and intervening with violent youth:

  ★★★ *Lost Boys* by James Garbarino

- On rescuing boys from the destructive myths of boyhood:

  ★★★★ *Raising Cain* by Dan Kindlon and Michael Thompson

  ★★★ *Real Boys* by William Pollack

Autobiographies

- On growing up in a tough neighborhood and in a violent juvenile home:

  ★★★ *Sleepers* by Lorenzo Carcaterra

Films

- On surviving a violent stepfather and a passive mother:

  ★★★ *This Boy's Life*

Internet Resources

- On youth violence in general:

  ★★★★★ *National Youth Violence Prevention Resource Center*
  http://www.safeyouth.org/pubs/inetmatcatselect.cfm

  ★★★★★ *Youth Violence: A Report of the Surgeon General*
  http://www.surgeongeneral.gov/library/youthviolence/

- On taking early action:

  ★★★★ *The Warning Signs*
  http://helping.apa.org/warningsigns

  ★★★★ *Early Warning, Timely Response: A Guide to Safe Schools*
  http://www.ed.gov/offices/OSERS/OSEP/Products/
  earlywrn.html

- On preventing bullying:

  ★★★ *Steps to Respect: A Bullying Prevention Program*
  http://www.cfchildren.org/str.shtml

changes through a system of praise, rewards, and mild punishment. The book clearly details what causes defiance, when it becomes a problem, and how it can be resolved. It also possesses assessment tools that will help evaluate a situation. This practical book is filled with charts, questionnaires, and checklists. An excellent, research-based resource for families and clinicians alike, *Your Defiant Child* tops the list of self-help books in this area according to the experts in our national studies.

★★★★ *The Explosive Child* (1999) by Ross Greene. New York: HarperCollins.

Greene attempts to explicate the dynamics of violent behavior in children. In a compassionate style, the author helps readers to reduce the child's meltdowns and parent's frustration. The text is long and serious, covering an enormous amount of ground. Excerpts from actual sessions with parents and children will help psychotherapists, families, and identified patients understand the origins of these violent acts and how a treatment plan is developed. The book addresses the education, psychotherapy, and medication of violent behavior. A splendid albeit lengthy resource.

Recommended

★★★ *The Defiant Child: A Parent's Guide to Oppositional Defiant Disorder* (2002) by Douglas A. Riley. Dallas, TX: Taylor.

Riley explains the mindset of children with ODD and thereby teaches parents how to recognize the signs and modify the behavior of their child's oppositional behavior. The author helps parents remain in control when their children are acting out. The book is written like a behavioral treatment plan for parents, filled with practical interventions, case examples, and family therapy techniques. This well-written, easy-to-read book is a perfect fit for parents who hunger for information about ODD. If it had been rated by a few more experts in our national studies, this book would have received at least a four-star rating.

★★★ *Raising Cain: Protecting the Emotional Life of Boys* (2000) by Daniel J. Kindlon and Michael Thompson. New York: Ballantine.

Two psychologists examine the "culture of cruelty" boys live in, the "tyranny of toughness," the disadvantages of being a boy in elementary school, the systematic squelching of boys' emotional lives, and the corrective actions that society can take without turning "boys into girls." The authors assert that boys need to become more "emotionally literate." They advance seven things that boys need to protect their emotional lives. Topics covered include harsh discipline, distance between father and sons, the connection between mother and sons, depression and suicide, the role of drugs and alcohol in attempting to fill the emotional void, relationship with girls, and anger/violence. For parents, teachers, and anyone working with violent children.

★★★ *Lost Boys: Why Our Sons Turn Violent and How We Can Save Them* (2000) by James Garbarino. New York: Anchor.

This author takes a look at violence in boys and explores the etiology and treatment of violent behavior. Garbarino delves into the social, psychological, and moral factors that lead boys into violence. He offers a clear and broad-spectrum approach to reclaiming these lost boys. He blends statistics, personal experiences, and clinical suggestions with compassion and reality.

★★★ *Real Boys: Rescuing Our Sons from the Myths of Boyhood* (1998) by William Pollack. New York: Henry Holt.

The author explores boys' feelings of sadness, loneliness, and confusion while they try to appear tough, cheerful, and confident. Pollack discusses how to let real boys be real men by revising the "Boys' Code" and still feeling connected. He writes about what boys are like, how to help them, and what happens if they aren't helped. Adults working with violent boys will probably find this book valuable. Also reviewed in Chapter 24, Men's Issues, where it received a higher, four-star rating.

Diamonds in the Rough

♦ *High Risk: Children without a Conscience* (1990) by Ken Magid and Carole A. McKelvey. New York: Bantam.

Children without a conscience are growing in number and increasingly at risk for becoming "trust bandits," con men, dance-away lovers, back stabbers, and even sociopathic killers. Magid and McKelvey discuss what attachment is and what happens when that bond does not occur in peoples' lives. On the book jacket, the authors ask, "Who are these children without a conscience?" They answer, "They are children who cannot trust, children who cannot love, and children who will not be loved." This book, highly but rarely rated in our national studies, leading to a Diamond in the Rough designation, is for parents and professionals alike.

♦ *Bullies and Victims: Helping Your Child Survive the Schoolyard Battlefield* (1998) by Suellen Fried and Paula Fried. New York: Evans.

The authors survived peer abuse themselves and provide suggestions for parental intervention and constructive reactions. This book defines different forms of bullying and different levels of response to the bullying. Punctuated by short case studies, *Bullies and Victims* presents individual, family, school and societal methods to reduce bullying. The book is characterized as a Diamond in the Rough because it was positively but infrequently evaluated in our national studies.

AUTOBIOGRAPHIES

Recommended

★★★ *Sleepers* (1996) by Lorenzo Carcaterra. New York: Ballantine.

As a young man growing up in a tough neighborhood, the author and his friends engaged in crime. When they were caught, the four teenagers were sent to a juvenile home, where they were assaulted and raped by brutal guards. Years later, now grown and one a lawyer, another a journalist (Carcaterra), and the other two murderers, the men take revenge against their tormenters. This fast-paced, emotional tale has been made into a movie, with names, dates, and places changed "to protect the innocent and the guilty." Questions have been raised about the authenticity of the story. Whether a true story or the invention of its journalist–author, the book describes brutal conditions of confinement and the vicious cycle of violence. Also reviewed in Chapter 2, Abuse.

Diamonds in the Rough

♦ *All Souls: A Family History from Southie* (2000) by Michael Patrick MacDonald. New York: Ballantine.

Gripping, gritty story of growing up in South Boston's poor Irish Catholic housing projects. The author was the seventh of nine children born to a single mom who worked hard to provide for her family. It describes neighborhood and family loyalty in the face of grinding poverty, rampant corruption (everyone hustles or is on the take), violent youth terrorizing the residents, unwanted pregnancies, and drug dealing. MacDonald lost half his siblings to violence or suicide. It is a story of resilience, survival, and redemption. The author is a neighborhood activist working on social programs in South Boston. A good book for understanding the scars, both visible and invisible, left by growing up in a brutal neighborhood. This book is not widely known in our national studies, thus qualifying as a Diamond in the Rough.

♦ *Monster: The Autobiography of an LA Gang Member* (1998) by Sanyika Shakur AKA Monster Kody Scott. New York: Viking Penguin.

Growing up in an urban war zone, initiated into the Crips at age 11, an Original Gangster and admitted killer for 16 years, the author found redemption in prison through radical black nationalism. In a graphic depiction of why some inner city youth join gangs and the angry mind-set of a gangbanger who commits unspeakable crimes, this insider account will have credibility for at-risk youth and those who work with them.

FILMS

Recommended

★★★ *This Boy's Life* (1993) directed by Michael Caton-Jones. R rating. 114 minutes.

After her divorce, a mother takes her son, played by Leonardo DeCaprio, and heads west. She settles in Concrete (Washington) and for a vicious but colorful man, Robert DeNiro, who makes DeCaprio's life miserable with his pretensions, bullying, lying, and violence. The mother, desperate for the paycheck DeNiro provides, remains neutral. As a consequence, DeCaprio is forced to accept the abuse and to grow up faster and become more independent. Based on a true story, the film is a realistic tale of a child surviving an abusive stepfather and a passive mother. Had this film been more frequently known by professionals in our studies, it would have probably garnered a four- or five-star rating.

★★★ *The Good Son* (1993) directed by Joseph Ruben. R rating. 87 minutes.

Macaulay Culkin plays an evil boy of about 10 who commits crimes, enjoys torture, kills his baby brother, and performs assorted psychopathic acts. His evil is unrecognized by the adults, including a psychiatrist, but is seen by Elijah Wood, who suffers from it as well. It is not a suitable film for children; its only redeeming value is the frightening presentation of unfettered violence.

INTERNET RESOURCES

Metasites

★★★★★   *National Youth Violence Prevention Resource Center*
            http://www.safeyouth.org/pubs/inetmatcatselect.cfm

The Center is sponsored by the Centers for Disease Control and Prevention and the Federal Working Group on Youth Violence, and serves a gateway to just about every paper, office, and program concerned with youth violence. The site listed above is the publications available from them and other government agencies. Here are hundreds of newsletters, fact sheets, and brochures for clients, parents, youth, and educators under headings such as Conflict Resolution, Bullying, Substance Abuse, Risk Factors, Dating Violence, Family Violence, Gangs, Firearms, Protective Factors/Parenting, Racial and Ethnic Minorities, School Violence, Hate Crimes, Media Violence, and Community-Based Programs. A collection of about 30 FAQs on youth violence is available at the site http://www.safeyouth.org/faq/index.htm.

★★★★★   *Youth Violence: A Report of the Surgeon General*
            http://www.surgeongeneral.gov/library/youthviolence

Might as well start at the top. Everything is here, including the developmental issues; demonstration programs; real data on gangs, arrests, and prevalence; risk factors; exposure of the myths of the "superpredator"; and the "epidemic"of school shootings. Highly recommended for a dose of reality.

Psychoeducational Materials for Clients and Families

★★★★   *The Warning Signs* http://helping.apa.org/warningsigns

The Warning Signs guide, produced by MTV and the American Psychological Association, was designed to help youth avoid violent situations and prevent violence before it happens. This guide covers topics such as reasons for violence, recognizing violence warning signs in others, what you can do if someone you know shows violence warning signs, dealing with anger, controlling your own risk for violent behavior, and violence against self.

★★★★   *Early Warning, Timely Response: A Guide to Safe Schools*
            http://www.ed.gov/offices/OSERS/OSEP/Products/earlywrn.html

This 50-page book offers "research-based practices designed to assist school communities identify these warning signs early and develop prevention, intervention and crisis response plans." The guide includes sections on Characteristics of a School that is Safe and Responsive to All Children; Early Warning Signs; Getting Help for Troubled Children; Developing a Prevention and Response Plan; and Responding to Crisis. A follow-up publication on implementation, entitled Safeguarding our Children: An Action

Guide, is 68 pages and available at http://www.ed.gov/offices/OSERS/OSEP/Products/ActionGuide/Action_Guide.pdf.

★★★★ *Project Achieve* http://www.coedu.usf.edu/projectachieve

Parents, citizens, and educators searching for effective interventions should look at this large-scale, research-based program to teach social and problem-solving skills to reduce violence in the schools and community. The Second Step program is similar and details are available at http://www.cfchildren.org.

★★★ *Checklist of Characteristics of Youth Who Have Caused School-Associated Violent Deaths* http://www.nssc1.org/reporter/checklist.htm

Twenty items developed by Dr. Ronald D. Stephens.

★★★ *Working Together to Create Safe Schools*
    http://www.nssc1.org/handouts/worktog.pdf

This six-page handout offers strategies on how schools can work together with school board members, school employees, students, parents, community leaders, service groups, business leaders, government representatives, law enforcers, and the media to create safer schools.

★★★ *NASP Fact Sheets* http://www.naspcenter.org/factsheets

The National Association of School Psychologists has two fact sheets of relevance: Bullying: What Schools and Parents Can Do, and Zero Tolerance and Alternative Strategies. To summarize, bullying is violence that provokes even more violence, and zero tolerance policies don't work.

Bullying

★★★★ *Bullying: Information for Parents and Teachers*
    http://www.lfcc.on.ca/bully.htm

A 14-page, comprehensive and intelligent paper here is part of a prevention project.

★★★★ *Bullying at School Information* http://www.scre.ac.uk/bully/index.html

Many linked pages in a thorough booklet.

★★★ *Steps to Respect: A Bullying Prevention Program*
    http://www.cfchildren.org/str.shtml

This comprehensive program is well described at the website.

See also Anger (Chapter 6), Child Development and Parenting (Chapter 13), and Teenagers and Parenting (Chapter 34).

CHAPTER 38

Strategies for Selecting Self-Help Resources

A massive and systemic revolution is occurring in mental health: self-help with or without professional treatment. This self-help revolution entails diverse activities: changing behavior by oneself, reading and applying self-help books, attending support and 12-step groups, watching films and incorporating their cinematic lessons, surfing the Internet for advice and treatments, and participating in alternative health care. All these and many other examples compellingly indicate that people are making concerted efforts to change themselves on their own (Norcross, 2000).

Self-help is big business. Americans spend almost $600 million on self-help books each year and surf more than 15,000 websites devoted to mental health (Paul, 2001). The use of self-help services and alternative treatments for mental health conditions is increasing steeply, according to the latest research (e.g., Druss & Rosenheck, 2000; Kessler et al., 1999). Some experts claim that self-help will become the nation's de facto treatment of choice for many behavioral disorders and life predicaments by the year 2010 or 2020 (Goodman & Jacobs, 1994).

When you select or recommend self-help materials, you obviously want those that are the most effective. You visit a bookstore, Internet site, or video store but are immediately confronted with dozens of choices that address your particular problem or life challenge (or that of a family member). And you would like guidelines to help you select the best.

Although self-help is big business, it is, alas, not scientific business. As the volume and accessibility of self-help information soar, the question of quality assumes urgency. Of the thousands of websites launched yearly and of the estimated 2,000 self-help books published annually, more than 95% are published without any controlled research documenting their accuracy or effectiveness. The Internet, in particular, is awash in snake oil.

The self-help market resembles a Persian bazaar with proliferating choices and without clear answers: Should you nurture others or nurture your inner child; seek success or simplicity; just say no or just do it; confront your fears or honor them (Albom, 1997)? Sorely needed are trustworthy and scientific means to determine the quality of self-help resources.

In the preceding chapters, we have tried to provide just that. The expert ratings and descriptions of self-help books, autobiographies, films, and Internet resources are designed to guide mental health professionals' recommendations to their clients, as well as consumers' selection of useful resources.

There is no magic key to the self-help kingdom, but several strategies can help you select the best resource and avoid the clunkers. By analyzing the mental health experts' comments in our eight national studies, and by reviewing the research literature on self-help, we have arrived at 11 strategies for selecting an effective self-help resource.

1. Don't select a self-help resource because of its cover, title, or glitzy advertising campaign. The old saying, "You can't tell a book by its cover," probably applies to self-help books more than to any other type of book. Publishers spend huge sums of money to create splashy covers with sensational titles and to develop attention-grabbing, Madison Avenue advertising campaigns. They describe each year's new crop of self-help books as "phenomenal breakthroughs" and "scientific revolutions" in understanding life's problems. Some good self-help books have fancy covers and catchy titles, but so do some bad ones. The same is true for expensive advertisements—the bad books are just as likely to have huge advertising outlays as the good books.

One category with especially flashy titles, huge advertising outlays, and good fodder for talk shows is love and marriage. Several of our Not Recommended books were, in fact, national best-sellers with huge advertising budgets and catchy titles. Based on what you hear and see on talk shows, book covers, and advertising, there isn't any way people can sort through titles in this category and tell that these books aren't good self-help books.

Publishers and bookstores influence self-help book purchases by how many books they display and where the books are located. However, this year's top-selling book that is stacked from floor to ceiling often finds its way to next year's wastebasket. Or something worse happens: Lavish advertising, expensive promotional campaigns, and support by national book chains enable some bad self-help books to sell extremely well. Without guidelines, consumers don't know that these books are bad. It is not unusual for bookstores to have only one or two copies of some of the best self-help books hidden on the bottom shelves or not to carry them at all.

When one area of self-help becomes popular, many authors jump on the bandwagon and quickly pump out books in rapid succession, hoping to exploit the latest "in" topic or movement. In the early 1990s, codependency, the inner child, and dieting were especially hot topics, and authors whipped out books on them at an astonishing pace. In the late 1990s, spirituality was in the ascendancy. Yet most of the books in these hot categories were not rated favorably by mental health experts.

In summary, be an intelligent consumer of psychological knowledge by going beyond the cover, the celebrity testimonials, the fancy ads, the author's appearance on talk shows, and the bookstore's elaborate display. Instead, make your choices based on the next 10 strategies.

2. Select a resource that makes realistic rather than grandiose claims. If you have a problem, you want to cope with it as effectively and painlessly as possible. The quicker you can fix the problem, the better. Unfortunately, the self-help resources that make extravagant claims are the most alluring and thus sell better than books that are more realistic. Most problems do not arise overnight, and most can't be solved overnight. Books that promise wondrous insights that can immediately solve problems should be avoided.

When a self-help claim appears too good to be true, it probably is not true. If a resource states that a "miraculous" new diet guarantees you lose a pound a day and keep the weight off permanently, don't buy it. The largest number of low-rated books in our national studies was in the weight management category. Most of these books made extravagant claims and took a very narrow approach to weight loss. More reasonable books are not as eye-catching and as sensational, but they present a more balanced approach to weight loss—and tend not to sell as well, even though they are far better self-help books.

Try to make a realistic judgment about the book's claims. Be skeptical of anything that sounds easy, magical, and wondrous. Overcoming depression, losing weight, improving relationships, and becoming more self-fulfilled are not easy tasks. They take a lot of effort. Coping effectively with any of life's important tasks or problems—anxiety, parenting, divorce, addiction, or career development—is a lifelong project.

3. Examine the evidence reported in the self-help resource. Many self-help resources are not based on reliable scientific evidence but rather on the author's anecdotal experiences or clients' testimonials. In some instances, evidence is gleaned from interviews with a narrow range of people or a few clients seen in therapy. Too much of what you read in the self-help literature is based on speculative intuition.

Most of the self-help resources highly rated by the mental health professionals were based on reliable research or clinical evidence. The cognitive therapy of depression advocated by Aaron Beck and David Burns (Chapter 17) has undergone careful scrutiny by the clinical and research community and been found to be effective for many people. The same is true for Herbert Benson's *The Relaxation Response* (Chapter 32), *Learned Optimism* by Martin Seligman, and *Changing for Good* by James Prochaska and associates (Chapter 29). These books are not based on the subjective opinions of the authors or the testimonials of others, but on years of sound research and clinical results.

Hardly any self-help resource contains elaborate research citations. This is by design, because lengthy citations make the books difficult to read. However, authors of the most effective resources typically describe the research evidence, the clinical evidence, or both, on which the book is based. And the good books often list sources in an appendix.

4. Select self-help materials that recognize problems are caused by a number of factors and have alternative solutions. It's not just your imagination. You are a complex being living in a complex world. Your problems are not so simple that they have a simple cause and a single solution. Yet the human mind is biased toward simple answers to complex problems. After all, solving a problem is easier if there is one simple solution than if you have to modify a number of factors in your life.

Consider stress and anxiety. Thinking positively may well help you cope more effectively with stress, but self-help resources that deal only with positive thinking often oversimplify the change process. Stress and anxiety reduction can be facilitated by thinking optimistically, rearranging your life, practicing relaxation, exercising regularly, eating healthfully, learning assertion skills, training your breathing, knowing your personality, and cultivating more interpersonal support.

Counter the "single trick" mentality by examining self-help materials for multiple causes and multiple sources of assistance. A variety of self-change methods in your repertoire will assuredly be more useful than a solitary technique.

5. Self-help resources that focus on a particular problem are better than those that claim to be a general solution for all of your problems. Effective self-help materials tend to concentrate on a specific problem rather than promising to cure all of life's ills. Materials that try to solve all problems are shallow and lack the detailed recommendations that are needed to improve a particular problem. When authors claim that their methods will solve all of your problems and will help everybody, don't buy it, figuratively and literally.

The more authors can convince the public that their books are for everyone, the greater their chances of selling millions of copies. And that is exactly what far too many self-help authors try to do—writing books that are so broad in scope that they will appeal to a huge audience. The concept of codependency (Chapter 3) initially applied to the specific problems of people married to alcoholics, especially women married to male alcoholics. But the concept spread rapidly to a host of other circumstances, and codependency authors now claim that codependency is in every relationship. That is far too broad and all encompassing to be useful.

Most of the leading self-help resources in our studies tackle specific disorders. Davis and associates' *The Relaxation and Stress Reduction Workbook* is a perfect illustration. As the title indicates, it is specific and detailed; it does not promise a panacea for all conditions. Bourne's *The Anxiety and Phobia Workbook* does likewise. *The Courage to Heal* addresses recovery from child sexual abuse, and Brazelton's *Infants and Mothers* focuses on a specific age—infants from birth to one year of age—and how parents should respond to active, average, or quiet infants. These books don't try to reel everyone in and don't pretend to be all things to all people. They focus on specific types of problems and offer specific solutions to those problems.

6. Select self-help resources that clearly explain their limitations and contraindications. A single self-help resource is only applicable for a limited range of behavioral disorders and life challenges. We do not expect, say, a self-help book on pregnancy or an Internet site on trauma to help effectively with career development. It sounds so obvious, but many self-help resources do not delineate the boundaries of their applicability. In an effort to reach millions of people and sell more copies, marketers are pushing products for everything that ails you.

Effective self-help materials clearly articulate their limits. Good books and sites will explain which people should not use them and describe when their usage is, in fact, contraindicated. Meritorious resources inform you about the potential downside of using the resource on your own and provide guidance for seeking professional treatment. Self-help materials that are not forthcoming about their limits are simply not honest.

7. Don't be conned by psychobabble and slick writing. In 1977, R. D. Rosen wrote *Psychobabble*, a sizzling attack on the psychological jargon that fills the space between the covers of many self-help resources. Unfortunately, 25 years later, psychobabble is still alive and well.

Psychobabble is a hip and vague language that will not improve your ability to cope with a problem. Too many self-help authors write in psychobabble, saying things like "You've got to get in touch with your feelings"; "Get with the program"; "You've got to get it"; "The real you"; "To solve your problem you need some high-energy experiences"; "You are sending off the wrong vibes"; and on and on. In a number of chapters, we specifically criticize some books for having too much psychobabble and praised others for being free of it.

Psychobabble is not the only semantic problem of poor self-help materials. Some disguise their inadequacies with slick writing that is so friendly that it seems as if the author is personally talking to you. After you have read only a few pages of the book or website, you say to yourself, "Wow! This can really help me." All too often, such slick books offer little more than one or two basic ideas that could be communicated in a few pages. The rest of the book is filled with polished writing and case examples that provide little additional knowledge. Such books lack the specific recommendations and sound strategies needed to cope more effectively with life's problems.

Self-help resources characterized by psychobabble and slick writing frequently resort to motivational cheerleading and inspirational sermons. This approach can get you pumped up to solve your problem, but then it lets you down by giving you no precise strategies. After a few weeks, the buzz wears off, because the author's recommendations lack depth. Examples of books characterized by this approach are Zig Zigler's *Steps to the Top* (in contrast to Steven Covey's *The 7 Habits of Highly Effective People*, which has detailed, effective strategies; Chapter 29) and Leo Buscaglia's *Loving Each Other* (in contrast to Aaron Beck's *Love Is Never Enough*, which examines the complexity of love and its many different avenues; Chapter 22).

We are not opposed to personal and fluid writing. However, it takes a lot more than an author's slick language to help you. Select self-help materials that are clearly written in language you can understand and that include detailed recommendations for how to change.

8. Check out the author's educational and professional credentials. Not all authors of self-help resources are mental health professionals who have gone through rigorous training at respected universities and have spent years rendering professional treatment. Just about anyone can get their self-help ideas onto the web if they have a modicum of computer skills, and most can get those ideas into print if they have the resources to self-publish or can convince a publisher that they will make money. But most of the best self-help books and Internet sites (excluding autobiographies) are written by mental health professionals, not writers.

In our national studies, the authors of 80–90% of the top self-help books have PhDs or MDs and have done extensive research or have had clinical training. Psychologists David Barlow and Edna Foa, the authors of excellent resources for anxiety disorders, are world-renowned researchers in their areas. Aaron Beck and David Burns, the authors of excellent books on depression and relationships, are respected psychiatrists and medical school professors. T. Berry Brazelton, author of four highly touted books, is an esteemed pediatrician who has experience working with parents and babies; he is affiliated with the Harvard Medical School. Harriet Lerner, author of *The Dance of Anger* and *The Dance of Intimacy*, is a psychologist on the staff of the famous Menninger Clinic.

Of course, the reverse can also happen. A PhD or an MD does not guarantee a wonderful self-help book. The consensus of the mental health experts in the national studies was that Phil McGraw, Joyce Brothers, and Wayne Dyer, all of whom have PhDs, and a large number of authors with MDs in the weight management category, have written self-help books that should be avoided.

9. Be wary of authors who reject the conventional knowledge of mental health professionals. Some self-help authors attack the mental health professions as being too conservative and overly concerned with scientific evidence. Consider such attacks a red flag, and avoid these authors. These antiestablishment, antiscience mavericks avow that their ideas are way ahead of their time and that it will take years for mental health professionals to catch up with their avant garde thinking. Many New Age and Scientology authors, such as L. Ron Hubbard, fall into this category.

There is nothing wrong with new ideas, of course. But there is something seriously wrong with new ideas uncritically promulgated in the absence of reliable evidence of their effectiveness and safety. For the most part, the materials of self-help authors who condemn the mental health establishment will not meaningfully assist you.

10. Distinguish between balanced information and subtle advertising. The Internet offers a wealth of information, but it is virtually uncontrolled. The traditional fire walls between reliable information on the one hand, and advertising on the other, are often blurred or absent altogether on the Web. Frequently, conflicts of interest are not disclosed, financial sponsors are hidden, and advertisements are not labeled as such.

Many health and consumer groups, including the Consumer Union, have launched programs to develop disclosure standards for the Internet and to report on the business practices of websites. But in the meantime, please cast a critical eye to Internet sites and realize that some sites charge for listings or are actually lengthy advertisements for drug companies and for-profit clinics, to take two common examples. Check the Who Are We? and the Privacy Notice sections of the sites; if these are sketchy or absent, let that be notice that the materials may be quite biased. Always "consider the (financial) source" and critically evaluate whether the resource provides balanced and comprehensive information.

11. Use the *Authoritative Guide to Self-Help Resources in Mental Health* as a guide. Even armed with the first 10 strategies for selecting an effective self-help resource, you may still experience difficulty in sorting through the jungle and picking the best one. With practice in using the strategies, you will become a more knowledgeable consumer.

For us, the most trustworthy strategy for selecting good self-help materials and avoiding the lemons is accessing the knowledge of the most highly trained mental health professionals in the United States. We have compiled and shared their knowledge in this book.

As explained in Chapter 1, our eight national studies have involved nearly 3,500 psychologists in evaluating self-help books, autobiographies, and films. Professional consensus is no guarantee, but it is superior to individual judgments, random selection, or best-seller lists. We trust and value the collective ratings of thousands of experts. Use their knowledge to help select effective self-help materials.

The Eight National Studies

Over the past 10 years, we have conducted a series of national studies to determine the most useful and most frequently recommended self-help resources for diverse problems. The resources we evaluated were self-help books, autobiographies, and films. In each case, the methodology and the samples were very similar: a lengthy survey mailed to clinical and counseling psychologists residing in the United States. The responding psychologists rated self-help resources with which they were sufficiently familiar on the same five-point scale:

+2	Extremely good	Outstanding; highly recommended book, best or among best in category
+1	Moderately good	Provides good advice, can be helpful; worth purchasing
0	Average	An average self-help book
−1	Moderately bad	Not a good self-help book; may provide misleading or inaccurate information
−2	Extremely bad	This book exemplifies the worst of the self-help books; worst, or among worst in its category

The precise wording was slightly altered, of course, for ratings of autobiographies and films. For example, the wording read "An average autobiographical account," "Outstanding; highly recommended film," and so on.

As authors of this book and lead researchers on the eight studies, we strove to avoid theoretical bias. Our theoretical orientations are explicitly eclectic or integrative; that is, we believe that a number of treatment approaches can be used to help people overcome disorders and cope effectively with life transitions. Something of value can be found among the dizzying diversity of treatments ranging from A to Z—analytical, behavioral, cognitive, all the way to Zen Buddhism.

Overall, the mental health experts were far more likely to rate the self-help resources positively than negatively. The stars (one to five) and the dagger assigned to the various resources were based primarily on the average rating of the resource, and secondarily on its frequency of rating. After extensive discussions and data analyses, we selected the cutoff points for one to five stars described in Chapter 1 and presented below:

★★★★★ Average rating of 1.25 or higher; the resource was rated by 30 or more mental health professionals

★★★★ Average rating of 1.00 or higher; rated by 20 or more mental health professionals

★★★ Average rating of .50 through .99; rated 10 or more times

★★ Average rating of .25 through .49; rated 10 or more times

★ Average rating of .00 through .24; rated 10 or more times

† Average negative rating; rated by 10 or more mental health professionals

The sole exception to this rating system was the autobiographies. There, we used a cutoff of 8 or more ratings, as opposed to 10, simply because fewer psychologists were sufficiently familiar with autobiographies than with self-help books or movies and because in one of our investigations (Study 2) we had previously used 8 as the minimum number of raters. Thus, the rating systems for autobiographies was:

★★★★★ Average rating of 1.25 or higher; rated by 24 or more mental health professionals

★★★★ Average rating of 1.00 or higher; rated by 16 or more mental health professionals

★★★ Average rating of .50 through .99; rated 8 or more times

★★ Average rating of .25 through .49; rated 8 or more times

★ Average rating of .00 through .24; rated 8 or more times

† Average negative rating; rated by 8 or more mental health professionals

Our recommendations in each chapter are guided by the collective judgment of the mental health experts in our studies. The Strongly Recommended self-help resources are those receiving five or four stars. The three-star resources receive the more modest designation of Recommended. Although the one- and two-star books were in the positive range, they were low positive and received a large number of 0 and even some negative ratings. Thus, we opted not to recommend them. And, as described in Chapter 1, the worst rating—the dagger (†)—was reserved for books, autobiographies, and films receiving a negative rating. This rating, it should be noted, was given to only 5% of all the self-help resources in our studies.

The individual ratings for all the self-help resources canvassed in our eight studies are detailed in Appendix B (self-help books), Appendix C (autobiographies), and Appendix D (films).

Across the eight studies, nearly 3,500 psychologists contributed their expertise and judgment to evaluate self-help resources. Below we briefly review the survey methodology and sample composition of each study.

STUDY 1: SELF-HELP BOOKS

The first study entailed mailing a questionnaire to 4,000 members of the clinical and counseling divisions of the American Psychological Association (APA). Almost 800 psychologists returned the questionnaires, but full ratings of the books were completed by just under 600. Some of the members had died, and their spouses returned the unanswered questionnaires with a note; more than 100 respondents filled out the first part of the questionnaire (demographic information and general items about self-help books) but did not rate individual books; and some respondents returned the forms unanswered. In many such studies, a follow-up mailing is conducted to increase the sample size. We considered this alternative but did not exercise it for a simple reason: inadequate funds. The results of the first national study formed the basis for *The Authoritative Guide to Self-Help Books* by John W. Santrock, Ann M. Minnett, and Barbara D. Campbell (1994).

The responding mental health professionals all held doctorates. They lived in every state and represented a broad cross-section of clinical and counseling psychologists in the United States. Although the respondents were members of the clinical and counseling divisions of the APA, their evaluations of self-help books in the study and in this book are not in any way endorsed by the APA itself.

STUDY 2: AUTOBIOGRAPHIES

A few years later, we expanded our focus to embrace autobiographies of people suffering from a behavioral or mental disorder. Our inclusion criteria were that they be first-person narrative accounts that dealt primarily or substantially with the author's disorder or treatment in book-length works. Excluded were fictional and second-person accounts. Brief articles, poetry collections, and film accounts were also excluded. Our aim was to obtain solid, national data on the published autobiographies that psychologists recommend to their clients.

We mailed a cover letter, a four-page questionnaire, and a stamped return envelope to 1,000 randomly selected members of the APA's Division of Psychotherapy living in the United States. Of these, 379 questionnaires (38%) were returned; however, 17 were not usable because the psychologists were retired or did not wish to participate. The final sample consisted of 362 psychologists who were demographically and geographically representative of the entire Division of Psychotherapy membership. Thirty-five percent of the psychologists were women, and 94% were Caucasian. Primary employment settings were private practice (66% of sample), universities (10%), hospitals (5%), and outpatient clinics (5%). Portions of these results were reported in a *Professional Psychology* article authored by Jennifer S. Clifford, John C. Norcross, and Robert Sommer (1999).

STUDY 3: SELF-HELP BOOKS

Study 3 canvassed self-help books published since Study 1 was performed and included self-help books on three additional disorders: schizophrenia, attention-deficit/hyperactivity disorder

(ADHD), and dementia/Alzheimer's disease. Two separate surveys were mailed to a total of 3,000 randomly selected members of the APA's clinical psychology and counseling psychology divisions. The first questionnaire was sent to 1,500 psychologists soliciting quality ratings on self-help books for 14 problem areas; the second questionnaire was sent to another 1,500 psychologists requesting ratings on self-help books on a different set of 15 problems. The first questionnaire was returned by 336 psychologists, and full ratings of the books were completed by 324. The total response rate was 22%. The second questionnaire was completed and returned by 376 psychologists; of these, 357 provided usable data. This yielded a total response rate of 25%. The psychologists returning the questionnaires were demographically, professionally, and geographically representative of the APA divisions of clinical psychology and counseling psychology (Bechtoldt, Norcross, Wyckoff, Pokrywa, & Campbell, 2001).

STUDY 4: AUTOBIOGRAPHIES

Study 4 assessed psychologists' knowledge and evaluations of autobiographies not covered in our earlier study. A lengthy questionnaire was mailed to 1,500 members of APA's clinical psychology division and counseling psychology division seeking their ratings on the value of autobiographies concerning 13 different problems. Of these, 328 were returned, but 21 were incomplete, leaving 307 usable questionnaires. As in the other studies, the primary reasons for returning an incomplete questionnaire were that the psychologists were not in clinical practice or had recently retired. The response rate for this study was 22%.

STUDY 5: FILMS

In Study 5 we entered new territory: psychologists' evaluations of commercial films as self-help resources. We sent a lengthy questionnaire concerning the value of specific movies to 1,500 members of the APA's clinical and counseling psychology divisions. Psychologists were asked to rate the quality of listed movies with which they were sufficiently familiar for 20 problem areas. A total of 417 surveys were returned, with usable data provided by 401 of the respondents, a 28% total response rate. As in the previous studies, the participating mental health experts were all doctoral-level psychologists of various genders, ethnicities, theoretical orientations, and work settings.

STUDY 6: SELF-HELP BOOKS

In preparation for this book, we conducted three new studies in 2002 covering self-help books, autobiographies, and films. For Study 6, we mailed a lengthy questionnaire requesting evaluations of self-help books for 15 behavioral disorders and life challenges to 1,666 members of the APA clinical and counseling divisions. A total of 257 questionnaires were retuned, with ratings of the books completed by 237 experts.

Table A.1 summarizes the demographic and professional characteristics of the psychologists participating in Study 6, as well as those participating in Studies 7 and 8 (described below). The responding psychologists constituted a broad sample of mental health experts. Hailing from ev-

Table A.1. Descriptive Summary of Responding Psychologists in the Three Latest Studies

Characteristic	Study 6 (N = 257)	Study 7 (N = 292)	Study 8 (N = 338)
Gender			
Male	53%	53%	59%
Female	47%	47%	41%
Ethnic/racial background			
Native American	1%	0%	1%
African American/black	1%	2%	2%
Caucasian/White	92%	94%	92%
Hispanic/Latino	3%	2%	2%
Asian American	1%	1%	1%
Multiple/Other	2%	1%	2%
Theoretical orientation			
Behavioral	7%	13%	12%
Cognitive	24%	20%	24%
Eclectic/integrative	37%	33%	35%
Humanistic/existential	9%	6%	4%
Interpersonal	3%	5%	4%
Psychodynamic/analytic	12%	12%	16%
Systems/family systems	3%	5%	2%
Other	5%	6%	3%
Employment setting			
Private practice	38%	40%	42%
General hospital	4%	3%	2%
Outpatient clinic/HMO	8%	9%	9%
Psychiatric hospital	4%	2%	3%
University	29%	23%	25%
Medical school	6%	7%	7%
Other	11%	16%	12%

ery state in the union, they all held doctoral degrees and averaged 19 years of postdoctoral experience. As shown in Table A.1, the psychologists represented diverse theoretical orientations and a variety of employment sites, largely private practice and academia.

STUDY 7: SELF-HELP BOOKS

The rapid proliferation of self-help books required yet another questionnaire on self-help books, simply to canvass the remaining behavioral disorders and life challenges covered in our book. Together, Studies 6 and 7 collected evaluative data on books in 36 areas, including the new chapters in this book devoted to trauma, obsessive–compulsive disorder, violent youth, borderline and narcissistic personality disorders, bipolar disorder, and suicide.

Specifically, we compiled a lengthy questionnaire on recent self-help books for 21 problem areas and mailed it to another 1,666 psychologists who belonged to the APA clinical psychology and counseling psychology divisions. A total of 292 psychologists participated, but 31 of them returned the questionnaire incomplete for various reasons.

STUDY 8: FILMS AND AUTOBIOGRAPHIES

Our final study involved a lengthy questionnaire concerning the value of specific films and autobiographies for particular disorders. Paralleling all of our previous studies, we mailed the questionnaire to a large sample of American psychologists who were members of APA's division of clinical psychology or division of counseling psychology. We sent 1,666 questionnaires and received 338 returns, for a total response rate of 20%. Of the returned questionnaires, 316 were usable, for a usable return rate of 19%.

Ratings
of Self-Help Books
in the National Studies

Only those self-help books rated five or more times in our national studies are included in this list. Some books appear on this list but were not included in the text because they were rated by fewer than 10 mental health experts. Please consult Appendix A for details on the methodology of the national studies and the meaning of the guide ratings.

Category and title	Author(s)	Study no.	Avg. rating	No. of raters	Guide rating
Abuse					
Abused No More	Ackerman & Pickering	1	0.48	57	★★
Allies in Healing	Davis	3	1.24	33	★★★★
Battered Wives	Martin	1	0.85	56	★★★
Battered Woman, The	Walker	1	1.22	121	★★★★
Beginning to Heal	Bass & Davis	3	0.84	43	★★★
Breaking Violence in a Relationship	Blue	3	1.00	6	—
Courage to Heal, The	Bass & Davis	1	1.53	244	★★★★★
Facing the Shadow	Carnes	6	1.17	6	—
Getting Free	NiCarthy	1	1.00	38	★★★★
Healing the Incest Wound	Courtois	6	1.31	54	★★★★★
Healing the Shame That Binds You	Bradshaw	1	0.56	192	★★★
Healing the Trauma of Abuse	Copeland & Harris	6	1.25	12	★★★
I Never Called It Rape	Warshaw	3	1.53	17	★★★
Invisible Wounds	Douglas	6	0.80	5	—

Category and title	Author(s)	Study no.	Avg. rating	No. of raters	Guide rating
Abuse (*cont.*)					
Me Nobody Knows, The	Bean & Bennett	6	1.13	8	—
Reclaiming the Inner Child	Abrams	1	0.20	97	★
Secret of Overcoming Verbal Abuse, The	Ellis & Grad-Powers	6	0.81	16	★★★
Secret Trauma, The	Russell	6	1.30	10	★★★
Sexual Healing Journey, The	Maltz	6	1.44	18	★★★
Toxic Parents	Forward	1	0.47	119	★★
Verbally Abusive Relationship, The	Evans	3	1.61	13	★★★
Victims No Longer	Lew	3	1.19	21	★★★★
Waking the Tiger: Healing Trauma	Levine & Frederick	3	0.83	6	—
When Your Child has Been Molested	Hagans & Case	6	1.30	10	★★★
Wounded Boys, Heroic Men	Sonkin	3	0.80	10	★★★
Wounded Heart, The	Allender & Crabb	6	0.86	7	—
You Are Not Alone	Rouse	6	1.40	5	♦
You Can't Say That to Me!	Elgin	3	1.00	9	—
Addictive Disorders					
Addiction and Grace	May	1	0.67	26	★★★
Addiction Workbook, The	Fanning & O'Neill	6	1.20	10	★★★
Adult Children of Alcoholics	Woititz	1	0.52	220	★★★
Alcoholic Man, The	Carey	1	0.35	17	★★
Alcoholics Anonymous	Alcoholics Anonymous	1	1.13	179	★★★★
Beyond Codependency	Beattie	3	0.90	61	★★★
Co-Dependence	Whitfield	1	0.04	52	★
Codependent No More	Beattie	1	0.84	197	★★★
Day at a Time, A	CompCare	1	0.72	52	★★★
Healing the Addictive Mind	Jampolsky	1	−1.05	20	†
How to Break Your Addiction to a Person	Halpern	1	0.49	72	★★
In the Shadows of the Net	Carnes	6	1.57	7	—
It Will Never Happen to Me	Black	1	1.61	14	★★★
Love Is a Choice	Helmfelt et al.	1	0.05	41	★
Miracle Method, The	Miller & Berg	3	−0.08	12	†
One Day at a Time in Al-Anon	Al-Anon Family Group	1	0.93	110	★★★
Out of the Shadows	Carnes	3	0.67	39	★★★
Recovery Book, The	Mooney et al.	3	0.86	21	★★★
Resisting 12-Step Coercion	Peele et al.	3	0.17	6	—
Sober and Free	Kettelhack	3	0.86	14	★★★
Sober for Good	Fletcher & Glaser	6	1.67	6	—
Time to Heal, A	Cermak	3	1.14	22	★★★★
Truth about Addiction and Recovery, The	Peele et al.	3	0.73	11	★★★
Twelve Steps and Twelve Traditions	Alcoholics Anonymous	1	1.02	180	★★★★
When AA Doesn't Work for You	Ellis & Velton	3	0.88	33	★★★

Category and title	Author(s)	Study no.	Avg. rating	No. of raters	Guide rating
Adult Development					
50+ Wellness Program, The	McIlwain et al.	1	0.24	17	★
Fly Fishing through the Midlife Crisis	Raines	3	1.00	5	—
How to Deal with Your Parents	Osterkamp	1	0.50	24	★★★
Making Peace with Your Parents	Bloomfield	1	0.99	69	★★★
Necessary Losses	Viorst	1	1.10	182	★★★★
Old Folks Going Strong	York	1	0.61	7	—
Passages	Sheehy	1	0.72	356	★★★
Seasons of a Man's Life	Levinson	1	1.05	222	★★★★
Silent Passage, The	Sheehy	3	0.81	73	★★★
What Do You Want to Do When You Grow Up	Cantor & Thompson	6	0.57	7	—
When You and Your Mother Can't Be Friends	Secunda	1	0.60	30	★★★
Aging					
Ageless Body, Timeless Mind	Chopra	3	0.77	43	★★★
Aging Well	Vaillant	6	1.29	14	★★★
Aging Well	Fries	1	0.84	16	★★★
Another Country	Pipher	6	1.36	11	★★★
Chicken Soup for the Golden Soul	Canfield	6	0.25	9	—
Complete Guide to Health and Well-Being after 50	Weiss & Subak-Sharpe	1	0.88	24	★★★
Enjoy Old Age	Skinner & Vaughan	6	1.00	15	★★★
Fountain of Age, The	Friedan	3	0.69	16	★★★
How to Live Longer and Feel Better	Pauling	1	0.53	46	★★★
It's Better to be Over the Hill Than under It	LeShan	3	1.18	11	★★★
Your Renaissance Years	Veninga	3	1.00	5	♦
Anger					
Anger at Work	Weisinger	3	1.33	6	—
Anger Control Workbook, The	McKay & Rogers	6	1.41	37	★★★★★
Anger: Deal with It, Heal with It, Stop It From Killing You	Defoore	1	0.38	24	★★
Anger: How to Live with and without It	Ellis	1	0.85	24	★★★
Anger Free: Ten Basic Steps to Managing Your Anger	Gentry	6	1.14	7	—
Anger Kills	Williams & Williams	3	1.44	9	♦
Anger: The Misunderstood Emotion	Tavris	1	1.18	83	★★★★
Anger Workbook, The	Bilodeau	3	1.13	31	★★★★
Angry All the Time	Potter-Efron	3	1.21	14	★★★
Angry Book, The	Rubin	1	0.52	95	★★★
Angry Men and the Women Who Love Them	Hegstrom	3	0.71	7	—
Angry Self, The	Gottlieb	6	1.33	9	♦
Beyond Anger: A Guide for Men	Harbin	6	1.14	7	—
Dance of Anger, The	Lerner	1	1.39	211	★★★★★

Category and title	Author(s)	Study no.	Avg. rating	No. of raters	Guide rating
Anger (*cont.*)					
How to Control Your Anger before It Controls You	Ellis & Tafrate	3	1.14	35	★★★★
Letting Go of Anger	Potter-Efron & Potter-Efron	3	1.30	23	★★★★
Prisoners of Hate	Beck	6	1.58	12	★★★
Volcano in My Tummy, A	Whitehouse & Pudney	3	1.33	6	◆
When Anger Hurts	McKay et al.	1	0.92	36	★★★
When Chicken Soup Isn't Enough	Barris	6	0.57	7	—
Anxiety Disorders					
Anxiety and Panic Attacks	Handly	1	0.81	27	★★★
Anxiety and Phobia Workbook, The	Bourne	3	1.58	117	★★★★★
Anxiety Disease, The	Sheehan	1	0.64	59	★★★
Anxiety Disorders and Phobias	Beck & Emery	1	1.18	172	★★★★
Beyond Anxiety and Phobia	Bourne	6	1.33	21	★★★★
Don't Panic	Wilson	1	1.04	82	★★★★
End to Panic, An	Zuercher-White	3	1.42	12	★★★
Feel the Fear and Do It Anyway	Jeffers	3	1.15	34	★★★★
Good News about Panic, Anxiety, and Phobias, The	Gold	1	0.59	45	★★★
Healing Fear	Bourne	6	1.00	5	—
How to Control Your Anxiety before It Controls You	Ellis	3	0.95	59	★★★
Life without Fear	Wolpe & Wolpe	3	0.85	33	★★★
Mastery of Your Anxiety and Panic III	Craske & Barlow	3	1.53	58	★★★★★
Overcoming Anxiety	Kennerley	6	0.88	9	—
Overcoming Generalized Anxiety Disorder	White	6	1.14	7	◆
Overcoming Shyness and Social Phobia	Rapee	6	1.46	13	★★★
Panic and Anxiety Disorder	Manassee-Buell	6	1.00	6	—
Panic Disorder	Rachman & de Silva	3	0.93	29	★★★
Peace from Nervous Suffering	Weekes	1	0.88	57	★★★
Shyness and Social Anxiety Workbook, The	Anthony & Swinson	6	1.21	24	★★★★
Sky Is Falling, The	Dumont	3	1.33	9	◆
Why Does Everything Have to Be Perfect?	Shackerman	6	1.00	6	—
Worry	Hallowell	6	1.40	10	★★★
Assertiveness					
Assert Yourself	Lendenfield	6	1.13	8	—
Asserting Yourself	Bower & Bower	3	1.10	20	★★★★
Assertive Woman, The	Phelps & Austin	3	1.35	43	★★★★★
Assertiveness Workbook, The	Peterson	6	1.17	18	★★★
Control Freaks	Piaget	1	0.00	11	★
Creative Aggression	Bach & Goldberg	1	0.43	72	★★

Category and title	Author(s)	Study no.	Avg. rating	No. of raters	Guide rating
Don't Say Yes When You Want to Say No	Fensterheim & Baer	1	0.91	150	★★★
Gentle Art of Verbal Self-Defense, The	Elgin	1	0.66	61	★★★
Good-Bye to Guilt	Jampolsky	1	0.77	31	★★★
How to be a Bitch with Style	Ashley	6	−0.20	5	—
Looking Out for Number One	Ringer	1	−0.73	67	†
Pulling Your Own Strings	Dyer	1	0.19	148	★
Stand Up, Speak Out, Talk Back	Alberti & Emmons	1	1.11	75	★★★★
Stick Up for Yourself	Kaufman & Raphael	3	0.67	3	◆
When I Say No, I Feel Guilty	Smith	1	1.00	223	★★★★
Winning through Intimidation	Ringer	1	−1.11	83	†
Your Perfect Right	Alberti & Emmons	1	1.37	283	★★★★★

Attention-Deficit/Hyperactivity Disorder

ADD and the College Student	Quinn	6	0.89	9	—
ADHD and Teens	Alexander-Roberts	3	1.17	12	★★★
Adventures in Fast Forward	Nadeau	6	1.30	9	◆
All about Attention Deficit Disorder	Phelan	6	1.00	8	—
Answers to Distraction	Hallowell & Ratey	6	1.25	12	★★★
Distant Drums, Different Drummers	Ingersoll	3	1.00	8	—
Driven to Distraction	Hallowell & Ratey	3	1.26	73	★★★★★
Learning to Slow Down and Pay Attention	Nadeau & Dixon	3	1.13	15	★★★
Living with ADD	Roberts & Jansen	6	1.40	5	—
Living with ADHD Children	Buntman	3	1.00	13	★★★
Putting on the Brakes	Quinn & Stern	6	1.31	29	★★★★
Ritalin Is Not the Answer	Stein	6	0.00	7	—
Ritalin Nation	DeGrandpre	3	0.00	6	—
Running on Ritalin	Diller	3	0.60	5	—
Taking Charge of ADHD	Barkley	3	1.41	65	★★★★★
Teenagers with ADD	Zeigler Dendy	6	1.20	5	◆

Bipolar Disorder

Bipolar Child, The	Papolos & Papolos	7	0.88	26	★★★
Bipolar Disorder	Mondimore	7	0.45	11	★★
Bipolar Survival Guide, The	Miklowitz	7	1.18	11	★★★
Depression Workbook, The	Copeland	7	0.93	42	★★★
New Hope for People with Bipolar Disorder	Fawcett	7	1.00	5	—
Overcoming Depression and Manic Depression	Wider	7	0.88	8	—

Borderline and Narcissistic Personality Disorders

Children of the Self-Absorbed	Brown	6	1.40	5	—
Culture of Narcissism, The	Lasch	6	1.00	16	★★★
Drama of the Gifted Child, The	Miller	6	1.41	58	★★★★★
Humanizing the Narcissistic Style	Johnson	6	1.00	7	—
I Hate You—Don't Leave Me	Kriesman	6	0.95	37	★★★
Narcissism: Denial of the True Self	Lowen	6	0.83	6	—
Shame: The Underside of Narcissism	Morrison	6	1.17	6	—

Category and title	Author(s)	Study no.	Avg. rating	No. of raters	Guide rating
Borderline and Narcissistic Personality Disorders (*cont.*)					
Skills Training Manual for Treating Borderline Personality Disorder	Linehan	6	1.70	53	★★★★★
Stop Walking on Eggshells	Mason & Kreger	6	0.80	10	★★★
Trapped in the Mirror	Golomb	6	1.40	5	◆
Career Development					
Career Anchors	Schein	3	1.20	5	—
Career Mastery	Levinson	3	0.80	5	◆
Diversity and Women's Career Development	Farmer et al.	3	1.28	7	—
Do What You Love, the Money Will Follow	Sinetar	1	0.57	38	★★★
Knock 'Em Dead	Yate	1	0.74	15	★★★
Life Choices: Problems and Solutions	Sharf	6	1.17	6	—
100 Best Companies to Work for in America, The	Levering & Moskowitz	1	0.27	33	★★
Portable MBA, The	Collins & Devanna	1	0.40	15	★★
Shifting Gears	Hyatt	1	0.85	20	★★★
Staying the Course	Weiss	1	1.06	33	★★★★
Upward Mobility	Edwards	1	0.00	6	—
What Color Is Your Parachute?	Bolles	1	1.32	324	★★★★★
Win–Win Negotiating	Jandt	1	1.02	47	★★★★
Child Development and Parenting					
Between Parent and Child	Ginott	1	1.30	261	★★★★★
Boys into Men	Boyd-Franklin et al.	6	1.38	8	—
Childhood	Konner	1	0.67	9	—
Children: The Challenge	Dreikurs	1	1.27	126	★★★★★
Common Sense Parenting	Burke & Herron	3	1.43	7	◆
Difficult Child, The	Turecki	6	1.21	28	★★★★
Dr. Spock on Parenting	Spock	1	1.05	114	★★★★
Drama of the Gifted Child, The	Miller	1	1.90	5	◆
Everyday Blessings: The Inner Work of Mindful Parenting	Kabat-Zinn & Kabat-Zinn	6	1.14	7	—
Helping the Child Who Doesn't Fit In	Nowicki & Duke	3	1.00	7	◆
How to Behave So Your Children Will Too	Severe	6	1.43	7	—
How to Discipline Your Six- to Twelve-Year-Old without Losing Your Mind	Wyckoff & Unell	1	0.57	22	★★★
How to Raise a Child with a High EQ	Shapiro	6	1.43	7	—
How to Talk So Kids Will Listen and Listen So Kids Will Talk	Faber & Mazlish	3	1.35	63	★★★★★
Hurried Child, The	Elkind	1	1.17	114	★★★★
Living with Children	Patterson	1	1.83	11	★★★
Mother Dance, The	Lerner	6	1.00	11	★★★
1-2-3 Magic	Phelan	3	1.27	33	★★★★★
Over-Scheduled Child	Rosenfeld et al.	6	0.60	5	—
Parent Effectiveness Training	Gordon	1	1.15	259	★★★★
Parenthood by Proxy	Schlessinger	6	-2.00	7	—

Category and title	Author(s)	Study no.	Avg. rating	No. of raters	Guide rating
Parenting the Strong-Willed Child	Forehand & Long	3	1.45	20	★★★★
Parenting Young Children	Dinkmeyer & McKay	1	1.96	8	◆
Parent Power!	Rosemond	3	0.27	11	★★
Positive Discipline A–Z	Nelsen et al.	3	0.94	16	★★★
Raising Resilient Children	Brooks & Goldstein	6	1.31	13	★★★
Tips for Toddlers	Beebe	1	0.71	7	—
Toddlers and Parents	Brazelton	1	1.37	101	★★★★★
To Listen to a Child	Brazelton	1	1.41	89	★★★★★
Touchpoints	Brazelton & Sparrow	6	1.38	16	★★★
Your Defiant Child	Barkley & Benton	6	1.55	38	★★★★★
Communication and People Skills					
Are You the One for Me?	DeAngelis	3	0.11	18	★
Body Language	Fast	1	0.20	113	★
Boundaries	Cloud & Townsend	3	1.44	23	★★★★
Coping with Difficult People	Bramson	1	0.87	62	★★★
Dance of Connection, The	Lerner	6	1.24	25	★★★★
Difficult Conversations	Stone et al.	6	1.40	5	—
Difficult People	Cava	3	0.91	22	★★★
Games People Play	Berne	1	0.62	350	★★★
Getting to Yes	Fisher & Ury	1	1.03	69	★★★★
How to Argue and Win Every Time	Spence	3	0.29	14	★★
How to Communicate	McKay et al.	3	1.17	23	★★★★
How to Start a Conversation and Make Friends	Gabor	1	0.42	12	★★
How to Win Friends and Influence People	Carnegie	1	0.24	161	★
Intimate Connections	Burns	1	1.08	46	★★★★
Intimate Strangers	Rubin	1	1.18	82	★★★★
Just Friends	Rubin	1	1.07	31	★★★★
Mars and Venus on a Date	Gray	3	-0.31	32	†
Men Are from Mars, Women Are from Venus	Gray	3	0.32	167	★★
New Peoplemaking, The	Satir	6	1.17	59	★★★★
Opening Up	Pennebaker	1	0.91	18	★★★
People Skills	Bolton	1	1.03	32	★★★★
Shyness	Zimbardo	1	1.14	164	★★★★
Stop! You're Driving Me Crazy	Bach & Deutsch	1	0.50	46	★★★
Talk Book, The	Goodman & Esterly	3	1.11	9	◆
That's Not What I Meant!	Tannen	1	0.99	61	★★★
You Just Don't Understand	Tannen	1	1.24	148	★★★★
Why Men Don't Listen and Women Can't Read Maps	Pease & Pease	6	-0.57	7	—
Women Can't Hear What Men Don't Say	Farrell	6	0.60	5	—

Category and title	Author(s)	Study no.	Avg. rating	No. of raters	Guide rating
Death and Grieving					
Ambiguous Loss	Boss	6	1.80	5	♦
Bereaved Parent, The	Schiff	1	2.00	5	—
Coming Back	Stern	1	0.78	9	—
Final Exit	Humphrey	1	-0.33	61	†
Grief Recovery Handbook, The	James & Cherry	3	1.46	26	★★★★
Healing Journey Through Grief, The	Rich	6	1.50	6	♦
Helping Children Grieve	Huntley	1	1.08	25	★★★★
How to Go on Living When Someone You Love Dies	Rando	1	1.25	31	★★★★★
How to Survive the Loss of a Love	Colgrove et al.	1	1.41	100	★★★★★
How We Die	Nuland	3	0.58	19	★★★
Learning to Say Good-Bye	LeShan	1	1.22	52	★★★★
Life after Loss	Volkan & Zintl	3	0.78	9	—
Life Lessons	Kübler-Ross & Kessler	6	1.45	22	★★★★
Living through Personal Crisis	Stearns	1	1.06	18	★★★
Needs of the Dying, The	Kessler	6	1.17	6	—
On Children and Death	Kübler-Ross	3	1.28	61	★★★★★
On Death and Dying	Kübler-Ross	1	0.99	355	★★★
Recovering from the Loss of a Child	Donnelly	1	1.15	27	★★★★
Sudden Infant Death	DeFrain et al.	1	1.00	16	★★★
Talking about Death	Grollman	1	1.23	40	★★★★
Time to Say Good-bye, A	Goulding	3	1.20	10	★★★
When Bad Things Happen to Good People	Kushner	3	1.29	150	★★★★★
When Children Grieve	James & Friedman	6	1.14	7	♦
Widowed	Brothers	1	-0.02	34	†
Widow's Handbook, The	Foehner & Cozart	1	0.54	13	★★★
Working It Through	Kübler-Ross	3	1.19	36	★★★★
Dementia/Alzheimer's					
Alzheimer's Caregiver, The	Hodgson	3	1.14	14	★★★
Hidden Victims of Alzheimer's Disease, The	Zarit et al.	3	1.18	11	★★★
36-Hour Day, The	Mace & Rabins	3	1.55	49	★★★★★
When Your Loved One Has Alzheimer's	Carroll	3	0.86	7	♦
Depression					
Breaking the Patterns of Depression	Yapko	7	0.69	13	★★★
Cognitive Therapy and the Emotional Disorders	Beck	1	1.16	198	★★★★★
Complete Idiot's Guide to Beating the Blues	McGrath & Kogan	7	0.13	8	—
Control Your Depression	Lewinsohn et al.	3	1.28	36	★★★★★
Feeling Good	Burns	1	1.51	254	★★★★★
Feeling Good Handbook, The	Burns	1	1.38	116	★★★★★
Getting Un-Depressed	Emery	1	0.93	42	★★★
Getting Your Life Back	Wright & Basco	7	0.50	6	—
Good News about Depression, The	Gold	1	0.01	50	★
Hand-Me-Down Blues	Yapko	7	0.80	10	★★★

Category and title	Author(s)	Study no.	Avg. rating	No. of raters	Guide rating
How to Cope with Depression	DePaulo & Ablow	1	0.65	20	★★★
How to Stubbornly Refuse to Make Yourself Miserable about Anything	Ellis	3	0.84	31	★★★
I Don't Want to Talk about It	Real	7	0.90	20	★★★
Listening to Prozac	Kramer	3	0.57	83	★★★
Mind over Mood	Greenberger & Padesky	3	1.43	61	★★★★★
Overcoming Depression	Gilson & Freeman	7	0.77	13	★★★
Overcoming Teen Depression	Kaufman	7	1.33	6	♦
Self-Coaching: How to Heal Anxiety and Depression	Luciani	7	0.33	6	—
Self-Help Guide to Managing Depression, A	Baker	3	1.13	8	—
Stop Depression Now	Brown et al.	7	−0.80	5	—
Understanding and Overcoming Depression	Bates	7	0.58	12	★★★
When Feeling Bad Is Good	McGrath	3	1.04	27	★★★★
When Living Hurts	Yapko	3	1.15	27	★★★★
When the Blues Won't Go Away	Hirschfield	1	0.62	13	★★★
Winter Blues	Rosenthal	7	1.06	16	★★★
You Can Beat Depression	Preston	3	1.23	13	★★★
You Mean I Don't Have to Feel This Way?	Dowling	1	0.44	16	★★
Zoloft, Paxil, Luvox, and Prozac	Sullivan	3	0.17	6	—
Divorce					
Boys and Girls Book about Divorce, The	Gardner	1	1.39	212	★★★★★
Coping with Divorce, Single Parenting, and Remarriage	Heatherington	7	1.05	20	★★★★
Crazy Time	Trafford	3	1.44	16	★★★
Creative Divorce	Krantzler	1	0.66	88	★★★
Custody Revolution, The	Warshak	3	0.60	5	—
Dinosaurs Divorce	Brown & Brown	1	1.42	44	★★★★★
Divorce: The Best Resources to Help You Survive	Wemhoff	3	1.33	6	—
Divorce Book, The	McKay et al.	7	0.90	10	★★★
Divorce Poison	Warshak	7	0.57	7	—
Does Wednesday Mean Mom's House or Dad's?	Ackerman	7	0.57	7	—
Don't Divorce Us!: Kids' Advice to Divorcing Parents	Sommers-Flannigan et al.	7	1.00	6	—
Dumped	Warren & Thompson	3	1.00	3	♦
For Better or for Worse: Divorce Reconsidered	Heatherington & Kelly	7	1.00	12	★★★
Forgive Your Parents, Heal Yourself	Grosskopf	7	0.80	5	—
Good Divorce, The	Ahrons	7	1.19	16	★★★
Growing Up with Divorce	Kalter	1	1.00	33	★★★★
Helping Children Cope with Divorce	Teyber	7	1.25	12	★★★
Helping Your Kids Cope with Divorce	Neuman & Romanowski	3	1.05	18	★★★

Category and title	Author(s)	Study no.	Avg. rating	No. of raters	Guide rating
Divorce (*cont.*)					
How It Feels When Parents Divorce	Krementz	1	1.09	70	★★★★
Mars and Venus Starting Over	Gray	3	0.09	22	★
My Parents Are Divorced Too	Blackstone-Ford et al.	7	0.71	7	—
Parents Book about Divorce, The	Gardner	7	0.87	52	★★★
Second Chances	Wallerstein & Blakeslee	1	0.99	102	★★★
Surviving the Breakup	Wallerstein & Kelly	7	1.03	38	★★★★
Unexpected Legacy of Divorce, The	Wallerstein et al.	7	1.08	37	★★★★
What Can I Do? A Book for Children of Divorce	Lowry	7	1.17	6	—
Eating Disorders					
Anatomy of Anorexia	Levenkron	7	0.88	8	♦
Binge No More	Nash	7	0.00	7	—
Body Betrayed, The	Zerbe	3	1.11	9	—
Bulimia: A Guide for Family and Friends	Sherman & Thompson	7	1.00	5	—
Bulimia/Anorexia	Boskind-White & White	7	0.92	12	★★★
Dying to Be Thin	Sacker & Zimmer	3	1.24	21	★★★★
Emotional Eating	Abramson	7	0.56	9	—
Fat Is a Family Affair	Hollis	1	0.88	41	★★★
Food for Thought	Hazelden Foundation	1	0.66	32	★★★
Golden Cage, The	Bruch	7	0.92	36	★★★
Good Enough	Bitter	7	0.57	7	—
Healing the Hungry Self	Price	3	1.10	10	★★★
Hunger Within, The	Migliore & Ross	3	1.36	11	★★★
Love Hunger	Minirth et al.	1	0.13	31	★
Love-Powered Diet, The	Moran	1	−0.91	11	†
Overcoming Binge Eating	Fairburn	3	1.06	18	★★★
Twelve Steps and Twelve Traditions of Inner Eating	Billigmeier	1	0.22	9	—
Twelve-Steps and Twelve Traditions of Overeaters Anonymous, The	Overeaters Anonymous	3	1.00	14	★★★
Weight Watchers Stop Stuffing Yourself	Weight Watchers	7	0.40	10	★★
When Food Is Love	Roth	1	0.66	32	★★★
When Your Child Has an Eating Disorder	Natenshon	7	0.33	6	—
Why Weight?	Roth	1	0.68	22	★★★
You Can't Quit Eating until You Know What's Eating You	LeBlanc	1	0.47	17	★★
Families and Stepfamilies					
Adult Children	Friel & Friel	1	0.52	49	★★★
Back to the Family	Guarendi	1	0.91	11	★★★
Blending Families	Shimberg	3	1.08	13	★★★
Bradshaw on the Family	Bradshaw	1	0.34	129	★★
Families	Patterson	1	1.78	12	★★★

Category and title	Author(s)	Study no.	Avg. rating	No. of raters	Guide rating
Family Crucible, The	Napier & Whitaker	1	1.04	108	★★★★
Love in the Blended Family	Clubb	1	1.23	13	★★★
Mom's House, Dad's House	Ricci	7	1.35	17	★★★
Old Loyalties, New Ties	Visher & Visher	1	1.28	42	★★★★★
Second Time Around, The	Janda & MacCormack	1	1.20	10	★★★
Shelter of Each Other, The	Pipher	3	1.43	14	★★★
Step by Step-Parenting	Eckler	1	1.30	20	★★★★
Stepfamilies	Bray & Kelly	7	1.00	11	★★★
Step-Fathering	Rosin	1	1.10	21	★★★★
Strengthening Your Stepfamily	Einstein & Albert	1	1.10	10	★★★

Infant Development and Parenting

Baby Book, The	Sears & Sears	7	1.13	16	★★★
Dr. Spock's Baby and Child Care	Spock & Parker	1	1.43	187	★★★★★
Father's Almanac, The	Sullivan	1	0.90	16	★★★
First Three Years of Life, The	White	1	1.34	102	★★★★★
First Twelve Months of Life, The	Caplan	1	1.33	60	★★★★★
Infants and Mothers	Brazelton	1	1.47	114	★★★★★
Secrets of the Baby Whisperer	Hogg & Blau	7	0.13	8	—
What Every Baby Knows	Brazelton	1	1.44	105	★★★★★
What to Expect the First Year	Eisenberg et al.	1	1.44	37	★★★★★
What to Expect: The Toddler Years	Eisenberg et al.	7	1.49	35	★★★★★
Your Baby and Child	Leach	1	1.32	32	★★★★

Love and Intimacy

Art of Loving, The	Fromm	1	1.05	257	★★★★
Couples	Dym & Glenn	3	0.86	7	—
Creating Love	Bradshaw	3	0.74	35	★★★
Dance of Connection, The	Lerner	7	1.21	43	★★★★
Dance of Intimacy, The	Lerner	1	1.23	145	★★★★
Do I Have to Give Up Me to Be Loved by You?	Paul & Paul	1	0.83	56	★★★
Fear of Intimacy	Firetone & Catlett	7	1.17	12	★★★
Going the Distance	Barbach & Geisinger	1	0.67	33	★★★
I Only Say This Because I Love You	Tannen	7	1.04	25	★★★★
In the Meantime	Vanzant	3	1.50	8	♦
Keeping the Love You Find	Hendrix	7	1.15	33	★★★★
Love Cycle	Cutler	1	0.60	5	—
Love Is Never Enough	Beck	3	1.36	67	★★★★★
Love the Way You Want It	Sternberg	3	0.67	6	—
Loving Each Other	Buscaglia	1	0.31	94	★★
Mars and Venus in the Bedroom	Gray	3	-0.16	38	†
Men Who Can't Love	Carter	1	0.27	141	★★
Men Who Hate Women and the Women Who Love Them	Forward	1	0.29	141	★★
Obsessive Love	Forward & Buck	1	0.94	18	★★★
Permanent Partners	Berzon	7	1.11	9	♦
Relationship Cure, The	Gottman & DeClaire	7	1.25	24	★★★★
Relationship Rescue	McGraw	7	0.43	14	★★

Category and title	Author(s)	Study no.	Avg. rating	No. of raters	Guide rating
Love and Intimacy (*cont.*)					
Return to Love, A	Williamson	3	0.60	15	★★★
Soul Mates	Moore	3	0.72	39	★★★
Triangle of Love, The	Sternberg	1	1.00	23	★★★★
What Every Woman Should Know about Men	Brothers	1	−0.94	48	†
What Smart Women Know	Carter & Sokol	1	0.09	11	★
When Someone You Love Is Someone You Hate	Arterburn & Stoop	1	0.10	10	★
Women Men Love, Women Men Leave	Cowan & Kinder	1	−0.17	29	†
Women Who Love Too Much	Norwood	1	0.64	194	★★★
Marriage					
Couple's Survival Workbook, The	Olsen & Stephens	7	1.25	8	—
Divorce Busting	Weiner-Davis	3	1.04	24	★★★★
Do I Stay or Do I Go?	Occhetti et al.	7	0.60	5	—
Fighting for Your Marriage	Markman et al.	7	1.00	18	★★★
Getting the Love You Want	Hendrix	3	1.05	63	★★★★
Getting Together and Staying Together	Glasser & Glasser	7	0.50	12	★★★
Husbands and Wives	Kinder & Cowan	1	0.55	10	★★★
I Love You, Let's Work It Out	Viscott	3	0.90	10	★★★
Intimate Partners	Scarf	1	1.06	87	★★★★
Love for a Lifetime	Dobson	3	1.14	7	♦
Power of Two, The	Heitler & Singer	7	0.60	5	—
Reconcilable Differences	Christensen & Jacobson	7	1.00	10	★★★
Seven Principles for Making Marriages Work, The	Gottman & Silver	7	1.51	53	★★★★★
Ten Stupid Things Couples Do to Mess Up Their Relationships	Schlessinger	7	−0.88	32	†
Too Good to Leave, Too Bad to Stay	Kirshenbaum	7	1.00	9	—
We Love Each Other but . . .	Wachtel	3	1.40	5	♦
Why Marriages Succeed or Fail	Gottman	3	1.59	34	★★★★★
Men's Issues					
Adonis Complex, The	Pope et al.	7	0.40	5	—
Being a Man	Fanning & McKay	3	1.56	16	★★★
Chicken Soup for the Father's Soul	Canfield et al.	7	0.64	14	★★★
FatherLoss	Chethik	7	1.00	5	♦
Fire in the Belly	Keen	1	0.61	86	★★★
Hazards of Being Male, The	Goldberg	1	0.81	63	★★★
Iron John	Bly	1	0.30	158	★★
Man Enough	Pittman	3	1.00	14	★★★
Masculinity Reconstructed	Levant & Kopecky	7	0.75	16	★★★
Measure of a Man, The	Shapiro	3	0.67	6	—
New Male, The	Goldberg	1	0.67	39	★★★
Real Boys	Pollack	7	1.37	27	★★★★
Seasons of a Man's Life	Levinson	1	1.05	222	★★★★
Straight Talk to Men	Dobson	7	0.45	11	★★

Category and title	Author(s)	Study no.	Avg. rating	No. of raters	Guide rating
Ten Stupid Things Men Do to Mess Up Their Lives	Schlessinger	3	−0.50	22	†
What Men Really Want	Bakos	1	−0.12	25	†
Why Men Don't Get Enough Sex and Women Don't Get Enough Love	Kramer & Dunaway	1	0.10	20	★
Obsessive–Compulsive Disorder					
Brain Lock	Schwartz & Beyette	6	1.40	15	★★★
Obsessive–Compulsive Disorders	Levenkron	1	1.00	31	★★★★
Obsessive–Compulsive Disorders	Penzel	6	1.50	6	◆
Obsessive–Compulsive Disorder: The Facts	de Silva & Rachman	6	1.20	5	◆
Overcoming Obsessive–Compulsive Disorder	Steketee	6	1.32	22	★★★★
S.T.O.P. Obsessing	Foa & Wilson	3	1.36	50	★★★★★
Posttraumatic Stress Disorder					
Coping with Trauma	Allen	7	1.00	5	—
Healing the Hurt Within	Sutton	7	0.86	7	—
I Can't Get Over It	Matsakis	7	1.27	26	★★★★
Life after Trauma	Rosenbloom et al.	7	1.18	11	★★★
Post-Traumatic Stress Disorder Sourcebook	Schiraldi	7	0.78	9	—
PTSD Workbook, The	Williams & Poijula	7	1.33	12	★★★
Rebuilding Shattered Lives	Chu	7	1.5	8	◆
Reclaiming Your Life after Rape	Rothbaum & Foa	7	1.53	15	★★★
Scared Child, The	Brooks & Siegel	7	0.50	6	—
Survivor Guilt	Matsakis	7	1.20	5	◆
Trauma and Recovery	Herman	7	1.42	50	★★★★★
Waking the Tiger	Levine & Frederick	7	0.75	8	—
Pregnancy					
Complete Book of Pregnancy and Childbirth, The	Kitzinger	1	1.41	39	★★★★★
Expectant Father, The	Brott & Ash	3	1.40	5	—
From Here to Maternity	Marshall	1	0.80	10	★★★
Girlfriend's Guide to Pregnancy, The	Iovine	7	1.14	7	◆
Pregnancy after 35	McCauley	1	0.90	20	★★★
Pregnancy, Childbirth, and the Newborn	Simkin	1	0.83	6	—
Well Pregnancy Book, The	Samuels & Samuels	1	0.87	15	★★★
What to Eat When You're Expecting	Eisenberg et al.	1	1.00	16	★★★
What to Expect When You're Expecting	Eisenberg et al.	3	1.56	43	★★★★★
Will It Hurt the Baby?	Abrams	1	1.00	5	—

Category and title	Author(s)	Study no.	Avg. rating	No. of raters	Guide rating
Schizophrenia					
Coping with Schizophrenia	Mueser & Gingerich	7	1.33	12	★★★
Helping Someone with Mental Illness	Carter & Golant	7	0.87	15	★★★
How to Cope with Mental Illness in Your Family	Marsh & Dickens	3	1.08	12	★★★
Surviving Schizophrenia	Torrey	3	1.25	40	★★★★★
Understanding Schizophrenia	Keefe & Harvey	7	1.50	6	◆
Self-Management and Self-Enhancement					
All I Really Needed to Know I Learned in Kindergarten	Fulghum	3	0.78	89	★★★
Art of Happiness, The	Dalai Lama & Cutler	7	0.96	23	★★★
Awaken the Giant Within	Robbins	3	0.00	14	★
Changing for Good	Prochaska et al.	3	1.17	23	★★★★
Chicken Soup for the Soul	Canfield & Hansen	3	0.72	100	★★★
Do It! Let's Get Off Our Butts	McWilliams	1	-0.06	9	—
Don't Blame Mother	Caplan	1	1.00	20	★★★★
Don't Sweat the Small Stuff . . . and It's All Small Stuff	Carlson	3	1.06	95	★★★★
Emotional Intelligence	Goleman	3	0.97	118	★★★
Feel the Fear and Do It Anyway	Jeffers	1	1.24	25	★★★★
Gentle Roads to Survival	Auw	1	0.70	10	★★★
How to Live 365 Days a Year	Schindler	1	0.58	12	★★★
How to Stop Worrying and Start Living	Carnegie	1	0.15	65	★
I'm OK, You're OK	Harris	1	0.60	318	★★★
Learned Optimism	Seligman	1	1.27	89	★★★★★
Life's Little Instruction Book	Brown	3	0.82	33	★★★
Life Strategies	McGraw	7	0.83	24	★★★
Making Life Right When It Feels All Wrong	Fensterheim	1	0.78	18	★★★
New Guide to Rational Living, A	Ellis & Harper	1	1.12	238	★★★★
Opening Up	Pennebaker	7	1.33	15	★★★
Overcoming Procrastination	Ellis & Knaus	1	1.00	69	★★★★
Positive Addiction	Glasser	1	0.82	89	★★★
Positive Illusions	Taylor	1	1.23	13	★★★
Power of Optimism, The	McGinnis	1	0.27	11	★★
Power of Positive Thinking, The	Peale	1	0.22	153	★
Self-Defeating Behaviors	Cudney & Hardy	1	0.80	10	★★★
Self-Directed Behavior	Watson & Tharp	7	1.15	13	★★★
Self Matters	McGraw	7	0.43	14	★★
7 Habits of Highly Effective People, The	Covey	1	1.28	67	★★★★★
Short Guide to a Happy Life, A	Quindlen	7	0.80	15	★★★
Simple Abundance	Ban Breathnach	7	0.72	29	★★★
60-Second Shrink, The	Lazarus & Lazarus	3	0.97	30	★★★
Spontaneous Healing	Weil	3	1.10	41	★★★★☆
Staying Rational in an Irrational World	Bernard	1	0.91	71	★★★

Category and title	Author(s)	Study no.	Avg. rating	No. of raters	Guide rating
Steps to the Top	Zigler	1	0.13	23	★
Success Is a Choice	Pitino & Reynolds	3	1.33	9	♦
Take Time for Your Life	Richardson	7	0.43	7	—
Talking to Yourself	Butler	1	0.80	18	★★★
Ten Days to Self-Esteem	Burns	7	1.16	45	★★★★
Tough Times Never Last but Tough People Do	Schuller	1	0.41	42	★★
Unlimited Power	Robbins	1	0.54	14	★★★
What to Say When You Talk to Yourself	Helmstetter	1	1.10	21	★★★★
What You Can Change and What You Can't	Seligman	3	1.27	59	★★★★★
Who Moved My Cheese?	Johnson	7	0.77	60	★★★
Winner Within, The	Riley	3	0.43	7	—
You Can't Afford the Luxury of a Negative Thought	John-Rogers & McWilliams	1	0.44	6	—
Your Erroneous Zones	Dyer	1	0.37	169	★★
Your Maximum Mind	Benson	1	0.47	25	★★

Sexuality

Category and title	Author(s)	Study no.	Avg. rating	No. of raters	Guide rating
Becoming Orgasmic	Heiman & LoPiccolo	7	1.69	32	★★★★★
Dr. Ruth's Guide to Erotic and Sensuous Pleasures	Westheimer & Lieberman	1	−0.42	47	†
Dr. Ruth's Guide to Good Sex	Westheimer	1	−0.66	65	†
Family Book about Sexuality, The	Calderone & Johnson	3	1.60	5	♦
For Each Other	Barbach	3	1.69	29	★★★★
For Women Only	Berman & Berman	7	1.00	11	★★★
For Yourself	Barbach	1	1.87	17	★★★
Illustrated Manual of Sexual Therapy	Kaplan	3	1.19	41	★★★★
Making Love: A Man's Guide	White	1	0.81	27	★★★
Making Love: A Woman's Guide	Davis	1	0.77	26	★★★
Male Sexual Awareness	McCarthy & McCarthy	7	1.13	8	♦
New Joy of Sex, The	Comfort	1	0.99	173	★★★
New Male Sexuality, The	Zilbergeld	1	1.89	18	★★★
Seven Weeks to Better Sex	Renshaw	3	1.00	8	-
Sexual Awareness	McCarthy & McCarthy	3	1.67	12	★★★
Soul of Sex, The	Moore	3	0.80	10	★★★
What Really Happens in Bed	Carter & Coopersmith	1	0.80	15	★★★

Spiritual and Existential Concerns

Category and title	Author(s)	Study no.	Avg. rating	No. of raters	Guide rating
American Paradox, The	Myers	7	1.80	5	♦
Be (Happy) Attitudes, The	Schuller	1	0.23	21	★
Care of the Soul	Moore	3	0.87	62	★★★
Celestine Prophecy, The	Redfield	3	0.28	76	★★
Clear Body, Clear Mind	Hubbard	1	−1.62	62	†
Dianetics	Hubbard	1	−1.77	187	†
Finding Flow	Csikszentmihalyi	3	1.32	25	★★★★

Category and title	Author(s)	Study no.	Avg. rating	No. of raters	Guide rating
Spiritual and Existential Concerns (*cont.*)					
Flow	Csikszentmihalyi	1	0.57	43	★★★
From Beginning to End	Fulghum	3	0.60	5	—
Further Along the Road Less Traveled	Peck	3	0.93	61	★★★
Illuminata	Williamson	7	0.55	11	★★★
Loving What Is	Katie & Mitchell	7	0.60	5	—
Man's Search for Meaning	Frankl	1	1.27	260	★★★★★
Peace, Love, and Healing	Siegel	1	1.13	66	★★★★
Power of Now, The	Tolle	7	1.08	12	★★★
Road Less Traveled, The	Peck	1	1.03	285	★★★★
Sacred Contracts	Myss	7	1.38	8	◆
Scientology	Hubbard	1	-1.88	173	†
Search for Significance, The	McGee	3	1.11	9	◆
Seven Spiritual Laws of Success, The	Chopra	3	0.63	32	★★★
Spiritual Healing	Grayson	3	1.20	5	—
Way of the Wizard, The	Chopra	3	-0.20	10	†
When All You Ever Wanted Isn't Enough	Kushner	1	1.20	72	★★★★
Your Sacred Self	Dyer	7	0.62	13	★★★
Stress Management and Relaxation					
Beyond Chaos	West	1	0.83	6	—
Beyond the Relaxation Response	Benson	1	1.22	135	★★★★
Cool Cats, Calm Kids	Willliams & Burke	3	0.83	6	—
Don't Sweat the Small Stuff . . . and Its All Small Stuff	Carlson	7	1.05	43	★★★★
Each Day a New Beginning	Casey	1	1.05	34	★★★★
Inner and Outer Peace through Meditation	Singh	3	1.60	5	◆
Learn to Relax	Walker	7	0.92	13	★★★
Male Stress Syndrome, The	Witkin-Lanoil	1	0.68	22	★★★
Minding the Body, Mending the Mind	Borysenko	3	1.21	48	★★★★
No Gimmick Guide to Managing Stress	Neidhart	1	0.88	8	—
Relaxation and Stress Reduction Workbook, The	Davis et al.	3	1.52	81	★★★★★
Relaxation Response, The	Benson	1	1.28	212	★★★★★
Staying on Top When Your World Is Upside Down	Cramer	1	1.50	8	—
Stress and Relaxation Handbook, The	Madders	3	1.36	47	★★★★★
Stresses	Curran	1	0.89	9	—
Touchstones	Hazelden Foundation	1	0.90	30	★★★
Wellness Book, The	Benson & Stuart	3	1.26	38	★★★★★
Wherever You Go, There You Are	Kabat-Zinn	3	1.45	53	★★★★★
Why Zebra's Don't Get Ulcers	Sapolsky	3	1.19	21	★★★★
Write Your Own Prescription for Stress	Matheny & McCarthy	7	0.67	6	—

Category and title	Author(s)	Study no.	Avg. rating	No. of raters	Guide rating
Suicide					
Choosing to Live	Ellis & Newman	7	1.70	10	★★★
Living When a Young Friend Commits Suicide	Grollman & Malikow	7	0.86	7	♦
No Time to Say Goodbye	Fine	7	0.63	8	—
Teenagers and Parenting					
All Grown Up and No Place to Go	Elkind	1	1.20	49	★★★★
Between Parent and Teenager	Ginott	1	1.34	181	★★★★★
Bringing Up Parents	Packer	3	1.25	8	♦
Chicken Soup for the Teenage Soul on Tough Stuff	Canfield et al.	7	0.86	14	★★★
Positive Parenting Your Teens	Joslin & Decher	3	1.54	11	★★★
Overcoming Teenage Depression	Kaufman	7	0.83	6	—
Preparing for Adolescence	Dobson	3	0.36	11	★★
Queen Bees and Wannabes	Wiseman	7	0.73	11	★★★
Reviving Ophelia	Pipher	3	1.42	87	★★★★★
Surviving Adolescence	Dumont	1	0.95	21	★★★
Toughlove	York et al.	1	0.54	124	★★★
What Teenagers Want to Know about Sex	Boston Children's Hospital et al.	3	1.00	6	♦
When Living Hurts	Gordon	3	1.25	12	★★★
You and Your Adolescent	Steinberg & Levine	3	1.00	11	★★★
Weight Management					
Beverly Hills Diet, The	Mazel	1	-1.35	61	†
Body for Life	Philips & D'Orso	7	0.40	10	★★
Carbohydrate Addict's Diet, The	Heller & Heller	1	-1.09	34	†
Diet Center Program, The	Ferguson	1	-0.83	35	†
Diet for a Small Planet	Lappe	1	0.44	78	★★
Dr. Abravanel's Anti-Craving Weight-Loss Diet	Abravanel & King	1	-1.05	22	†
Dr. Atkins' Diet Revolution	Atkins	1	-0.97	58	†
Dr. Atkins' New Diet Revolution	Atkins	3	0.00	28	★
Eat More, Weigh Less	Ornish	3	0.92	25	★★★
Eating Well for Optimum Health	Weil	7	0.96	28	★★★
Eight Weeks to Optimum Health	Weil	3	1.30	27	★★★★
Fat Is a Feminist Issue	Orbach	3	1.12	41	★★★★
5-Day Miracle Diet, The	Puhn	3	-1.20	15	†
Get with the Program	Green	7	-0.17	6	—
LEARN Program for Weight Control, The	Brownell	3	1.58	12	★★★
Lifetime Weight Control	Fanning	7	0.17	6	—
Make the Connection	Greene & Winfrey	3	1.07	14	★★★
New Fit or Fat, The	Bailey	1	0.69	65	★★★
One Meal at a Time	Katahn	1	0.00	21	★
Pritikin Program for Diet and Exercise, The	Pritkin	1	0.02	80	★
Rotation Diet, The	Katahn	1	-0.62	47	†
Sugar Busters	Steward et al.	3	0.58	12	★★★

Category and title	Author(s)	Study no.	Avg. rating	No. of raters	Guide rating
Weight Management (*cont.*)					
Suzanne Somers' Eat, Cheat, and Melt the Fat Away	Somer	7	−0.67	9	—
T-Factor Diet, The	Katahn	1	−0.22	41	†
35-Plus Diet for Women, The	Spodnik & Gibbons	1	−0.90	19	†
Zone, The	Sears	3	0.33	27	★★
Women's Issues					
Backlash	Faludi	1	0.87	47	★★★
Body Traps	Rodin	3	1.18	17	★★★
Chicken Soup for the Woman's Soul	Canfield et al.	3	1.00	25	★★★★
Juggling	Crosby	1	0.75	8	—
Life Preservers	Lerner	7	1.08	12	★★★
Making It Work	Houston	1	1.00	6	—
Menopause and the Mind	Warga	7	0.60	5	—
Mismeasure of Woman, The	Tavris	7	1.25	20	★★★★
My Mother/My Self	Friday	1	0.59	187	★★★
New Our Bodies, Ourselves, The	Boston Women's Collective	3	1.54	81	★★★★★
Seasons of a Woman's Life, The	Levinson & Levinson	3	1.20	25	★★★★
Second Shift, The	Hochschild	1	1.39	28	★★★★
Secrets about Men Every Woman Should Know	DeAngelis	1	−0.42	19	†
Silent Passage, The	Sheehy	3	0.96	67	★★★
Too Good for Her Own Good	Bepko & Krestan	1	1.26	16	★★★
We Are Our Mother's Daughters	Roberts	3	0.81	26	★★★
Wisdom of Menopause	Northrup	7	1.14	14	★★★
Women on Top	Friday	3	0.25	8	—
Women Who Run with the Wolves	Estes	3	0.95	58	★★★
Violent Youth					
Bullies and Victims	Fried & Fried	7	1.20	5	♦
Defiant Child, The	Riley	7	1.44	16	★★★
Explosive Child, The	Greene	7	1.50	20	★★★★
High Risk	Magid & McKelvey	7	1.40	5	♦
Lost Boys	Garbarino	7	0.86	14	★★★
Raising Cain	Kindlon & Thompson	7	1.08	13	★★★
Real Boys	Pollack	7	1.11	18	★★★
Savage Spawn	Kellerman	7	1.00	9	—
Your Defiant Child	Barkley & Benton	7	1.32	44	★★★★★

Ratings of Autobiographies in the National Studies

Only those autobiographies rated five or more times in our national studies are included in this list. Some books appear on this list but were not included in the text because they were rated by fewer than eight mental health experts. Please consult Appendix A for details on the methodology of the national studies and the meaning of the guide ratings.

Category and title	Author(s)	Study no.	Avg. rating	No. of raters	Guide rating
Abuse					
Call Me Crazy	Heche	8	−1.29	7	—
Child Called "It," A	Pelzer	4	1.00	9	★★★
Daddy's Girl	Allen	4	0.92	25	★★★
Lost Boy, The	Pelzer	8	1.40	20	★★★★
Man Named Dave, A	Pelzer	8	1.41	22	★★★★
Secret Life	Ryan	2	0.54	13	★★★
Sleepers	Carcaterra	4	0.78	9	★★★
Surviving Domestic Violence	Weiss & Magill	8	0.83	6	—
Triumph over Darkness	Wood	4	0.60	5	—
Addictive Disorders					
Both Sides of Recovery	Harrison & Harrison	4	1.00	5	—
Broken Cord	Dorris	8	1.40	20	★★★★

Category and title	Author(s)	Study no.	Avg. rating	No. of raters	Guide rating
Addictive Disorders (*cont.*)					
Codependent No More	Beattie	2	1.00	142	★★★★
Drinking: A Love Story	Knapp	2	1.00	16	★★★
Drinking Life, A	Hamill	2	1.07	29	★★★★
Getting Better: Inside AA	Robertson	2	1.10	28	★★★★
Go Ask Alice	Anonymous	8	1.06	33	★★★★
Note Found in a Bottle	Cheever	8	1.38	8	★★★
Now You Know	Dukakis	2	0.60	32	★★★
Portraits of Recovery	Gaynor	4	1.00	6	—
Terry	McGovern	8	1.33	9	★★★
Adult Development					
Fly Fishing through the Midlife Crisis	Raines	8	0.80	10	★★★
Tuesdays with Morrie	Albom	4	1.58	59	★★★★★
Aging					
Changing Places	Kramer	8	1.11	9	★★★★
Fountain of Age, The	Friedan	4	0.96	23	★★★
Getting over Getting Older	Pogrebin	8	0.25	7	◆
Last Gift of Life, The	Heilbrun	8	1.00	9	★★★
No More Words	Lindbergh	8	1.00	5	—
Virtues of Aging, The	Carter	4	1.24	17	★★★★
Anxiety Disorders					
Afraid of Everything	Woods	2	0.89	9	★★★
Earl Campbell Story	Campbell	8	1.33	6	—
Flock, The	Casey & Wilson	4	0.71	7	—
Memoirs of an Amnesiac	Levant	2	0.93	14	★★★
Mind of My Own, A	Sizemore	2	1.00	8	★★★★
Panic Attack Recovery Book, The	Swede & Jaffe	4	1.25	12	★★★
Phantom Illness	Cantor & Fallon	2	0.89	9	★★★
Sybil	Schreiber	4	0.32	91	★★
When Rabbit Howls	Chase	2	0.48	48	★★
Attention-Deficit/Hyperactivity Disorder					
ADHD Handbook for Families	Weingartner	4	1.15	13	★★★
Maybe You Know My Kid	Fowler	4	1.14	7	◆
Parenting a Child with ADHD	Boyles & Contadino	4	1.06	16	★★★★
What Makes Ryan Tick	Hughes	8	0.67	6	—
Bipolar Disorder					
Breakdown	Sutherland	2	0.62	8	★★★
Brilliant Madness, A	Duke & Hochman	2	1.08	48	★★★★
Call Me Anna	Duke	2	0.85	39	★★★
Daughter of the Queen of Sheeba	Lyden	4	1.14	7	◆
His Bright Light	Steel	8	0.40	5	—
Loony-Bin Trip, The	Millett	2	0.07	13	★
Pain	Anderson	2	0.93	14	★★★
Unquiet Mind, An	Jamison	2	1.39	49	★★★★★

Category and title	Author(s)	Study no.	Avg. rating	No. of raters	Guide rating
Borderline and Narcissistic Personality Disorders					
Girl, Interrupted	Kaysen	2	1.22	41	★★★★
Welcome to My Country	Slater	8	0.60	5	◆
Death and Grieving					
After the Death of a Child	Finkbeiner	4	1.30	10	★★★
Death Be Not Proud	Gunther	8	1.52	50	★★★★★
Eric	Lund	8	1.43	7	◆
Grief Observed, A	Lewis	4	1.58	36	★★★★★
Letting Go	Schwartz	8	1.64	55	★★★★★
Hannah's Gift	Housden	8	1.43	7	◆
Motherless Daughter	Edleman	4	1.35	23	★★★★
Wheel of Life, The	Kübler-Ross & Gold	8	1.37	19	★★★★
Dementia/Alzheimer's					
Alzheimer's, A Love Story	Davidson	8	1.71	7	◆
Diminished Mind, The	Tyler & Anifantakis	1	0.87	23	★★★
Elegy for Iris	Bayley	8	1.53	17	★★★★
Depression					
Beast, The	Thompson	8	1.50	8	★★★
Bell Jar, The	Plath	4	0.86	87	★★★
Behind the Smile	Osmond	8	0.86	7	—
Darkness Visible	Styron	2	1.34	71	★★★★★
Holiday of Darkness	Endler	8	1.17	6	—
Leaves from Many Seasons	Mowrer	2	1.06	16	★★★★
Noonday Demon, The	Solomon	8	1.31	13	★★★
On the Edge of Darkness	Cronkite	8	1.07	14	★★★
Prozac Nation	Wurtzel	2	0.49	37	★★
Undercurrents	Manning	2	1.11	25	★★★★
Eating Disorders					
Am I Still Visible?	Heater	2	1.09	11	★★★
Good Enough	Bitter	4	0.86	7	◆
Holy Hunger	Bullitt-Jonas	8	1.20	5	—
Inner Hunger	Apostolides	4	0.60	5	—
Starving for Attention	O'Neill	2	0.91	22	★★★
Wasted	Hornbacher	4	0.33	6	—
Obsessive–Compulsive Disorder					
Memoirs of an Amnesiac	Levant	2	0.93	14	★★★
Schizophrenia					
Angel at My Table, An	Frame	2	0.70	10	★★★
Autobiography of a Schizophrenic Girl	Sechehaye	4	0.67	9	★★★
Beyond All Reason	Coate	2	0.75	12	★★★
Day the Voices Stopped, The	Steele	8	1.20	5	—
Eden Express, The	Vonnegut	2	0.89	53	★★★
Father, Have I Kept My Promise?	Weisskopf-Joelson	2	0.88	8	★★★

Category and title	Author(s)	Study no.	Avg. rating	No. of raters	Guide rating
Schizophrenia (*cont.*)					
I Never Promised You a Rose Garden	Greenberg	8	1.33	156	★★★★★
Memoirs of My Nervous Illness	Shreber	8	0.83	6	—
Nobody's Child	Balter & Katz	2	0.90	29	★★★
Out of the Depths	Boisen	2	1.27	22	★★★★
Quiet Room, The	Schiller & Bennett	4	0.64	11	★★★
Too Much Anger, Too Many Tears	Gotkin & Gotkin	2	1.12	16	★★★★
Welcome, Silence	North	2	1.08	12	★★★
When the Music's Over	Gates & Hammond	2	0.88	8	★★★
Suicide					
His Bright Light	Steel	8	0.50	6	◆
Night Falls Fast	Jamison	8	1.52	33	★★★★★
Violent Youth					
Sleepers	Carcaterra	4	0.78	9	★★★
Weight Management					
Breaking Free from Compulsive Eating	Roth	4	1.59	22	★★★★
Diary of a Fat Housewife	Green	2	1.00	14	★★★
Feeding the Hungry Heart	Roth	4	1.35	37	★★★★★
Wake Up, I'm Fat	Manheim	8	1.50	6	◆
You Can't Quit until You Know What's Eating You	Leblanc	4	0.20	5	—
Women's Issues					
Deborah, Golda, and Me	Pogrebin	4	1.09	11	★★★
Heart of a Woman	Angelou	8	1.38	24	★★★★★
Mothers: A Celebration	Stoddard	4	1.00	5	◆
Reason for Hope	Goodall	8	1.63	8	★★★

Ratings of Films in the National Studies

Only those films rated five or more times in our national studies are included in this list. Some films appear on this list but were not included in the text because they were rated by fewer than 10 mental health experts. Please consult Appendix A for details on the methodology of the national studies and the meaning of the guide ratings.

Category and title	Study no.	Avg. rating	No. of raters	Guide rating
Abuse				
Apostle, The	8	0.78	59	★★★
Color Purple, The	5	1.24	245	★★★★
Dolores Claiborne	8	0.93	58	★★★
Enough	8	−0.17	6	—
Matilda	8	0.31	29	★★
Mommie Dearest	5	0.34	149	★★
Prince of Tides, The	5	−0.02	245	†
Radio Flyer	5	1.00	41	★★★★
Sleeping with the Enemy	5	0.60	134	★★★
Thelma and Louise	5	0.40	229	★★
This Boy's Life	5	1.14	49	★★★★
Thousand Acres, A	8	1.00	37	★★★★
What's Love Got to Do with It?	5	0.88	83	★★★
Addictive Disorders				
Blow	8	0.88	49	★★★
Bright Lights, Big City	8	0.90	10	★★★
Cat on a Hot Tin Roof	5	0.99	171	★★★

Category and title	Study no.	Avg. rating	No. of raters	Guide rating
Addictive Disorders (*cont.*)				
Clean and Sober	5	1.19	90	★★★★
Days of Wine and Roses	5	1.37	167	★★★★★
Drugstore Cowboy	5	0.75	76	★★★
Gambler, The	5	0.53	30	★★★
Gia	8	0.60	10	★★★
Ironweed	8	1.00	26	★★★★
Jungle Fever	5	0.61	54	★★★
Leaving Las Vegas	5	0.88	154	★★★
Lost Weekend, The	8	1.38	77	★★★★★
Mask	5	0.89	121	★★★
My Name is Bill W.	5	1.22	54	★★★★
Postcards from the Edge	5	0.68	108	★★★
Traffic	8	1.03	121	★★★★
28 Days	8	0.73	55	★★★
When a Man Loves a Woman	5	1.03	80	★★★★
Adult Development				
Christmas Carol, A	5	0.89	170	★★★
Doctor, The	5	1.28	88	★★★★★
Field of Dreams	5	0.96	252	★★★
It's a Wonderful Life	5	1.22	246	★★★★
Mr. Holland's Opus	8	1.14	184	★★★★
Trip to the Bountiful, The	5	1.42	124	★★★★★
Aging				
Cocoon	5	0.92	247	★★★
Grumpy Old Men	8	0.32	179	★★
On Golden Pond	5	1.47	307	★★★★★
Space Cowboys	8	0.44	91	★★
Wrestling Ernest Hemingway	8	1.00	16	★★★
Anxiety Disorders				
High Anxiety	5	−0.03	127	†
Sybil	5	0.79	159	★★★
What about Bob?	5	0.15	244	★
Borderline and Narcissistic Personality Disorders				
After Hours	8	0.00	11	★
Fatal Attraction	8	0.84	188	★★★
Girl, Interrupted	8	1.07	103	★★★★
Great Santini, The	8	1.23	115	★★★★
Groundhog Day	8	0.21	164	★
In the Company of Men	8	0.28	18	★★
Like Water for Chocolate	8	1.00	109	★★★★
Misery	8	0.89	76	★★★
Murder by Numbers	8	−0.25	12	†
Sunset Boulevard	8	1.20	60	★★★★

Category and title	Study no.	Avg. rating	No. of raters	Guide rating
Child Development and Parenting				
Baby Boom	8	0.32	41	★★
Big	5	0.71	192	★★★
I Am Sam	8	1.00	38	★★★★
Little Man Tate	5	1.02	94	★★★★
Parenthood	5	0.69	115	★★★
Searching for Bobby Fischer	5	1.19	108	★★★★
Communication and People Skills				
Children of a Lesser God	5	1.26	182	★★★★★
Dead Poets Society	5	1.11	284	★★★★
He Said, She Said	5	0.44	57	★★
Death and Grieving				
Accidental Tourist, The	5	0.84	146	★★★
Corrina, Corrina	8	1.32	41	★★★★★
Ghost	5	0.37	209	★★
In the Bedroom	8	1.15	47	★★★★
Lion King, The	5	0.62	176	★★★
Message in a Bottle	8	0.44	75	★★
My Girl	5	0.50	30	★★★
My Life	5	0.93	40	★★★
Ordinary People	5	1.49	281	★★★★★
River Runs through It, A	5	1.15	214	★★★★
Steel Magnolias	5	1.18	220	★★★★
Summer of '42, The	5	0.77	170	★★★
Truly, Madly, Deeply	8	1.14	28	★★★★
Unstrung Heroes	8	1.08	12	★★★
Dementia/Alzheimer's				
Do You Remember Love?	5	1.20	10	★★★
Iris	8	1.62	40	★★★★★
Memories of Me	5	0.90	10	★★★
Depression				
Call Me Anna	8	1.00	7	—
Woman Under the Influence, A	8	1.24	34	★★★★
Divorce				
Bye Bye Love	5	0.53	17	★★★
First Wives' Club, The	5	0.19	196	★
Four Seasons, The	5	0.93	115	★★★
Good Mother, The	5	0.88	40	★★★
Husbands and Wives	8	0.76	21	★★★
Kramer vs. Kramer	5	1.24	280	★★★★
Mrs. Doubtfire	5	0.57	266	★★★
Starting Over	8	0.68	37	★★★
Unmarried Woman, An	5	1.02	94	★★★★
War of the Roses, The	5	−0.05	203	†

Category and title	Study no.	Avg. rating	No. of raters	Guide rating
Eating Disorders				
Best Little Girl in the World	5	1.19	31	★★★★
Eating	5	1.00	25	★★★★
For the Love of Nancy	5	0.64	11	★★★
Karen Carpenter Story, The	5	1.25	76	★★★★★
Families and Stepfamilies				
Family Man	8	1.24	35	★★★★
Father of the Bride, The	5	0.67	169	★★★
Fly Away Home	5	1.15	62	★★★★
Joy Luck Club, The	5	1.43	196	★★★★★
Life as a House	8	1.35	46	★★★★★
Radio Flyer	5	1.02	43	★★★★
Rain Man	5	1.15	274	★★★★
Stepmom	8	1.06	65	★★★★
Terms of Endearment	5	1.19	256	★★★★
What's Eating Gilbert Grape	5	1.14	133	★★★★
Love and Intimacy				
Four Seasons, The	5	0.97	116	★★★
9½ Weeks	5	-0.67	127	†
Pretty in Pink	5	0.36	103	★★
Serendipity	8	0.03	35	★
Sleepless in Seattle	5	0.55	259	★★★
Story of Us, The	8	0.61	31	★★★
Way We Were, The	5	0.73	174	★★★
When Harry Met Sally	5	0.94	289	★★★
Men's Issues				
American Beauty	8	0.68	196	★★★
Billy Elliot	8	1.46	104	★★★★★
City Slickers	5	0.67	208	★★★
Disney's The Kid	8	0.83	23	★★★
Fields of Dreams	5	1.11	245	★★★★
Glengarry Glen Ross	8	0.96	82	★★★
I Never Sang for My Father	5	1.48	80	★★★★★
Nothing in Common	5	0.90	40	★★★
October Sky	5	1.31	48	★★★★★
Rape of Richard Beck, The	5	0.50	20	★★★
Tootsie	5	0.66	246	★★★
Obsessive–Compulsive Disorder				
As Good As It Gets	5	1.16	267	★★★★
Posttraumatic Stress Disorder				
Accused, The	8	1.20	45	★★★★
Angel Eyes	8	0.23	13	★
Beloved	8	0.42	45	★★
Born on the Fourth of July	5	0.97	148	★★★
Client, The	8	0.69	91	★★★
Deer Hunter, The	5	0.76	175	★★★

Category and title	Study no.	Avg. rating	No. of raters	Guide rating
Fearless	8	1.17	12	★★★
Fisher King, The	8	0.97	100	★★★
Full Metal Jacket	5	0.52	103	★★★
Legend of Bagger Vance, The	8	0.37	86	★★
Pregnancy				
Baby M.	5	0.00	13	★
Father of the Bride II	5	0.12	92	★
Next Best Thing, The	8	-0.56	9	—
Nine Months	5	0.02	41	★
Steel Magnolias	5	0.77	168	★★★
Where the Heart Is	8	0.92	12	★★★
Schizophrenia				
Beautiful Mind, A	8	1.29	214	★★★★★
Benny and Joon	5	0.97	93	★★★
Birdy	5	1.18	66	★★★★
Fisher King, The	5	1.02	150	★★★★
Mad Love	5	0.06	17	★
Shine	5	1.14	149	★★★★
Sexuality				
Boys in the Band, The	5	0.77	107	★★★
Carnal Knowledge	5	0.51	123	★★★
Eyes Wide Shut	8	-0.44	87	†
Kissing Jessica Stein	8	1.19	26	★★★★
9½ Weeks	5	-0.22	112	†
Paris Is Burning	5	0.80	46	★★★
Torch Song Trilogy	5	1.22	81	★★★★
Suicide				
Dead Poets Society	8	1.14	218	★★★★
Field, The	8	1.20	5	—
Hospital, The	8	1.00	21	★★★★
Last Tango in Paris	8	0.15	92	★
'Night, Mother	5	1.10	42	★★★★
Ordinary People	8	1.56	229	★★★★★
Slender Thread, The	5	0.94	16	★★★
Virgin Suicides, The	8	1.00	23	★★★★
Teenagers and Parenting				
Breakfast Club, The	5	1.16	198	★★★★
Bronx Tale, A	8	1.17	29	★★★★
Circle of Friends	5	1.11	71	★★★★
Dead Poets Society	5	1.23	275	★★★★
Good Will Hunting	5	1.03	275	★★★★
Little Women	5	1.10	156	★★★★
My Bodyguard	5	0.83	93	★★★
Pretty in Pink	5	0.63	102	★★★
Powder	5	0.66	47	★★★
St. Elmo's Fire	5	0.49	121	★★

Category and title	Study no.	Avg. rating	No. of raters	Guide rating
Teenagers and Parenting (*cont.*)				
Sixteen Candles	5	0.62	97	★★★
Splendor in the Grass	5	0.71	82	★★★
Stand by Me	5	1.35	185	★★★★★
Women's Issues				
Eating	5	1.00	26	★★★★
Fried Green Tomatoes	8	1.19	223	★★★★
How to Make an American Quilt	5	1.02	102	★★★★
League of Their Own, A	5	1.18	190	★★★★
My Breast	5	0.70	10	★★★
Piano, The	5	0.88	235	★★★
Thelma and Louise	5	0.63	244	★★★
Turning Point, The	8	1.16	97	★★★★
Working Girl	8	0.69	126	★★★
Violent Youth				
Good Son, The	8	0.50	16	★★★
This Boy's Life	8	1.15	13	★★★

References

Ackerson, J., Scogin, F., McKendree-Smith, N., & Lyman, R. D. (1998). Cognitive bibliotherapy for mild and moderate adolescent depressive symptomatology. *Journal of Consulting and Clinical Psychology, 66*, 685–690.

Albom, M. (1997). *Tuesdays with Morrie.* New York: Doubleday.

Barlow, S. H., Burlingame, G. M., Nebeker, R. S., & Anderson, E. (1999). Meta-analysis of medical self-help groups. *International Journal of Group Psychotherapy, 50*, 53–69.

Bechtoldt, H., Norcross, J. C., Wyckoff, L. A., Pokrywa, M. L., & Campbell, L. F. (2001). Theoretical orientations and employment settings of clinical and counseling psychologists: A comparative study. *Clinical Psychologist, 54*(1), 3–6.

Carlbring, P., Westling, B. E., & Andersson, G. (2000). A review of published self-help books for panic disorder. *Scandinavian Journal of Behaviour Therapy, 29*, 5–13.

Clifford, J. S., Norcross, J. C., & Sommer, R. (1999). Autobiographies of mental health clients: Psychologists' uses and recommendations. *Professional Psychology: Research and Practice, 30*, 56–59.

Cuijpers, P. (1997). Bibliotherapy in unipolar depression: A meta-analysis. *Journal of Behavior Therapy and Experimental Psychiatry, 28*, 139–147.

Cuijpers, P. (1998). A psychoeducational approach to the treatment of depression: A meta-analysis of Lewinsohn's "Coping with Depression" course. *Behavior Therapy, 29*, 521–533.

Davis, R., & Miller, L. (July 15, 1999). Millions comb the web for medical information. *USA Today.*

DiBlassio, J., Simonin, D., DeCarolis, A., Morse, L., Jean, J., Vassalotti, L., Franks, K., & Chambliss, C. (1999, April). *Assessing the quality of psychological healthcare sites available on the Internet.* Poster presented at the 70th annual meeting of the Eastern Psychological Association, Providence, RI.

Druss, B. G., & Rosenheck, R. A. (2000). Use of practitioner-based complementary therapies by persons reporting mental conditions in the United States. *Archives of General Psychiatry, 57*, 708–714.

Eisenberg, D. M., Davis, R. B., Ettner, S. L., Appel, S., Wilkey, S., Rompay, M. V., & Kessler, R. C. (1998). Trends in alternative medicine use in the United States, 1990–1997. *Journal of the American Medical Association, 280*, 1575–1589.

Fried, S. B., & Schultis, G. A. (1995). *The best self-help and self-awareness books.* Chicago: American Library Association.

Gabbard, G. O., & Gabbard, K. (1999). *Psychiatry and the cinema* (2nd ed.). Washington, DC: American Psychiatric Press.

Gergen, K. (1991). *The saturated self.* New York: Basic Books.

Goodman, G., & Jacobs, M. (1994). The self-help, mutual support group. In A. Fuhriman & G. Burlingame (Eds.), *Handbook of group psychotherapy* (pp. 489–526). New York: Wiley.

Gould, R. A., & Clum, G. A. (1993). A meta-analysis of self-help treatment approaches. *Clinical Psychology Review, 13,* 169–186.

Grohol, J. M. (1999) *The insider's guide to mental health resources online.* New York: Guilford Press.

Hesley, J. W., & Hesley, J. G. (2001). *Rent two films and let's talk in the morning: Using popular movies in psychotherapy* (2nd ed.). New York: Wiley.

Joshua, J. M., & DiMenna, D. (2000). *Read two books and let's talk next week.* New York: Wiley.

Kessler, R. C., Zhao, S., et al. (1999). Past-year use of outpatient services for psychiatric problems in the National Comorbidity Survey. *American Journal of Psychiatry, 156,* 115–123.

Kownacki, R. J., & Shadish, W. R. (1999). Does Alcoholics Anonymous work?: The results from a meta-analysis of controlled experiments. *Substance Use and Misuse, 34,* 1897–1916.

Kurtz, L. F. (1997). *Self-help and support groups.* Thousand Oaks, CA: Sage.

Kurtzweil, P. L., Scogin, F., & Rosen, G. M. (1996). A test of the fail-safe N for self-help programs. *Professional Psychology: Research and Practice, 27,* 629–630.

Latner, J. D., Wilson, G. T., Stunkard, A. J., & Jackson, M. L. (2002). Self-help and long-term behavior therapy for obesity. *Behaviour Research and Therapy, 40,* 804–812.

Lawrence, S., & Giles, C. L. (1999). Accessibility of information on the web. *Nature, 400,* 107–109.

Lezak, M. D. (1995). *Neuropsychological assessment.* New York: Oxford University Press.

Lissman, T. L., & Boehnlein, J. K. (2001). A critical review of Internet information about depression. *Psychiatric Services, 52,* 1046–1050.

Marrs, R. W. (1995). A meta-analysis of bibliotherapy studies. *American Journal of Community Psychology, 23,* 843–870.

Morgenstern, J., Labouvie, E., McCrady, B. S., Kahler, C. W., & Frey, R. M. (1997). Affiliation with alcoholic anonymous after treatment: A study of its therapeutic effects and mechanisms of action. *Journal of Consulting and Clinical Psychology, 65,* 768–777.

Norcross, J. C. (2000). Here comes the self-help revolution in mental health. *Psychotherapy, 37,* 370–377.

Ouimette, P. C., Finney, J. W., & Moos, R. H. (1997). Twelve-step and cognitive-behavioral treatment for substance abuse: A comparison of treatment effectiveness. *Journal of Consulting and Clinical Psychology, 65,* 230–240.

Paul, A. M. (2001, March/April). Self-help: Shattering the myths. *Psychology Today,* pp. 58–68.

Project MATCH Research Group. (1997). Matching alcoholism treatments to client heterogeneity: Project MATCH posttreatment drinking outcomes. *Journal of Studies on Alcohol, 58,* 7–29.

Reissman, F., & Caroll, D. (1995). *Redefining self-help: Policy and practice.* San Francisco: New Resources for Human Services.

Rosen, G. M. (1987). Self-help treatment books and the commercialization of psychotherapy. *American Psychologist, 42,* 46–51.

Rosen, G. M. (1993). Self-help or hype?: Comments on psychology's failure to advance self-care. *Professional Psychology: Research and Practice, 24,* 340–345.

Rosen, R. D. (1977). *Psychobabble.* New York: Atheneum.

Santrock, J. W., Minnett, A. M., & Campbell, B. D. (1994). *The authoritative guide to self-help books.* New York: Guilford Press.

Scogin, F. (1998). Bibliotherapy: A nontraditional intervention for depression. In P. E. Hartman-Stein (Ed.), *Innovative behavioral healthcare for older adults: A guidebook for changing times* (pp. 129–144). San Francisco: Jossey-Bass.

Scogin, F., Bynum, J., Stephens, G., & Calhoun, S. (1990). Efficacy of self-administered treatment programs: Meta-analytic review. *Professional Psychology: Research and Practice, 21,* 42–47.

Scogin, F., Floyd, M., Jamison, C., Ackerson, J., Landreville, P., & Bissonnette, L. (1996). Negative outcomes: What is the evidence on self-administered treatments? *Journal of Consulting and Clinical Psychology, 64,* 1086–1089.

Scogin, F., Hamblin, D., & Beutler, L. (1987). Bibliotherapy for depressed older adults: A self-help alternative. *Gerontologist, 27,* 383–387.

Seligman, M. E. P. (1995). The effectiveness of psychotherapy. *American Psychologist, 50,* 965–974.

Skow, J. (1999, June). Lost in cyberspace. *Time,* p. 61.

Solomon, G. (1995). *The motion picture prescription.* Santa Rosa, CA: Aslan.

Sommer, R., Clifford, J. S., & Norcross, J. C. (1998). A bibliography of mental patients' autobiographies: An update and classification system. *American Journal of Psychiatry, 155,* 1261–1264.

Stamps, R. F., & Barach, P. M. (2001). *The therapist's internet handbook.* New York: Norton.

Tonigan, J. S., Toscoova, R., & Miller, W. R. (1995). Meta-analysis of the literature on alcoholic anonymous: Sample and study characteristics moderate findings. *Journal of Studies on Alcohol, 57,* 65–72.

U.S. Department of Justice Bureau of Statistics: Profile of State Prisoners under Age 18, 1985–97 [Online]. (June 16, 2002) (http://www.ojp.usdoj.gov/bjs/abstract/pspa1897.htm)

van Lankveld, J. J. D. M. (1998). Bibliotherapy in the treatment of sexual dysfunctions: A meta-analysis. *Journal of Consulting and Clinical Psychology, 66,* 702–708.

Walters, G. D. (2000). Behavioral self-control training for problem drinkers: A meta-analysis of randomized clinical studies. *Behavior Therapy, 31,* 135–149.

Watson, A. L., & Sher, K. J. (1998). Resolution of alcohol problems without treatment: Methodological issues and future directions of natural recovery research. *Clinical Psychology: Science and Practice, 5,* 1–18.

Wedding, D., & Boyd, M. A. (1999). *Movies and mental illness: Using films to understand psychopathology.* New York: McGraw-Hill.

Weekes, C. (1996). Bibliotherapy. In C. G. Lindemann (Ed.), *Handbook of the treatment of the anxiety disorders* (2nd ed., pp. 375–384). Northvale, NJ: Jason Aronson.

White, B. J., & Madara, E. J. (1995). *The self-help sourcebook* (5th ed.). Denville, NJ: American Self-Help Clearinghouse.

Zaccaria, J. S., & Moses, H. A. (1968). *Facilitating human development through reading.* Champaign, IL: Stipes.

Author and Title Index

Subject Index